Mitral Stenosis

Mitral Stenosis

Edited by
Neeraj Parakh
Ravi S. Math
Vivek Chaturvedi

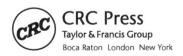

CRC Press
Taylor & Francis Group
Boca Raton London New York

CRC Press is an imprint of the
Taylor & Francis Group, an **informa** business

CRC Press
Taylor & Francis Group
6000 Broken Sound Parkway NW, Suite 300
Boca Raton, FL 33487-2742

First issued in paperback 2020

ISBN-13: 978-0-367-57139-9 (pbk)
ISBN-13: 978-1-138-89635-2 (hbk)

Library of Congress Cataloging-in-Publication Data

Names: Parakh, Neeraj, editor. | Math, Ravi S., editor. | Chaturvedi, Vivek, editor.
Title: Mitral stenosis / [edited by] Neeraj Parakh, Ravi S. Math, Vivek Chaturvedi.
Other titles: Mitral stenosis (Parakh)
Description: Boca Raton, Fl.: CRC Press/Taylor & Francis Group, [2018] | Includes bibliographical references and index.
Identifiers: LCCN 2018000781| ISBN 9781138896352 (hardback : alk. paper) | ISBN 9781315166735 (ebook)
Subjects: | MESH: Mitral Valve Stenosis--physiopathology | Mitral Valve Stenosis--therapy
Classification: LCC RC685.V2 | NLM WG 262 | DDC 616.1/25--dc23
LC record available at https://lccn.loc.gov/2018000781

Visit the Taylor & Francis Web site at
http://www.taylorandfrancis.com

and the CRC Press Web site at
http://www.crcpress.com

Contents

Foreword

Once something of an afterthought in cardiology, valvular heart disease has now become a focal point of interest. This change in emphasis has been spurred on by an aging population in which valve disease has increasing prevalence and also by the advent of less invasive and easier-applied percutaneous treatments for these diseases. These tenets especially influence the literary treatment of aortic stenosis and mitral regurgitation, where countless articles and many textbooks have been devoted to their discussion. In contrast, less has been recently written about mitral stenosis. This disease, largely a product of rheumatic fever, is now relatively rare in developed countries, where its primary cause, acute rheumatic fever, has become even rarer. Yet, in the developing world, rheumatic fever—and its primary exponent, mitral stenosis—are the centerpiece of valvular heart disease.

With this textbook, Ravi S. Math, Neeraj Parakh, and Vivek Chaturvedi fill this void comprehensively, covering the waterfront of mitral stenosis from epidemiology to mechanical therapy. Few diseases in cardiology have a more glittering presentation; from its exciting physical findings and its manifold images to its (now very effective) therapies, this text covers them all in an in-depth, logical, and opulent fashion.

I congratulate the authors on a much-needed text that should grace the shelves of any student of valvular heart disease. It should be read not just by providers practising in endemic areas but especially by students of cardiology because the pathophysiology of mitral stenosis is a lesson in how the heart works as a pump—a lesson often overlooked in other texts.

Blase A. Carabello
John "Jack" Rose Distinguished Professor
of Medicine
Brody School of Medicine
East Carolina University

It is a little-known fact that it was the Indian delegation to the World Health Assembly that, in the mid-1950s, pressed for the establishment of a Cardiovascular Diseases Unit at the Geneva headquarters of the World Health Organization. The impetus for that appeal came from the recognition that rheumatic heart disease (RHD) was maiming many young hearts by mangling cardiac valves, in many developing countries like India. The call for prevention and control of RHD was loud and clear, built around the clinical recognition that treatment was unavailable or unaffordable to many patients.

The remarkable diagnostic and therapeutic advances over the past six decades have made RHD a much more manageable problem. Throughout this period, mitral stenosis (MS) stood out as the classic prototype of RHD. Indian cardiology has made outstanding contributions to the study of pathology, clinical spectrum, non-invasive diagnosis, hemodynamics, medical management, interventional cardiac procedures, and surgical treatment related to MS. The description of "juvenile MS" documented the young age of presentation of MS in India, in distinction to the delayed evolution of natural history of MS in western patients, as described in the classic work of Paul Wood. This was not just a puzzling clinical curiosity but also a poignant human tragedy of a ravaged young heart, most often from a poor family.

It is surprising, therefore, that no attempt has been made earlier to systematically compile all aspects of MS into a single scientific monograph. Perhaps the all too familiar nature of MS lacked the excitement of an exotic subject. That regrettable neglect has now been redressed by Parakh, Chaturvedi, and Math in this comprehensive monograph that captures all the dimensions of MS. Not only is the rheumatic form detailed, but also presentations of MS within the spectrum of congenital heart disease and degenerative heart disease are well described.

Every student of heart disease, from the neophyte undergraduate student to the specialist who chooses to be a lifelong learner, will find this monograph eminently readable and immensely useful. I hope the authors will keep us supplied with periodic revisions as science advances, even as RHD recedes as a public health challenge and serious threat to personal health.

K. Srinath Reddy
President, Public Health Foundation of India
Former Head of Cardiology
All India Institute of Medical Sciences
Past President, World Heart Federation

Preface

Mitral stenosis continues to affect the younger population residing in lower income countries. Although uncommon in the developed world, it is seen among their immigrant and aging populations. Thus, while mitral stenosis remains an important public health problem in the developing world, it still commands much interest among cardiologists worldwide given its unique hemodynamics, classic clinical findings, and highly effective interventional therapy. While the disease has been extensively researched and documented, this data has not been systematically compiled and composed. As a result, interested readers are left with a vast sea of scattered academic and research material, from which relevant information has to be dug out. This book attempts to provide a standard updated reference for mitral stenosis in a concise manner. Most of the developments in the field of mitral stenosis predate the era of evidence-based medicine. They are based on detailed studies, often over prolonged periods of time, by a single or small groups of dedicated individuals. It is in fact a fascinating story, and possibly a reflection of the field of medicine as a whole. For example, mitral valvotomy was once considered a pariah, as it was believed that the stenosis was not primarily responsible for the symptoms. Subsequently, there were numerous failed attempts by courageous surgeons, followed finally by the fruits of success—all this even before the advent of cardiopulmonary bypass. Equally exciting and inspiring were the later developments in the field of percutaneous therapy.

Each topic has been dealt with extensively, making every effort to keep the content interesting, practical, and relevant. The contributing authors have substantial practical experience in dealing with mitral stenosis and have contributed years of research in this field. With their experience and knowledge, this book can serve as an authentic reference book for cardiology fellows and researchers, whereas for practising cardiologists it will be a ready reckoner. We wish to thank our teachers, colleagues, and fellows for their constant support and encouragement for the book. Special thanks go to Shivangi Pramanik from Taylor and Francis for sowing the seeds for this book. Last, but not least, this book would not have seen the light of day without the wholehearted support and sacrifices of our families.

**Neeraj Parakh, Ravi S. Math,
and Vivek Chaturvedi**

Glossary

AF	atrial fibrillation	NOAC	newer oral anticoagulant
AFl	atrial flutter	NVAF	non-valvular atrial fibrillation
AoV	aortic valve	OMC	open mitral commissurotomy
AR	aortic regurgitation	OMV	open mitral valvotomy
AS	aortic stenosis	PA	pulmonary artery
BMV	balloon mitral valvotomy	PAH	pulmonary artery hypertension
BNP	brain natriuretic peptide	PH	pulmonary hypertension
CABG	coronary artery bypass grafting	PA(S)P	pulmonary artery (systolic) pressure
CCB	calcium channel blocker	PCI	percutaneous coronary intervention
CMV	closed mitral valvotomy	PCWP	pulmonary capillary wedge pressure
CO	cardiac output	PMV	parachute mitral valve
DFP	diastolic filling period	PR	pulmonary regurgitation
DOMV	double orifice mitral valve	PS	pulmonary stenosis
DVR	double valve replacement	PTMC	percutaneous transvenous mitral
ECM	extra-cellular matrix		commissurotomy
GAS	group A beta hemolytic streptococcus	PV	pulmonary vein
HR	heart rate	PVI	pulmonary vein isolation
IE	infective endocarditis	PVR	pulmonary vascular resistance
LA	left atrium	RA	right atrium
LAA	left-atrial appendage	RAS	renin angiotensin system
LAP	left-atrial pressure	RHD	rheumatic heart disease
LV	left ventricle	RV	right ventricle
LVEDP	left-ventricular end diastolic pressure	SEC	spontaneous echo contrast
MAC	mitral annular calcification	SVD	subvalvular disease
MDG	mean diastolic gradient	TEE	transesophageal echocardiography
MDM	mid-diastolic murmur	TPG	transpulmonary gradient
MR	mitral regurgitation	TR	tricuspid regurgitation
MRI	magnetic resonance imaging	TS	tricuspid stenosis
MS	mitral stenosis	TTE	transthoracic echocardiography
MV	mitral valve	TV	tricuspid valve
MVA	mitral valve area	VKA	vitamin K antagonist
MVR	mitral valve replacement	WU	Wood Units

Contributors

Sudheer Arava
Associate Professor
Department of Cardiac Pathology
All India Institute of Medical Sciences
New Delhi, India

Raghav Bansal
Senior Resident
Department of Cardiology
All India Institute of Medical Sciences
New Delhi, India

Kanika Bhambri
Senior Resident
Department of Cardiovascular Radiology
and Endovascular Interventions
All India Institute of Medical Sciences
New Delhi, India

Balram Bhargava
Professor
Department of Cardiology
All India Institute of Medical Sciences
New Delhi, India

Amol Bhoje
Assistant Professor
Department of Cardiovascular
and Thoracic Surgery
All India Institute of Medical Sciences
New Delhi, India

Senguttuvan Nagendra Boopathy
Consultant General and Interventional
Cardiologist, and Assistant Professor of Cardiology
Sri Ramachandra Medical Centre
Chennai, India

Vivek Chaturvedi
Professor
Department of Cardiology
GB Pant Institute of Medical Education
and Research
New Delhi, India

Shiv Kumar Choudhary
Professor
Department of Cardiovascular
and Thoracic Surgery
All India Institute of Medical Sciences
New Delhi, India

Gurpreet S. Gulati
Professor
Department of Cardiovascular Radiology
and Endovascular Interventions
All India Institute of Medical Sciences
New Delhi, India

Anunay Gupta
Senior Resident
Department of Cardiology
All India Institute of Medical Sciences
New Delhi, India

Saurabh Kumar Gupta
Associate Professor
Department of Cardiology
All India Institute of Medical Sciences
New Delhi, India

Kusuma Harisha
Senior Resident
Department of Anatomy
All India Institute of Medical Sciences
New Delhi, India

Rajnish Juneja
Professor
Department of Cardiology
All India Institute of Medical Sciences
New Delhi, India

Ganesan Karthikeyan
Professor
Department of Cardiology
All India Institute of Medical Sciences
New Delhi, India

Danny Manglani
Senior Resident
Department of Cardiology
All India Institute of Medical Sciences
New Delhi, India

Cholenahally Nanjappa Manjunath
Director
Sri Jayadeva Institute of Cardiovascular
Sciences and Research
Bangalore-Karnataka, India

Ravi S. Math
Associate Professor
Department of Cardiology
Sri Jayadeva Institute of Cardiovascular
Sciences and Research
Bangalore-Karnataka, India

Arima Nigam
Associate Professor
Department of Cardiology
Govind Ballabh Pant Institute of Postgraduate
Medical Education and Research
New Delhi, India

Neeraj Parakh
Associate Professor
Department of Cardiology
All India Institute of Medical Sciences
New Delhi, India

Sivasubramanian Ramakrishnan
Professor
Department of Cardiology
All India Institute of Medical Sciences
New Delhi, India

Ruma Ray
Professor
Department of Cardiac Pathology
All India Institute of Medical Sciences
New Delhi, India

Ambuj Roy
Professor
Department of Cardiology
All India Institute of Medical Sciences
New Delhi, India

Anita Saxena
Professor
Department of Cardiology
All India Institute of Medical Sciences
New Delhi, India

Arun Sharma
DM Senior Resident
Department of Cardiovascular Radiology
and Endovascular Interventions
All India Institute of Medical Sciences
New Delhi, India

Sandeep Singh
Professor
Department of Cardiology
All India Institute of Medical Sciences
New Delhi, India

Kikkeri Hemannasetty Srinivas
Professor
Department of Cardiology
Sri Jayadeva Institute of Cardiovascular
Sciences and Research
Bangalore-Karnataka, India

Anand Subramaniam
Associate Professor
Department of Cardiology
Sri Jayadeva Institute of Cardiovascular
Sciences and Research
Bangalore-Karnataka, India

Jaganmohan A. Tharakan
Former Professor of Cardiology
Sree Chitra Tirunal Institute of Medical Sciences
and Technology
Trivandrum, India
and
Professor of Cardiology
PK Das Institute for Medical Sciences
Kerala, India

Preeti Yadav
Associate Consultant
Department of Gynecology and Obstetrics
Sant Parmanand Hospital
New Delhi, India

PART 1

Pathophysiology and clinical features

The history of mitral stenosis

BALRAM BHARGAVA AND NEERAJ PARAKH

THE MITRAL VALVE AND MITRAL STENOSIS

The existence of the mitral valve is as old as the human race, but its nomenclature and clinico-pathological recognition are no older than five centuries. The anatomical left atrioventricular valve was named the "mitral valve" by the Father of modern anatomy—Andreas Vesalius. In the second edition of *De Humani Corporis Fabrica*, published in 1555, he wrote that the mitral valve, when turned upside down, resembles a bishop's miter (a two-flapped angled hat) (Figure 1.1) and gave an accurate description of mitral valve anatomy.[1] In 1668, John Mayow from the Oxford school described the first patient of mitral stenosis with detailed clinical and pathological findings and was able to correlate clinical features with autopsy findings. Further, in 1705, Raymond de Vieussens scientifically detailed the clinical findings of a 30-year-old male patient of mitral stenosis.[2] Later, when this patient died, he documented various pathological findings of mitral stenosis in his magnificent engravings:

> I opened the left ventricle and I discovered here first that which I have just pointed out: namely the substance of the mitral valves has become bony and that it had very markedly diminished, and indeed changed the natural appearance of the lumen.

In 1806, Jean-Nicolas Corvisart described the thrill associated with mitral stenosis; he was the father of chest auscultation as well as the physician to Napoleon Bonaparte. Subsequently, in 1819, his pupil Rene H. T. Laennec, inventor of the stethoscope, described the murmur of mitral stenosis as *"bruit de soufflet"* (soft bellows).[3] Many years later, Sulpice Antoine Fauvel, a French epidemiologist, described the precise timing and nature of the presystolic murmur in mitral stenosis.[4] In 1862, Austin Flint provided precise and accurate

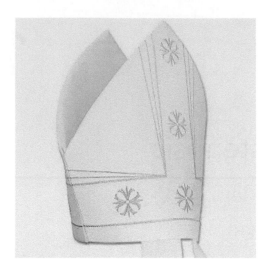

Figure 1.1 Bishop's miter.

descriptions of various cardiac murmurs,[5] in particular a similar presystolic murmur at the apex in severe aortic regurgitation and a normal mitral valve, eponymously described as an Austin Flint murmur. In 1877, Paul Louis Duroziez described congenital mitral stenosis and made an etiological

distinction between mitral stenosis of rheumatic and of congenital origin. He is also remembered for describing the Duroziez's murmur in severe aortic regurgitation (Table 1.1).[6]

THE SURGICAL ERA

The idea of surgically opening the mitral valve was first visualized by Frederick Alexander Samways in 1898 (Figure 1.2),[7] supported by Sir Lauder Brunton in 1902.[8] In Samways' own words, for the surgical treatment of mitral stenosis:

> I anticipate that with the progress of cardiac surgery some of the severest cases of mitral stenosis will be relieved by slightly notching the mitral orifice and trusting the auricle to continue its defence.

However, strong disapproval from contemporary physicians enforced a hasty retreat from the idea of surgery, which remained in cold storage for nearly 20 years. In 1923, an 11-year-old girl with mitral stenosis was successfully operated on by partial

Table 1.1 The history of mitral stenosis: The anatomical and clinical era

Contribution	Physician/surgeon/scientist	Year
Named mitral valve	Andreas Vesalius	1555
First description of mitral stenosis	John Mayow	1668
First scientific description of mitral stenosis	Raymond de Vieussens	1706
Described thrill of mitral stenosis	Jean Nicolas Corvisart	1806
Described murmur of mitral stenosis	Rene Theophile Hyacinthe Laennec	1819
Characterized presystolic timing of murmur in mitral stenosis	Sulpice Antoine Fauvel	1843
Described presystolic murmur of aortic regurgitation	Austin Flint	1862
Described congenital mitral stenosis	Paul Louis Duroziez	1877
Described juvenile mitral stenosis	Sujoy B. Roy	1963

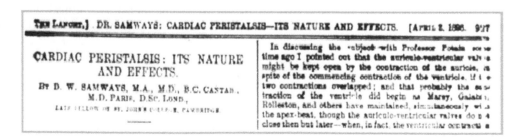

Figure 1.2 Samways' landmark paper in *The Lancet*, 1896.

valve excision. She survived for nearly 5 years after the operation; however, the next five patients operated on by the same technique died,[9] with the exception of one 15-year-old girl, operated on by Henry Souttar by digital commissurotomy in 1925.[10] Very high surgical mortality and strong opposition by contemporary physicians forced Souttar and other surgeons to abandon the idea of surgery, which, in Souttar's own words, was ahead of its time. The next two decades were years of introspection for surgeons. In 1948, four surgeons reported successful closed mitral commissurotomy (CMV) for mitral stenosis.[11–14] Although the respective years of publication vary, Horace Smithy from South Carolina performed the first successful CMV on January 18, 1948 with a valvulotome. He himself suffered from rheumatic heart disease and died of congestive heart failure the same year (age 34 years), unable to convince Alfred Blalock to operate on him with his own valvulotome. Incidentally, he diagnosed his valve disease, while testing his new stethoscope (bought as a medical student) on himself. Subsequently, CMV was successfully performed by Charles Philamore Bailey on June 10, 1948 at the Hahnemann Hospital in Philadelphia, after having performed two unsuccessful CMVs in 1945 and 1946. The first paper on CMV was published by Dwight Harken from Boston, a close friend of Joseph Garland, who at the time was the editor of the New England Journal of Medicine. Harken enjoyed 40 years of adulation, before confessing:

> When I performed my first valvuloplasty, I heard almost immediately that Dr. Bailey

had done his first successful commissurotomy 4 days earlier on June 10, 1948. I rushed to my friend Dr. Joseph Garland, Editor of the New England Journal of Medicine, and told him to get it published as soon as possible. He did and it was published in November 1948.[15]

Across the Atlantic in the same year, Sir Russell Brock also performed a successful CMV at Guys Hospital, London. Brock is now well-known for Brock's Procedure—a subpulmonic infundibular resection of the muscle by Brock's punch.

In the ensuing years, the CMV technique saw further refinement and became an established technique as a cure for mitral stenosis (Figure 1.3). The procedure became popular throughout the world, with the largest series being published by Stanley John, from Vellore in India, with excellent results.[16] As CMV underwent worldwide development, Roy and colleagues from New Delhi, India described a novel entity of juvenile mitral stenosis with very early pulmonary artery hypertension and pulmonary venous hypertension with fibrosis.[17]

The first open-heart surgical procedure, mitral valve repair, was performed by Dr. Forest Dewey Dodrill on July 3, 1952 at the Harper Hospital in Detroit, Michigan. Dodrill performed the surgery on the left ventricle of Henry Opitek by using the Dodrill-GMR, a machine developed by himself and researchers at General Motors and considered to be the first operational mechanical heart used while performing open-heart surgery.[18] Charles Walton Lillehei and colleagues from Minneapolis performed the first open mitral commissurotomy

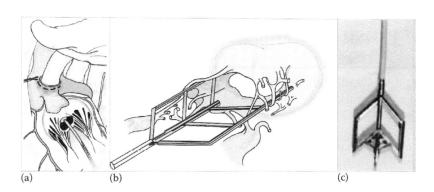

(a)   (b)   (c)

Figure 1.3 The evolution of mitral commissurotomy. **(a)** Finger commissurotomy; **(b)** Surgical commissurotomy; **(c)** Percutaneous metallic commissurotomy.

Table 1.2 The history of mitral stenosis: The surgical era

Contribution	Physician/surgeon/scientist	Year
Proposed surgical treatment	D. W. Samways	1898
Experimental valvotomy	Thomas Lauder Brunton	1902
Cardiotomy	E. C. Cutler and S. A. Levine	1923
Digital commissurotomy	Henry Sessions Souttar	1925
Tenotomy knife	E. C. Cutler and C. S. Beck	1929
Closed mitral valvotomy	Horace Smithy	January 18, 1948
	Charles Philamore Bailey	June 10, 1948
	Dwight Emary Harken	June 16, 1948
	Russel Brock and C. Baker	September 16, 1948
Open-heart mitral valve repair	Forest Dewey Dodrill	July 3, 1952
M-mode echocardiogram for mitral valve	Inge Edler and Carl Hellmuth Hertz	1953
Open mitral commissurotomy	Clarence Walton Lillehei	1956
Mitral valve replacement with metallic ball valve prosthesis	Albert Starr and Lowell Edwards	1960
Bioprosthetic valve and mitral valve repair	Alain Carpentier	1969
Bioprosthetic valve	Warren D. Hancock	1970

in 1956.[19] Charles Lillehei trained notable cardiac surgeons Charles Schumway and Christian Barnard, who, in turn, pioneered cardiac transplant. In 1957, Lillehei, along with engineer Earl Bakken, developed and implanted the first external-powered pacemaker. While Lillehei went on to become the medical director of St. Jude's Medical, Inc., Earl Bakken formed Medtronic, Inc. In 1967, the youngest brother of C.W. Lillehei, noted transplant surgeon Richard C. Lillehei, performed the first pancreas transplant.

Alain Carpentier further improvized and revolutionized mitral valve repair in 1969, and established a world-class heart institute in Vietnam in 1992 (Table 1.2).[20]

THE ERA OF PROSTHETIC MITRAL VALVES

The introduction of cardiopulmonary bypass opened the era of replacement of diseased mitral valves. In the 1950s, Harken defined "Ten Commandments" for the prosthetic valve.[21] In 1960, Nina Starr Braunwald (1928–1992) (the classmate and wife of Eugene Braunwald) successfully replaced the mitral valve using polyurethane.[22] Albert Starr, a cardiothoracic surgeon, collaborated with Lowell Edwards, a mechanical engineer, to design the first caged ball valve prosthesis

for the mitral valve. After studies on animals, the first valve was implanted at the mitral position on August 25, 1960 at the University of Oregon Medical Center.[23] Although the Starr-Edwards valve was the "gold standard," its high thromboembolic tendency led to the development of several prosthetic valves. Of these, the most successful were the tilting-disc Bjork-Shiley prosthesis and the bi-leaflet St. Jude's Medical valve.[24,25] The first commercially available bioprosthetic valves were developed in 1970 by Hancock in the United States and Carpentier in Paris.[26,27]

THE ADVENT OF ECHOCARDIOGRAPHY

The use of ultrasound for live imaging of the heart and its structure was another milestone in the history of mitral stenosis. Carl Helmuth Hertz, son of Gustav Hertz (winner of the Nobel Prize for experiments on electron collisions in gases), a soldier in the German army, was captured and imprisoned as a prisoner of war in the United States from 1943–1946 due to his father's history of research in the Soviet Union. On October 29, 1953, Inge Edler and Hertz recorded the first M-mode ultrasonic moving images of the heart.[28] Hellmuth Hertz also invented inkjet technology. Inge Edler further innovated 2D ultrasonic imaging of the heart, and for his pioneering work is known as the "father of echocardiography." The advent of echocardiography has been a major advance for the assessment and management of mitral stenosis, and its discovery was considered to be a major omission of the Nobel Prize Committee.

THE CATHETER ERA

In 1960, Edwin C. Brockenbrough, along with his colleagues, performed and studied left heart catheterization by the transseptal route (Table 1.3).[29] The advent of balloon atrial septostomy by Rashkind paved the way for left heart intervention through the transseptal route.[30] Much later, Charles E. Mullins refined the technique of transseptal puncture by using a very long sheath (Mullin's sheath).[31] The most revolutionary work for percutaneous management of mitral stenosis was done by the Japanese surgeon Kanji Inoue. He demonstrated the usefulness of a new balloon catheter for atrial septostomy in nine dogs and five pigs. The very next year he performed the first human transseptal mitral commissurotomy using this balloon catheter.[32–34] While Inoue's technique required surgical cut-down, a truly percutaneous transvenous mitral commissurotomy (PTMC) was performed in 1985 by James E. Lock and colleagues while visiting India. Between January and April 1985, eight patients underwent successful PTMC.[35] Many more modifications of the PTMC technique followed in

the next few years.[36] Al Zaibag from Saudi Arabia introduced double balloon mitral valvotomy, which offered a better valve area, albeit with higher complications.[37] Babic and colleagues from Beograd (then in Yugoslavia) established the railroad technique of performing valvuloplasty by the transarterial route.[38] Esteves and colleagues from Sao Paolo, Brazil established the efficacy of balloon mitral valvuloplasty during pregnancy with minimal fluoroscopy.[39] Stefanadis and colleagues from Greece successfully demonstrated the technique of retrograde nontransseptal mitral valvuloplasty in a series of 86 patients.[40] Shrivastava and colleagues from New Delhi, India compared the three techniques—single balloon, double balloon, and CMV—and demonstrated comparable results.[41] A more systematic catheterization follow-up comparison of surgery with balloon valvuloplasty was carried out on patients in Hyderabad, India by Somaraju and colleagues along with Zoltan Turi.[42] Alain Cribier from France used a metallic device for mitral commissurotomy in India and Pakistan with the promise of reduced cost and better valve area, as well as advantages in calcific valves. This device had potential for multiple uses and thus a major cost advantage over expensive single-use balloon catheters.[43] However, its use remained restricted due to complications of severe regurgitation and ventricular rupture. Jui-Sung Hung described various advantages and pitfalls in the PTMC technique.[44] George Joseph from Vellore, India improvized the

Table 1.3 The history of mitral stenosis: The percutaneous catheter era

Contribution	Physician/surgeon/scientist	Year
Transseptal puncture	Edwin C. Brockenbrough	1962
Balloon atrial septostomy	William J. Rashkind	1966
Percutaneous balloon mitral commissurotomy	Kanji Inoue	1982
Mullins sheath for transseptal puncture	Charles E. Mullins	1983
Percutaneous balloon mitral commissurotomy	James E. Lock	1985
Transarterial railroad technique	U. U. Babic	1986
Double balloon technique	M. Al Zaibag	1986
Retrograde non-transseptal technique	C. Stefanadis	1990
Percutaneous balloon mitral commissurotomy during pregnancy	C. A. Esteves and J. E. Sousa	1991
Metallic commissurotome	Alain Cribier	1997
Jugular approach	George Joseph	1997
Difficult PTMC approaches	C. N. Manjunath	1998
Mitral valve in valve	Multiple operators	2012

percutaneous mitral valvotomy technique by the jugular approach. This technique facilitates early mobilization and same-day discharge and was found to be useful in patients with interrupted inferior vena cava.[45] C. N. Manjunath from Bengaluru, India further improvized the technique for difficult cases, including those with left-atrial appendage clot.[46] By the end of the twentieth century, PTMC with the Inoue technique was mastered in India, with more than 30 centers performing about 15,000 procedures every year.

The latest weapon in the percutaneous treatment of stenotic degenerated mitral valve is percutaneous mitral valve-in-valve technique. As of now, six transcatheter mitral valve devices are available and have been implanted in humans.[47] This technique has a promising future for sick patients with high surgical risk. Further research and studies are underway for the treatment of mitral stenosis and its sequelae. These include newer anticoagulants for atrial fibrillation, pulmonary vein isolation for rheumatic atrial fibrillation, and device closure for the left-atrial appendage to decrease stroke risk.[48] Simultaneous PTMC and left-atrial appendage closure has been performed successfully.[49]

The ongoing saga of mitral stenosis has been through many peaks and troughs. The pioneers of yesteryear paved the way for the newer generation to effectively and safely treat this disease and modify its course. As we see a decline in rheumatic mitral stenosis in many parts of the world, this century may witness another turn in this journey.[50–52]

REFERENCES

1. Garrison D, Hast M. On the fabric of the human body: An annotated translation of the 1543 and 1555 editions of Andreas Vesalius' *De Humani Corporis Fabrica*. Illinois: Northwestern University; 2003.
2. Kellett CE. Raymond de Vieussens on mitral stenosis. *Br Heart J* 1959;21:440–4.
3. Rolleston H. The history of mitral stenosis. *Br Heart J* 1941;3:1–12.
4. Sulpice Antoine Fauvel (1813–1884), French epidemiologist. *JAMA* 1970;214:585–6.
5. Flint A. Classics in cardiology: On cardiac murmurs. *Heart Views* 2012;13:26–8.
6. Duroziez PL. Du rétrécissement mitral pur. *Archives générales de médecine* 1877;30:32–54, 184–97.
7. Samways DW. Cardiac peristalsis: Its nature and effects. *Lancet* 1898;1:927.
8. Brunton L. Preliminary note on the possibility of treating mitral stenosis by surgical methods. *Lancet* 1902;1:352.
9. Cutler EC, Levine SA. Cardiotomy and valvulotomy for mitral stenosis; experimental observations and clinical notes concerning an operated case with recovery. *Boston Med Surg J* 1923;188:1023–7.
10. Souttar HS. The surgical treatment of mitral stenosis. *Br Med J* 1925;2:603–6.
11. Smithy HG, Boone JA, Stallworth JM. Surgical treatment of constrictive valvular disease of the heart. *Surg Gynec Obst* 1950;90:175–92.
12. Bailey CP. The surgical treatment of mitral stenosis (mitral commissurotomy). *Dis Chest* 1949;15:377–97.
13. Harken DE, Ellis LB, Ware PF, Norman LR. The surgical treatment of mitral stenosis. 1. Valvuloplasty. *N Engl J Med* 1948; 239:801–9.
14. Baker C, Brock RC, Campbell M. Valvotomy for mitral stenosis: Report of six successful cases. *Br Med J* 1950;1:1283–93.
15. Harken DE. The emergence of cardiac surgery. I. Personal recollections of the 1940s and 1950s. *J Thorac Cardiovasc Surg* 1989; 98:805–13.
16. John S, Bashi VV, Jairaj PS et al. Closed mitral valvotomy: Early results and long-term follow-up of 3724 consecutive patients. *Circulation* 1983;68:891–6.
17. Roy SB, Bhatia ML, Lazaro EJ, Ramalingaswami V. Juvenile mitral stenosis in India. *Lancet* 1963;2(7319):1193–5.
18. Stephenson LW, Arbulu A, Bassett JS et al. Forest Dewey Dodrill: Heart surgery pioneer. Michigan Heart, Part II. *J Cardiac Surg* 2002;17:247–57.
19. Cherian KM, Vaijyanath P. Advances in the management of valvular heart diseases. *Asia-Pacific Cardiology* 2008;1:62–3.
20. Carpentier A. Cardiac valve surgery—The "French correction." *J Thorac Cardiovasc Surg* 1983;86:323–7.
21. Harken DE. Heart valves: Ten commandments and still counting. *Ann Thorac Surg* 1989;48 (Suppl. 3):S18–S19.
22. Edmunds LH, Jr. Evolution of prosthetic heart valves. *Am Heart J* 2001;141(5):849–55.

23. Starr A, Edwards ML. Mitral replacement: Clinical experience with a ball valve prosthesis. *Ann Surg* 1961;154:726–40.

24. Bjork VO. The central flow tilting disc valve prosthesis (Björk-Shiley) for mitral valve replacement. *Scand J Thorac Cardiovasc Surg* 1970;4:15–23.

25. Emery RW, Nicoloff DM. St Jude Medical cardiac valve prosthesis: In vitro studies. *J Thorac Cardiovasc Surg* 1979;78:269–76.

26. Kaiser GA, Hancock WD, Lukban SB, Litwak RS. Clinical use of new design stented xenograft heart valve prosthesis. *Surg Forum* 1969;20:137–8.

27. Carpentier A. Principles of tissue valve transplantation. In: Ionescu MI, Ross N, Wooler GH. *Biological Tissue in Heart Valve Replacement.* London: Butterworths; 1971;49–82.

28. Edler I, Hertz CH. The use of ultrasonic reflectoscope for the continuous recording of the movements of heart walls. *Clin Physiol Funct Imaging* 2004;24:118–36.

29. Brockenbrough EC, Braunwald E. A new technique of left ventricular angiocardiography and transseptal left heart catheterization. *Am J Cardiol* 1960;6:1062–4.

30. Rashkind WJ, Miller WW. Creation of an atrial septal defect without thoracotomy. A palliative approach to complete transposition of the great arteries. *JAMA* 1966;196:991–2.

31. Mullins CE. Transseptal left heart catheterization: Experience with a new technique in 520 pediatric and adult patients. *Pediatr Cardiol* 1983;4:239–45.

32. Inoue K, Nakamura T, Chikusa H et al. Atrial septostomy by a new balloon catheter. *Jpn Circ J* 1981;45:730–8.

33. Inoue K, Nakamura T, Kitamura F. Non operative mitral commissurotomy by a new balloon catheter [abstract]. *Jpn Circ J* 1982;46:877.

34. Inoue K, Owaki T, Nakamura T, Kitamura F, Miyamoto N. Clinical application of transvenous mitral commissurotomy by a new balloon catheter. *J Thorac Cardiovasc Surg* 1984;87:394–402.

35. Lock JE, Khalilullah M, Shrivastava S, Bahl V, Keane JF. Percutaneous catheter commissurotomy in rheumatic mitral stenosis. *N Engl J Med* 1985;313:1515–8.

36. Bhargava B, Gupta D, Agarwal R, Manchanda SC. A century of evolution in the treatment of mitral stenosis. *Indian Heart J* 1999;51:445–9.

37. Al Zaibag M, Ribeiro PA, Al Kasab S, Al Fagih MR. Percutaneous double-balloon mitral valvotomy for rheumatic mitral-valve stenosis. *Lancet* 1986;1:757–61.

38. Babic UU, Pejcic P, Djurisic Z, Vucinic M, Grujicic SM. Percutaneous transarterial balloon valvuloplasty for mitral valve stenosis. *Am J Cardiol* 1986;57:1101–4.

39. Esteves CA, Ramos AI, Braga SL, Harrison JK, Sousa JE. Effectiveness of percutaneous balloon mitral valvotomy during pregnancy. *Am J Cardiol* 1991;68:930–4.

40. Stefanadis C, Stratos C, Pitsavos C et al. Retrograde nontransseptal balloon mitral valvuloplasty. Immediate results and long-term follow-up. *Circulation* 1992;85:1760–7.

41. Shrivastava S, Mathur A, Dev V, Saxena A, Venugopal P, Sampath Kumar A. Comparison of immediate hemodynamic response to closed mitral commissurotomy, single-balloon, and double-balloon mitral valvuloplasty in rheumatic mitral stenosis. *J Thorac Cardiovasc Surg* 1992;104:1264–7.

42. Reyes VP, Raju BS, Wynne J et al. Percutaneous balloon valvuloplasty compared with open surgical commissurotomy for mitral stenosis. *N Engl J Med* 1994;331:961–7.

43. Cribier A, Rath PC, Letac B. Percutaneous mitral valvotomy with a metal dilator. *Lancet* 1997;349:1667–8.

44. Hung JS, Lau KW. Pitfalls and tips in Inoue balloon mitral commissurotomy. *Cathet Cardiovasc Diagn* 1996;37:188–99.

45. Joseph G, Baruah DK, Kuruttukulam SV, Chandy ST, Krishnaswami S. Transjugular approach to transseptal balloon mitral valvuloplasty. *Cathet Cardiovasc Diagn* 1997;42:219–26.

46. Manjunath CN, Srinivasa KH, Patil CB, Venkatesh HV, Bhoopal TS, Dhanalakshmi C. Balloon mitral valvuloplasty: Our experience with a modified technique of crossing the mitral valve in difficult cases. *Cathet Cardiovasc Diagn* 1998;44:23–6.

47. Krishnaswamy A, Mick S, Navia J, Gillinov AM, Tuzcu EM, Kapadia SR. Transcatheter mitral valve replacement: A frontier in cardiac intervention. *Cleve Clin J Med* 2016;83(11 Suppl 2):S10–S17.

48. Investigation of rheumatic AF treatment using vitamin K antagonists, rivaroxaban or aspirin studies, Non-Inferiority (INVICTUS-VKA). 2016. Available at https://clinicaltrials .gov/ct2/show/NCT02832544.

49. Gemma D, Moreno Gómez R, Fernández de Bobadilla J et al. Percutaneous balloon mitralvalvuloplasty and closure of the left atrial appendage: Synergy of two proce-duresin one percutaneous intervention. *Rev Port Cardiol* 2016;35:617.e1–617.e7. doi: 10.1016/j.repc.2016.01.008.

50. Ramakrishnan S, Kothari SS, Juneja R, Bhargava B, Saxena A, Bahl VK. Prevalence of rheumatic heart disease: Has it declined in India? *Natl Med J India* 2009;22(2):72–4.

51. Saxena A, Ramakrishnan S, Roy A et al. Prevalence and outcome of subclinical rheu-matic heart disease in India: The RHEUMATIC (Rheumatic Heart Echo Utilisation and Monitoring Actuarial Trends in Indian Children) study. *Heart* 2011;97:2018–22.

52. Watkins DA, Johnson CO, Colquhoun SM et al. Global, regional, and national burden of rheumatic heart disease, 1990–2015. *N Engl J Med* 2017;377:713–22.

2

Epidemiology and the natural history of mitral stenosis

ANITA SAXENA

INTRODUCTION

Rheumatic heart disease (RHD) affects over 32 million people worldwide, a vast majority of whom are in low- and middle-income countries.[1] According to a summary report commissioned by the World Health Organization, as many as 471,000 cases develop acute rheumatic fever (RF) every year.[2] About 275,000 patients die prematurely due to RHD, predominantly in low- and middle-income countries.[3] Although RHD has virtually disappeared from the Western world, it continues to be a major public health problem in developing countries, including India. Consequently, the burden of mitral stenosis (MS) is also high in these regions. India contributes to about 25%–50% of newly diagnosed cases of RHD.[4] It is estimated that a decline in RHD has occurred for less than 20% of the world's population. RHD remains a leading cause

of premature mortality in children and young adults living in endemic regions.[5]

RF and RHD affect young children and adolescents, mostly from poor families living in unhygienic conditions associated with overcrowding. It is important to note that over three-quarters of children worldwide live in high-prevalence regions[6] and RHD accounts for the greatest cardiovascular-related loss of disability-adjusted-life-years (DALYS) among children aged 10 to 14 years worldwide.[7] Inconsistent diagnostic criteria and methods of diagnosis, and limited access to appropriate diagnostic tests, may not allow estimation of the true prevalence of MS secondary to RHD, especially in developing countries. The actual burden may be much more than what has been published in the literature.

RHD is the most common etiology of MS worldwide. The development of MS is associated with a number of episodes, though not necessarily with the severity of carditis during RF reoccurrences.[9,10] MS is more common in women. Interestingly, a number of patients with pure chorea without clinical carditis have been seen to develop MS on long-term follow-up.[11,12]

RF occurs at a relatively younger age in developing countries, affecting children as young as 3 years. The incidence of carditis is also higher during an episode of RF. This has also been reported in some other countries where the prevalence of RF and RHD is high. MS can develop very quickly following RF. Further, 40%–50% of patients with significant mitral obstruction do not have a history to suggest RF. This indicates that acute RF remains unrecognized, possibly because in these patients RF occurs with subclinical carditis but without arthritis, arthralgia, subcutaneous nodules, and chorea.[8] In a study from Ethiopia, only 24.9% of patients with MS could recall a symptomatic episode of RF.[13] The most likely explanation by these authors of this study: that RF may escape attention if it is not associated with migratory polyarthritis or Sydenham's chorea, especially in medically unsophisticated regions.

EPIDEMIOLOGY

RF follows the classic epidemiologic triad, where all three components—namely agent, host, and environment—interact to result in the development of disease. These three components are important determinants of the disease's distribution in the population. However, even today our understanding of how these factors influence the occurrence of RF is incomplete. A genetic predisposition has been previously suggested based on the association of RHD with certain haplotypes, such as HLA DR2, DR4, DR1, and DRw6; however, this has not been convincingly proven.[14] A meta-analysis of twin studies showed a concordance risk of RF of 44% in monozygotic and 12% in dizygotic twins.[15]

DETERMINANTS OF DISEASE DISTRIBUTION

Interaction between the infecting agent, namely group-A β-hemolytic streptococcus (GAS), the susceptible host, and the environment is very complex and incompletely understood. Pharyngo-tonsillitis is one of the most prevalent infections caused by GAS. It accounts for up to one-third of throat infections in children, and up to one-tenth in adults. Although streptococcal infections are very frequent, only a few individuals develop rheumatic fever. It is calculated that, under endemic conditions, 0.3% of untreated infections, and 3% in epidemics, will lead to a first episode of rheumatic fever. So, obviously, host and environment play an important role in the epidemiology of RF. These three components are described below in more detail.

The agent

The agent responsible for RF has been well recognized for many decades, although the exact pathogenetic mechanism responsible for the development of RF secondary to GAS infection remains unclear. In most instances, RF follows tonsillopharyngitis due to GAS. This has been proven by the fact that penicillin given for bacterial pharyngitis reduces initial attack as well as recurrences of RF. Despite the fact that GAS has continued to constitute about 30% of all pharyngitis in children over the past five decades, the occurrence of RF in industrialized countries has fallen to a great extent. This may be linked to a change in the epidemiology of GAS pharyngitis with a shift from rheumatogenic to non-rheumatogenic strains.

The age group most commonly affected by GAS pharyngitis (5–15 years) is similar to the age group in which RF is far more common. In some of the aboriginal population of the Northern Territory, Australia, RF has occurred secondary to pyoderma, rather than pharyngitis.[16] Other streptococci belonging to group C and G, rather than GAS, are also thought to play an important role in some regions.[17] An analysis of "emm"-type distribution shows a variation in the molecular epidemiology of GAS infections in Africa and the Pacific in comparison with that observed in high-income countries. These issues have important implications for streptococcal vaccine development.

The host

Age: Initial attacks of RF most commonly affect children aged 5–15 years, although first episodes have been described in younger children. The peak incidence of RF occurs around the ages of 8–9 years. These ages coincide with the peak of streptococcal pharyngo-tonsillitis in school-aged children, this infection being less common in late adolescence and in adults. Rheumatic fever has been reported in children as young as 2–3 years of age.[16,17] Initial episodes can also occur in older adolescents and adults, although cases in people over 30 years of age are rare. On the other hand, recurrent episodes in those with previous rheumatic fever often affect older children, adolescents, and young adults but are rarely observed beyond the age of 35–40 years. Multiple episodes of RF or a single severe RF episode results in cumulated heart valve damage. Therefore, the prevalence of RHD peaks in adulthood, usually between the ages of 20–30 years. Survival is going to be influenced by compliance to secondary prophylaxis to prevent recurrence of RF, severity of valvular damage and access to specialist management and surgery.

In developed countries, the initial symptomatic presentation of MS is usually in the fourth to sixth decades of life. The disease shows slow progression and patients present after a latency period of 20–40 years after RF. On the other hand, patients in developing countries have a quickly progressive course and often present with symptomatic MS in the late teenage years or in early adulthood.[18] This issue of rapid progression of MS in developing countries will be discussed further in a later part of the chapter.

Gender: RF is equally common in both males and females, although chorea is very uncommon in postpubertal males. RHD occurs more commonly in females with a relative risk of 1.6–2.0 compared with males. These sex differences might be stronger in adolescents and adults than in children.[6,20] The reason for female preponderance is not clear. It may be related to intrinsic factors such as greater autoimmune susceptibility, as seen in systemic lupus erythematosus.[21] Other factors such as greater exposure to GAS infection due to closer proximity to children during child rearing may also play some part. In many developing countries, girls and women may have reduced access to health care as compared to boys and men and this could also contribute to differences in RHD rates between females and males.

MS is particularly more common in females, but the reasons for this preponderance are not clear. Two-thirds of all patients with rheumatic MS are females. In one echocardiographic study, MS was significantly more prevalent in women (1.6% vs. 0.4%, $p < 0.001$). The prevalence of mitral regurgitation was similar between the two sexes (24.4% in women vs. 25% in men).[22] Further, girls and women are more severely affected than men.[22,23] A number of the female patients are diagnosed for the first time during pregnancy. Data from many developing countries, including India, South Africa, and Senegal, suggest that RHD is a leading cause of indirect obstetric death, which in turn accounts for 25% of all maternal deaths in developing countries.[24–27] This may be related to the lack of early detection as the access to health services is limited in developing countries.

Race and ethnicity: It may be difficult to separate ethnic influences from environmental factors as socioeconomic status and access to health care are known to influence the occurrence of RF. Some studies have implicated one race or the other as being more predisposed to RF and RHD, but no race or ethnic group is immune from developing RF. In a study from New Zealand, Māori and Pacific ethnicity were seen to be strongly associated with RF incidence independent of deprivation.[28] Similarly, wide differences in the prevalence of chronic RHD have been documented in Hawaii in Samoan school children when compared with Caucasian Hawaiians.[29] Race and ethnicity may also be responsible for the rapid progression of MS in some countries.

Genetic influence: Robust evidence for genetic influence is lacking. However, it is well known that, for those who develop RF once, there is a 50% recurrence rate following GAS pharyngitis, although the initial attack of RF occurs only in 0.3%–3% of individuals after a GAS infection. Genetic predisposition has been previously suggested based on the association of RHD with certain haplotypes such as HLA DR2, DR4, DR1, and DRw6; however, this has not been convincingly proven.[14] A meta-analysis of twin studies showed a concordance risk of RF of 44% in monozygotic and 12% in dizygotic twins.[15] Genetic influences have also been implicated in the rapid progression of MS in certain families.

Environmental factors

RF has initially been reported as a disease of temperate climates, but currently it is more prevalent in warm tropical climates, especially in developing countries. The influence of seasonal variation on the incidence rates of RF is less well defined, but in general follows that of streptococcal infections, which are most commonly observed in late winter and early spring. However, seasonal variations in RF incidence are not pronounced in tropical countries. Environment plays a significant part as the vast majority of differences in risk between populations around the world can be explained by it. Environmental risk factors include household overcrowding,[30] poor and unhygienic living conditions, and poor access to medical care. The relative contribution of each of these individual risk factors is difficult to assess since many of them overlap and are associated with poverty and deprivation.[31–33] Crowded living conditions allow for the rapid spread of virulent streptococci and a lack of access to health care leads to these infections remaining untreated. RF and RHD are common, both in rural and urban communities. Improvements in these environmental factors are primarily responsible for the almost complete disappearance of RF and RHD in developed countries.

Other, less-well-studied environmental risk factors include under-nutrition, social instability, and the health-seeking behavior of the community. Poor nutrition may lead to a decreased immune response and perhaps a more severe or virulent disease.

NATURAL HISTORY

MS is a progressive disease consisting of a stable course in the early years followed by an accelerated course. The symptoms may progress rapidly during pregnancy. An increase in heart rate and cardiac output can increase the transmitral gradient, leading to symptoms in a previously asymptomatic patient or exacerbation of symptoms in an already-symptomatic patient.

Data from developed countries

In studies from developed countries, the progression of MS due to RHD has been considered to be very slow as presentation with clinical symptoms usually occurs after a latency period of 20–40 years after an episode of RF.[34,35] In one prospective study, the mean interval between the occurrence of RF and the appearance of symptoms was 16 ± 5 years. Progression from mild to severe disability took another 9 years. This inference was supported by echocardiography-based longitudinal studies that have estimated the average decrease in mitral valve area to be as low as 0.09 cm^2/year.[36,37] Survival among patients with MS is related to their symptomatic status. Rowe et al. followed a group of 250 patients with pure MS for 20 years, or until death. Of these patients, 52% were asymptomatic at initial assessment.[38] Among the asymptomatic patients, at 10 years, 84% were alive and 59% remained asymptomatic. After the first decade, there was a progressive deterioration of symptomatic status in this asymptomatic group, with only 24% remaining asymptomatic at 20 years and death occurring in 62% of cases. Overall, in this study, 39% of patients were dead at 10 years and 79% at 20 years. The prognosis dramatically worsens once the patient with MS develops symptoms. The progression from mild symptoms to severe symptoms may occur very rapidly even in developed countries. Among 271 symptomatic, unoperated patients, the 10-year survival rates for patients in functional classes II, III, and IV were 69%, 33%, and 0% respectively in the study by Olesen.[39] Of the patients with class II symptoms, 49% were alive at 20 years, compared to 0% of the class III symptomatic patients. Overall, in this study (with a follow-up 26 years after initial presentation), 10-year survival was 34% and 20-year survival was only 14%. Similarly, survival was 44% at 5 years and 32% at 10 years in patients in whom valve surgery was recommended but refused.[43] A combined analysis of 759 unoperated patients from three series with 10-year follow-up noted a survival rate of slightly over 50%.[38] In the asymptomatic or minimally symptomatic patients, survival was greater than 80% at 10 years but, when limiting symptoms occur, 10-year survival drops down to less than 15% if MS is not treated.[41,42]

Echocardiographic studies have shown variable rates of narrowing in individual patients with rheumatic MS. According to Gorden et al., the initial valve area did not correlate with the rate of progression of MS. However, patients with higher peak (>10 mmHg) and mean transmitral gradients and those with higher echocardiographic scores for mitral valve morphology (>8) were more likely to exhibit a more progressive course.[36] However, these factors were not found to be useful predictors in a later study.[37] In their study, the rate of progression was significantly greater among patients with a larger initial mitral valve area and milder MS (0.12 vs. 0.06 vs. 0.03 cm^2/year for mild, moderate, and severe stenosis, respectively) ($p < 0.01$). However, the natural history of moderate MS may be different from that of mild and severe stenosis. In another echocardiographic study from Israel, where 36 patients with moderate MS were followed for approximately 6 years, the rate of progression of mitral valve narrowing was variable and could not be predicted by the patient's age, past commissurotomy, valve score, or gradient. In many patients, the valve area did not change on follow-up.[40] These studies have implications for the frequency of follow-up and prognosis in patients with MS.

Data from developing countries

In contrast to data from developed countries, studies from developing countries document rapid progression of MS leading to serious disability early in life requiring interventional treatment.[13,44–49] The disease progresses very rapidly with an almost-malignant course producing MS at a very young age.[23,24] In a more recent report from Ethiopia, 26.5% of 365 patients with MS were between 6 to 10 years of age.[13] The factors that determine this progression are not clearly understood, but appear to be multifactorial. Success of treatment with antibiotics for GAS pharyngitis, pattern of living conditions, severity of the initial episode, access to health care, recurrence of RF episode, and immune response of the host may be responsible for rapid progression of valve injury. A genetic predisposition and other as-yet-unknown factors could also contribute.

The recurrence of RF is a common problem in developing regions. This is due to the persistence of predisposing factors to recurrent RF and the non-availability of prophylactic penicillin. Disease progression is often not detected. A number of RHD patients lack access or fail to adhere to secondary prophylaxis.[48,50] The rates for secondary prophylaxis are abysmally low, even in those who are aware of their diagnosis.[51]

JUVENILE MITRAL STENOSIS

The term "Juvenile MS" was coined by Sujoy B. Roy in 1963.[23] This article reported for the first time the rapid progression of MS in the Indian subcontinent. Authors wrote that it does not take over 20 years to become symptomatic and it is not infrequent to see critical MS in patients under the age of 20 years. They emphasized that MS can lead to congestive heart failure and that the presence of congestive failure was not sine qua non with active RF and carditis in children and adolescents in India. Mitral valve calcification is uncommon in these patients and most are in sinus rhythm indicating relatively shorter duration of disease due to which changes in the left atrium may not have occurred. However, severe pulmonary hypertension is present in more than one-third of patients. This picture of juvenile MS remains unchanged even today in clinical practice in India and several other developing countries with a high burden of RF and RHD. Echocardiography often demonstrates severe, grade 3, or grade 4 subvalvular deformity of the mitral apparatus in addition to thick mitral valve with critical stenosis.[52]

The reasons for the accelerated progression of MS are not clear but frequent, clinical, or subclinical recurrences of RF, which remain unrecognized and untreated, may play a role. It is possible that the host factors may also be contributing. Early intervention, mostly in the form of percutaneous transvenous mitral commissurotomy, is required in most of these patients. The results of percutaneous transvenous mitral commissurotomy have been shown to be as good as in adult patients, though the likelihood of restenosis may be higher.[53]

COMPLICATIONS IN THE NATURAL HISTORY OF MITRAL STENOSIS

Atrial fibrillation: The most common complication in MS; overall incidence in untreated patients is 40%.[54] Atrial fibrillation is less common in younger patients. The natural history of MS is profoundly affected by the onset of atrial fibrillation, disabling the patient due to a lowering of cardiac output. A rapid ventricular rate is further detrimental as it raises left-atrial pressure due to a reduction in diastolic filling time. According to the study by Olesen, 10-year and 20-year survival rates are only 25% and 0% as against 46% and 29% respectively for those in sinus rhythm.[39] The usual risk factors for atrial fibrillation include increasing age and severe MS.[55] It is believed that left-atrial enlargement is the result of atrial fibrillation rather than its cause.[56,57] Atrial fibrillation also increases the probability of systemic embolism.

Pulmonary hypertension: In a series of 586 patients with MS, 48 patients (8.2%) had severe pulmonary hypertension with resting systolic pulmonary artery pressure of >80 mmHg and pulmonary vascular resistance of 10 Wood units or more.[58] The mean survival of patients with severe pulmonary hypertension who did not undergo surgery was 2.4 ± 0.5 years. One-fourth of these patients had died within 6 months and half by 12 months after catheterization, indicating the markedly poor prognosis in this subgroup. These patients often develop functional tricuspid regurgitation and, subsequently, right-ventricular failure.

Systemic embolism: The risk of systemic embolism is 9%–14% in patients with MS. The majority have cerebral embolism (60%–75%) and are in atrial fibrillation. Surprisingly, cerebrovascular stroke may be the first presentation in some of these patients as MS is mild or moderate. Increasing age and the presence of atrial fibrillation are main predictors of systemic embolism with previous thromboembolism being positively correlated.

Other complications include infective endocarditis, pulmonary hemorrhage, pulmonary embolism, respiratory infections, etc.

Causes of death in MS

Death is due to a progressive increase in pulmonary venous pressure leading to right-sided heart failure and/or pulmonary edema in over 60% of cases. Remaining deaths are due to systemic thromboembolism (11%–22%), hemorrhagic complications, and rarely are due to infective endocarditis (3.6%). Sudden cardiac death is noted in a significant proportion of cases (14%).[39,40]

THE PREVENTION OF RHEUMATIC FEVER AND RHEUMATIC HEART DISEASE

Considering that RF follows a bacterial infection, it should be possible to prevent it as long as the organism remains susceptible to the available antibiotics. Fortunately, GAS continue to remain sensitive to penicillin. So, theoretically, it should be possible to eradicate RHD. In fact, RHD is the only heart disease that is preventable. That RF and RHD can be eliminated has been proven by the fact that high-income countries hardly have any new cases of RF or RHD. On the other hand, RHD remains a devastating illness in developing parts of the world that produces considerable morbidity and mortality. Once valvular damage is severe, balloon intervention or heart surgery is often required to repair or replace the damaged valve; both of these procedures are palliative. Surgery is expensive and most developing countries in which RHD is rampant do not have the resources to provide this facility. Further, patients with prosthetic mechanical valves continue to have adverse events due to valve thrombosis, bleeding, stroke, etc. Their survival is less frequent than in the control population. Keeping in mind the limited resources available in most areas with high prevalence rates, preventive programs should cater to the high-risk population as the returns will be much more beneficial. Extensive research continues into developing a vaccine for the prevention of RF but, as of today, no vaccine is available for clinical use. The prevention of RF and RHD can be undertaken at four different levels. All four levels are important; however, a combination of primary and secondary prevention seems to be most cost-effective.

Primordial prevention

This refers to the prevention of general risk factors, e.g., social, economic, and environmental initiatives to reduce the burden and impact transmission of group A streptococcal infection in a population. The various measures include: (1) creating awareness about RF and RHD and its link with bacterial sore throat; (2) better access to health-care facilities; and (3) education of the community about the importance of maintaining hygiene and sanitation. Improvements in housing and living conditions have contributed significantly to the decline of RF and RHD in the West. However, the feasibility of measures such as better housing, proper waste disposal, etc., is limited as these measures take a long time and are dependent on local policy makers and administrators.

Primary prevention

This term refers to any action that aims to prevent a first episode of RF. This is primarily achieved by the treatment of GAS throat infections in a timely and proper manner. Primary prevention can be quite challenging for various reasons. Since viral sore throats are very common, people with a sore throat may not attend a health-care facility. As many as 25%–30% of sore throats may be bacterial in origin, especially in the age group of 5–15 years. Staff at primary health centers and district hospitals may not be fully trained to recognize the bacterial nature and significance of a sore throat and its association with RHD, a serious sequel. Poor microbiological infrastructure for the confirmation of streptococcal sore throats by throat cultures and poor compliance with a full course of antibiotics are other reasons for the failure of primary prevention. It is also well known that many patients of RHD do not present with a history of sore throat. Therefore, the feasibility of primary prevention strategy remains low in developing countries. However, all efforts must be made to diagnose and treat streptococcal infections whenever feasible, as diagnosis and treatment are an important part of the control strategy.[59] Young patients with sore throats should be referred to a health facility early and health staff should be trained to differentiate a bacterial sore throat from a viral sore throat, and educated about the importance of treating sore throats. Throat swabbing and culture facilities will further help recognize GAS infection, although the low availability of this facility and the long time taken for the report to be ready are its major limitations. A rapid antigen diagnostic test for recognizing GAS pharyngitis may be better, if available, as it will obviate this delay. For treatment of GAS sore throat/skin infection, one can use a single intramuscular injection of long-acting penicillin, benzathine penicillin (BPG), or a full 10-day course of oral penicillin. Alternate antibiotics such as amoxicillin, erythromycin, etc., can also be used, but a full 10-day course is to be ensured. Treatment should be started promptly; however, the initiation of antibiotics as late as by the ninth day of infection is effective in preventing the attack of RF.

Secondary prevention

Secondary prevention aims at preventing recurrent episodes of RF in a person who already has had RF in the past or has RHD. Secondary prevention is primarily achieved by the long-term administration of antibiotics (long-acting penicillin in most cases), regularly (every three weeks). Secondary prevention with long-term penicillin (BPG) injections has been shown to prevent development of

RHD in those who have had RF. It also prevents the progression of heart damage and, in 50%–70% of cases, penicillin given over a 10-year period has been shown to regress valve disease.[60,61] Community health workers should work with families to ensure compliance with BPG injections in a timely fashion. Patients and their families should be educated about the importance of long-term secondary prophylaxis. Secondary prevention with BPG prophylaxis is the most cost-effective strategy in the prevention of RF and RHD.

Tertiary prevention

Tertiary prevention refers to interventions in patients who already have RHD to reduce symptoms and disability from associated complications. It is the least effective strategy. The aim is to prevent premature death from rheumatic heart disease. Treatments include medicines to treat heart failure and abnormal heart rhythms, etc. Performing percutaneous transvenous mitral commissurotomy in patients with MS remains a palliative treatment and all such patients need further follow-up to look for any complications, including restenosis. Surgery is very expensive and is not curative in nature. Management after surgery is also complicated because most patients need to be treated with blood-thinning drugs. Penicillin prophylaxis with BPG should also continue after surgery.

Prevention of RF and RHD is very challenging, particularly in regions with a high disease burden. This may be related to the lack of awareness in the community, socioeconomic factors, a lack of training of health professionals, poor access to health care, and health-seeking behavior of the local community. Other challenges include the poor availability of penicillin, the declining interest of the medical fraternity, fractured basic health systems, and an absence of interest amongst health policy makers in government. RF and RHD are diseases of poverty and social injustice and do not get priority in fund allocation for health at a national level.

CONCLUSION

RF results from interaction between the agent (GAS bacteria), a susceptible host, and an adverse environment. This disease has virtually disappeared from the Western world. The burden of RF and RHD continues to be high in developing countries where the vast majority of all patients with RHD live. RF commonly affects children between the ages of 5 and 15 years and is equally common in both sexes. MS secondary to RHD has a female preponderance. Natural history studies published in the 1950s and 1960s from Western countries describe a slow progression of the severity of MS. However, a number of studies from India and other developing countries have reported a much more rapid progression of MS leading to severe or critical MS at a very young age. These children and young adults have disabling symptoms, have severe pulmonary hypertension, and require early intervention. MS is also an important cause of maternal morbidity and mortality in India and many developing countries. RF and RHD are preventable diseases. The preventive strategies need to be multipronged but are challenging in those very countries where RF and RHD are rampant.

BIBLIOGRAPHY

1. Global Burden of Disease Study 2013 Collaborators. Global, regional, and national incidence, prevalence, and years lived with disability for 301 acute and chronic diseases and injuries in 188 countries, 1990–2013: A systematic analysis for the Global Burden of Disease Study 2013. Lancet 2015;386 (9995):743–800.
2. Carapetis JR. Rheumatic heart disease in developing countries. N Engl J Med 2007;357:439–41.
3. Global Burden of Disease 2013 Mortality and Causes of Death Collaborators. Global, regional, and national age-sex specific all cause and cause-specific mortality for 240 causes of death, 1990–2013: A systematic analysis for the Global Burden of Disease Study 2013. Lancet 2015;385:117–71.
4. World Health Organization. Rheumatic fever and rheumatic heart disease: Report of a WHO expert consultation. Geneva, 29 Oct–1 Nov 2001. World Health Organ Tech Rep Ser 2004;923:1–122.
5. Carapetis JR, Steer AC, Mulholland EK, Weber M. The global burden of group A streptococcal diseases. Lancet Infect Dis 2005;5:685–94.
6. Rothenbuhler M, O'Sullivan CJ, Stortecky S, Stefanini GG, Spitzer E, Estill J, Shrestha NR, Keiser O, Jüni P, Pilgrim T. Active surveillance for rheumatic heart disease in endemic regions: A systematic review and meta-analysis of prevalence among children and adolescents. Lancet Glob Health 2014;2:e717–26.
7. Global Burden of Disease Study 2010 Collaborators. Disability-adjusted life years (DALYs) for 291 diseases and injuries in 21 regions, 1990–2010: A systematic analysis for the Global Burden of Disease Study 2010. Lancet 2012;380:2197–223.
8. Kumar RK, Tandon R. Rheumatic fever and rheumatic heart disease: The last 50 years. Indian J Med Res 2013;137:643–58.
9. Bland EF, Jones DT. Rheumatic fever and rheumatic heart disease; A twenty-year report on 1000 patients followed since childhood. Circulation 1951;4:836–43.
10. Walsh BJ, Nestor JO. Rheumatic fever with heart disease. Clinical Proceedings – Children's Hospital of the District of Columbia 1956;12:68–74.
11. Bland EF. Chorea as a manifestation of rheumatic fever: A long-term perspective. Trans Am Clin Climatol Assoc 1961;73:209–13.
12. Aron AM, Freeman JM, Carter S. The natural history of sydenham's chorea. Review of the literature and long-term evaluation with emphasis on cardiac sequelae. Am J Med 1965;38:83–95.
13. Tadele H, Mekonnen W, Tefera E. Rheumatic MS in children: More accelerated course in sub-Saharan patients. BMC Cardiovasc Disord 2013;13:95. doi: 10.1186/1471-2261-13-95.
14. Ayoub EM, Barrett DJ, Maclaren NK, Krischer JP. Association of class II human histocompatibility antigens with rheumatic fever. J Clin Invest 1986;77:2019–26.
15. Engel ME, Stander R, Vogel J, Adeyemo AA, Mayosi BM. Genetic susceptibility to acute rheumatic fever: A systematic review and meta-analysis of twin studies. PLoS One 2011;6:e25326.
16. Carapetis JR, Currie BJ. Group A streptococcus, pyoderma, and rheumatic fever. Lancet 1996;347:1271–2.
17. Haidan A, Talay SR, Rohde M, Sriprakash KS, Currie BJ, Chhatwal GS. Pharyngeal carriage of group C and group G streptococci and acute rheumatic fever in an Aboriginal population. Lancet 2000;356:1167–9.

18. Lawrence JG, Carapetis JR, Griffiths K, Edwards K, Condon JR. Acute rheumatic fever and rheumatic heart disease: Incidence and progression in the Northern Territory of Australia, 1997 to 2010. *Circulation* 2013;128:492–501.
19. Parnaby MG, Carapetis JR. Rheumatic fever in indigenous Australian children. *J Paediatr Child Health* 2010;46:527–33.
20. Chandrashekhar Y, Westaby S, Narula J. Mitral stenosis. *Lancet* 2009;374(9697):1271–83.
21. Yacoub WSZ. Gender differences in systemic lupus erythematosus. *Gend Med* 2004;1:12–17.
22. Movahed MR, Ahmadi-Kashani M, Kasravi B, Saito Y. Increased prevalence of MS in women. *J Am Soc Echocardiogr* 2006;19:911–13.
23. Roy SB, Bhatia ML, Lazaro EJ, Ramalingaswami V. Juvenile MS in India. *Lancet* 1963;ii:1193–6.
24. Cherian G, Vytilingam KI, Sukumar IP, Gopinath M. Mitral valvotomy in young patients. *Br Heart J* 1964;26:157–66.
25. Diao M, Kane A, Ndiaye MB, Mbaye A, Bodian M, Dia MM, Sarr M, Kane A, Monsuez JJ, Ba SA. Pregnancy in women with heart disease in sub-Saharan Africa. *Arch Cardiovasc Dis* 2011;104:370–4.
26. Say L, Chou D, Gemmill A, Tunçalp Ö, Moller AB, Daniels J, Gülmezoglu AM, Temmerman M, Alkema L. Global causes of maternal death: A WHO systematic analysis. *Lancet Glob Health* 2014;2:e323–e333.
27. Soma-Pillay P, MacDonald AP, Mathivha TM, Bakker JL, Mackintosh MO. Cardiac disease in pregnancy: A 4-year audit at Pretoria Academic Hospital. *S Afr Med J* 2008;98:553–6.
28. Milne RJ, Lennon DR, Stewart JM, Vander Hoorn S, Scuffham PA. Incidence of acute rheumatic fever in New Zealand children and youth. *J Paediatr Child Health* 2012;48:685–91.
29. Chun LT, Reddy VD, Yamamoto LG. Rheumatic fever in children and adolescents in Hawaii. *Pediatrics* 1987;79:549–52.
30. Jaine R, Baker M, Venugopal K. Acute rheumatic fever associated with household crowding in a developed country. *Pediatr Infect Dis J* 2011;30:315–9.
31. Steer AC, Carapetis JR, Nolan TM, Shann F. Systematic review of rheumatic heart disease prevalence in children in developing countries: The role of environmental factors. *J Paediatr Child Health* 2002;38:229–34.
32. Brown A, McDonald MI, Calma T. Rheumatic fever and social justice. *Med J Aust* 2007;186:557–8.
33. Riaz BK, Selim S, Karim MN, Chowdhury KN, Chowdhury SH, Rahman MR. Risk factors of rheumatic heart disease in Bangladesh: A case–control study. *J Health Popul Nutr* 2013;31:70–7.
34. Carapetis JR, McDonald M, Wilson NJ. Acute rheumatic fever. *Lancet* 2005;366:155–68.
35. Selzer A, Cohn KE. Natural history of MS: A review. *Circulation* 1972;45:878–90.
36. Gordon SPF, Douglas PS, Come PC, Manning WJ. Two-dimensional and doppler echocardiographic determinants of the natural history of mitral valve narrowing in patients with rheumatic MS: Implications for follow-up. *J Am Coll Cardiol* 1992;19:968–73.
37. Sagie A, Freitas N, Padial LR, Leavitt M, Morris E, Weyman AE, Levine RA. Doppler echocardiographic assessment of long-term progression of MS in 103 patients: Valve area and right heart disease. *J Am Coll Cardiol* 1996;28:472–9.
38. Rowe JC, Bland EF, Sprague HB, White PD. Course of MS without surgery: Ten and twenty perspectives. *Ann Intern Med* 1960;52:741–9.
39. Olesen KH. The natural history of 271 patients with MS under medical treatment. *Br Heart J* 1962;24:349–57.
40. Horstkotte D, Niehues R, Strauer BE. Pathomorphological aspects, aetiology and natural history of acquired mitral valve stenosis. *Eur Heart J* 1991;12 Suppl B:55–60.
41. Bonow RO, Carabello BA, Kanu C et al. ACC/AHA 2006 guidelines for the management of patients with valvular heart disease: A report of the American College of Cardiology/American Heart Association Task Force on Practice Guidelines (writing committee to revise the 1998 Guidelines for the Management of Patients with Valvular Heart Disease): Developed in collaboration with the Society of Cardiovascular Anesthesiologists: Endorsed by the Society for Cardiovascular Angiography and Interventions and the Society of Thoracic Surgeons. *Circulation* 2006;114:e84–231.
42. Bonow RO, Carabello BA, Chatterjee K et al. 2008 focused update incorporated into the ACC/AHA 2006 guidelines for the

management of patients with valvular heart disease: A report of the American College of Cardiology/American Heart Association Task Force on Practice Guidelines (Writing Committee to revise the 1998 guidelines for the management of patients with valvular heart disease). Endorsed by the Society of Cardiovascular Anesthesiologists, Society for Cardiovascular Angiography and Interventions, and Society of Thoracic Surgeons. *J Am Coll Cardiol* 2008;52:e1–142.

43. Rinkevich D, Lessick J, Mutlak D, Markiewicz W, Reisner SA. Natural history of moderate mitral valve stenosis. *Isr Med Assoc J* 2003;5:15–8.

44. Tandon HD, Kasturi J. Pulmonary vascular changes associated with isolated MS in India. *Br Heart J* 1975;37:26–36.

45. Shrivastava S, Tandon R. Severity of rheumatic MS in children. *Int J Cardiol* 1991;30:163–7.

46. Borman JB, Stern S, Shapira T, Milvidsky H, Braun K. Mitral valvotomy in children. *Am Heart J* 1961;61:763–9.

47. Al-Bahrani IR, Thamer MA, Al-Omeri MM, Al-Namaan YD. Rheumatic heart disease in the young in Iraq. *Brit Heart J* 1966;28:824–8.

48. Marcus RH, Sareli P, Pocock WA et al. Functional anatomy of severe mitral regurgitation in active rheumatic carditis. *Am J Cardiol* 1989;63:577–84.

49. Reale A, Colella C, Bruno AM. MS in childhood: Clinical and therapeutic aspects. *Amer Heart J* 1963;66:15–28.

50. Ahmad S, Hayat U, Naz H. Frequency of severe MS in young female patients having pure MS secondary to rheumatic heart disease. *J Ayub Med Coll Abbottabad* 2010;22:19–22.

51. Rizvi SF, Khan MA, Kundi A, Marsh DR, Samad A, Pasha O. Status of rheumatic heart disease in rural Pakistan. *Heart* 2004;90:394–9.

52. Wilkins GT, Weyman AE, Abascal VM, Block PC, Palacios I. Percutaneous balloon dilatation of the mitral valve: An analysis of echocardiographic variables related to outcome and the mechanism of dilatation. *Br Heart J* 1988;60:299–308.

53. Kothari SS, Kamath P, Juneja R, Bahl VK, Airan B. Percutaneous transvenous mitral commissurotomy using Inoue balloon in children less than 12 years. *Cathet Cardiovasc Diagn* 1998;43:408–11.

54. Wood P. An appreciation of MS. *Brit Med J* 1954;1(4870):1051–63.

55. Kim HJ, Cho GY, Kim YJ et al. Development of atrial fibrillation in patients with rheumatic mitral valve disease in sinus rhythm. *Int J Cardiovasc Imaging* 2015;31:735–42.

56. Probst P, Goldschlager N, Selzer A. Left atrial size and atrial fibrillation in MS. Factors influencing their relationship. *Circulation* 1973;48:1282–7.

57. Sanfilippo AJ, Abascal VM, Sheehan M et al. Atrial enlargement as a consequence of atrial fibrillation. A prospective echocardiographic study. *Circulation* 1990;82:792–7.

58. Ward C, Hancock BW. Extreme pulmonary hypertension caused by mitral valve disease. Natural history and results of surgery. *Br Heart J* 1975;37:74–8.

59. Denny FW, Wannamaker LW, Brink WR, Rammelkamp CH Jr, Custer EA. Prevention of rheumatic fever; treatment of the preceding streptococcal infection. *J Am Med Assoc* 1950;143;151–3.

60. Feinstein A, Stern EK, Spagnuolo M. The prognosis of acute rheumatic fever. *Am Heart J* 1964;68:817–34.

61. Majeed H, Batnager S, Yousof AM, Khuffash F, Yusuf AR. Acute rheumatic fever and the evolution of rheumatic heart disease: A prospective 12 year follow up report. *J Clin Epidemiol* 1992;45:871–5.

3

The etiology of mitral stenosis

ANUNAY GUPTA AND SANDEEP SINGH

INTRODUCTION

Mitral stenosis (MS) causes obstruction to the blood flow from the left atrium to the left ventricle, leading to an increase in left-atrium pressure and, subsequently, increased pulmonary capillary wedge pressure. Over time, the patient develops pulmonary artery hypertension and eventually right-heart failure. Table 3.1 shows important causes of MS. Rheumatic heart disease (RHD) remains the most common cause of MS. Other causes are uncommon and are encountered rarely in clinical practice. In a study with 1051 consecutive patients with pure or predominant MS requiring surgical intervention, aetiology was rheumatic in 76.9%, infective in 3.3%, degenerative (severe annular and leaflet calcification) in 2.7%, and Lutembacher's syndrome (an association of atrial septal defect and rheumatic MS) was present in 1.2% of cases. Other causes, such as systemic lupus erythematosus, carcinoid heart disease, endomyocardial fibrosis, and rheumatoid arthritis, were seen in less than 1% of cases. In approximately 15% of cases, the aetiology remained unclassified.[1] This chapter reviews various aetiologies of MS.

RHEUMATIC HEART DISEASE

RHD is the most common cause of MS. Histopathology of excised valves having MS reveal changes suggestive of RHD in 99% of cases. RHD is a chronic sequela of either a single severe attack or recurrent episodes of acute rheumatic fever. However, only 50%–70% of patients with MS report a history of rheumatic fever. The time lag for development of clinically evident MS after an initial episode of rheumatic fever is variable, ranging between a few years and two decades. It is a slowly progressive disease with the progress of valve narrowing being 0.09 ± 0.21 cm^2 per year.[2]

The inflammatory process in the valve is due to the cross-reactivity of streptococcal cell wall proteins and enzymes against the heart valve tissue. Valve leaflets do not show any evidence of active infection. Carditis during an episode of rheumatic fever usually leads to the formation of multiple inflammatory foci in the valve tissue. With time, the valve apparatus becomes thickened, contracted, and calcified. There is commissural adhesion and fibrosis, ultimately resulting in stenosis of the mitral valve. These anatomical changes lead to the typical appearance of rheumatic MS.

Table 3.1 The etiology of mitral stenosis

Rheumatic heart disease (commonest cause)
Congenital mitral stenosis
Mitral annular calcification
Radiation-induced
Rare causes
- Drug-induced valvular disease: methysergide, pergolide, fenfluramine, or dexfenfluramine
- Connective tissue disorders: rheumatoid arthritis, systemic lupus erythematosus
- Carcinoid syndrome
- Mucopolysaccharidosis
- Whipple's disease
- Hyper-eosinophilic syndrome, endomyocardial fibrosis
- External compression: tumors, chronic constrictive pericarditis, hematoma

Iatrogenic causes
- Transcatheter aortic valve replacement
- MitraClip
- Alfieri surgical repair
- Impella device

Prosthetic heart valve thrombosis of mitral valve
Bioprosthetic valve degeneration

Table 3.2 Causes of congenital mitral stenosis

Abnormalities of leaflet
- Double-orifice mitral valve
- Supramitral ring associated with Shone's complex

Abnormalities of tensor apparatus
- Arcade or hammock valve
- Straddling mitral valve

Abnormalities of the papillary muscles
- Parachute mitral valve

Abnormalities of mitral annulus
- Hypoplasia of mitral annulus

In initial stages of the disease, there is a restriction of motion at the leaflet tips leading to diastolic doming, which is most evident in the motion of the anterior leaflet. With the progress of disease and in elderly patients, doming becomes less prominent as the leaflets become more fibrotic and calcified.

CONGENITAL MITRAL STENOSIS

Congenital causes of MS are rare. Its reported incidence in patients with congenital heart disease is 0.4% in clinical and 0.6% in autopsy series.[3] Developmental abnormalities of mitral valve leaflets, commissures, interchordal spaces, papillary muscles, mitral annulus, or supravalvular structures can produce obstruction to left-ventricular filling. Usually, there is involvement of multiple segments of the mitral valve apparatus in varied forms and severity. The most frequently observed pathology is fusion or poor development of commissures, short or even absent chordae, and tethering of the papillary muscle to the left-ventricle free wall. There can be associated involvement of other cardiac valves. Table 3.2 summarizes various mechanisms of congenital MS. Based on the histopathology of autopsy specimens of mitral valve apparatus, four types of congenital MS are known. These are typical MS caused by short chordae tendineae along with obliteration of the interchordal space and reduction of inter-papillary distance; hypoplastic congenital MS associated with hypoplastic left-heart syndrome; supramitral ring; and parachute mitral valve, in which the chordal apparatus is inserted into a single papillary muscle or a muscle group.

Patients with congenital MS usually present during infancy and early childhood. Their clinical presentation depends upon the severity of obstruction, presence of mitral regurgitation, severity of pulmonary artery hypertension, and presence of other associated lesions like hypoplastic left heart, aortic stenosis, and coarctation of aorta.

MITRAL ANNULAR CALCIFICATION

Mitral annular calcification (MAC) is a chronic, progressive, and degenerative process causing dystrophic calcification in the mitral valve annulus. Usually, it is detected as an incidental finding in the elderly age group. Rarely, it becomes clinically significant due to the impairment of normal diastolic annular dilation along with restricted mitral valve leaflet motion causing left-ventricular inflow obstruction. The prevalence of this condition is increasing due to a better life expectancy, a higher population of elderly individuals, and an increasing number of patients having risk factors such as hypertension. According to the European Heart Survey, degenerated MS accounted for approximately 10%, 30%, and 60% of all cases of

MS in the age groups of 60–70, 70–80, and more than 80 years, respectively.[4] This condition is also known as senile MS. Degeneration becomes accelerated and can occur even in younger age groups in patients with chronic kidney disease, hypertension, diabetes mellitus, hypercalcemia, hypercholesterolemia, and congenital abnormalities like Marfan and Hurler syndromes. Diagnosis of rheumatic mitral stenosis should be considered if commissural calcium and fusion is seen. In fewer than 1% of cases, the calcified mass may contain a radiolucent core. This finding has been termed "caseous" calcification of the mitral valve annulus, or mitral annular calcification with central softening. In a study of 100 patients of more than 62 years of age with MAC, only 6% had a mean gradient of more than 5 mmHg and mitral valve area of less than 1.8 cm^2.[5] It is hypothesized that due to the presence of concurrent diastolic abnormalities during relaxation, mitral valve area calculated by pressure half-time on echocardiography may be underestimated. MAC can be associated with conduction system diseases, atrial fibrillation, and an increased risk of coronary and vascular disease. It can serve as a nidus for secondary infective endocarditis.

RADIATION-INDUCED MITRAL STENOSIS

The heart was initially considered to be a radio-resistant organ; however, with the introduction of high-voltage radiotherapy, it is now considered to be a radiosensitive organ that undergoes pathological changes because of radiation. Radiation exposure is now considered a definite risk factor for the development of clinically significant valvular heart disease, especially of the aortic valve.[6] Survivors of Hodgkin's lymphoma, non-Hodgkin's lymphoma, and breast cancer and patients receiving mediastinal radiotherapy require vigilance and screening for any valvular heart disease, even after 15 to 20 years of curative treatment. The risk is related to radiotherapy dose and progressively increases with time following the initial exposure.[7] The majority of patients develop valvular regurgitation and are usually asymptomatic. Radiation-induced development of MS is uncommon.[8] It occurs late and is characterized by leaflet thickening predominantly involving the base and mid-body of the valve with the absence of commissural fusion. The predominant pathology is chronic valve inflammation, fibrosis, and calcification.[9]

RARE CAUSES

Drug-induced valvular disease: there is sufficient evidence to support an association between fibrotic valve disease and certain drugs. The implicated drugs are methysergide, an ergot alkaloid; pergolide, an ergot-derived dopaminergic agonist used for the treatment of parkinsonism; and anti-obesity drugs such as fenfluramine or dexfenfluramine. These drugs have been shown to have a common pharmacological action on specific serotonin (5HT$_{2B}$) receptors. These receptors are concentrated in the valvular tissue. The changes in the valves are similar to those observed in carcinoid heart disease, a neuro-endocrine serotonin producing disorder. Clinically, a variable degree of valve regurgitation is seen. Typically, there is only mild to moderate valve thickening. Severe valve stenosis is usually not observed.[10] In contrast with rheumatic MS, there is an absence of any calcification or commissural fusion. The morphological and histological features include tissue thickening and the formation of an extracellular matrix of glycosaminoglycan and collagen with a proliferation of myofibroblasts and smooth muscle cells. The underlying valve structure usually remains unchanged.

Fabry disease is a rare X-linked lysosomal storage disorder leading to an accumulation of glycosphingolipids in all tissues and organs including the heart. Usually, there is valve regurgitation. Rarely, it can lead to the development of MS.[11]

Connective tissue disorders such as rheumatoid arthritis and systemic lupus erythematous can cause myocardial, valvular, pericardial, and conduction system abnormalities. Cardiac involvement in these chronic diseases varies from asymptomatic or mild to severe life-threatening conditions. Rarely, there can be development of MS.[12]

Metastatic carcinoid tumors usually involve the right side of the heart. Left-sided valvular involvement leading to MS is uncommon.[13] The carcinoid lesion consists of deposits of fibrous tissue devoid of elastic fibers known as carcinoid plaque. The deposits are seen on the endocardial surface on the ventricular aspect of the tricuspid or mitral leaflets

Table 3.3 Hemodynamic mimics of mitral stenosis

1. Large left-atrial myxoma
2. Large vegetation on mitral valve
3. Ball valve thrombus in left atrium

and on the arterial aspect of the pulmonary or aortic valve cusps.

Whipple disease is a rare infection, affecting the gastrointestinal system. Chronic valvular deformity mimicking the presentation of MS has been reported in these patients.[14]

Mucopolysaccharidosis syndromes (MPS) are inherited diseases characterized by increased tissue glycosaminoglycans concentrations as a result of decreased enzymatic activity of degrading enzymes. There are case reports of MS in MPS requiring mitral valve replacement due to accumulation of glycosaminoglycans in cardiac valves.[15]

HEMODYNAMIC MIMICS

Many conditions can produce hemodynamic abnormalities similar to valvular MS (Table 3.3). A large atrial myxoma may mimic the clinical presentation of MS due to the obstruction of the mitral valve orifice by tumor mass. Other conditions that can mimic MS are large vegetations on the mitral valve, ball-valve thrombus in the left atrium, prosthetic heart valve thrombosis of the mitral valve, and degenerative bioprosthetic mitral valve.

IATROGENIC CAUSES

Transcatheter aortic valve replacement can cause iatrogenic MS.[16] There are case reports of mitral stenosis after MitraClip implantation.[17,18] The edge-to-edge repair, also known as "Alfieri's stitch," is an effective technique in the restoration of mitral valve competence. It leads to the formation of two orifices and the effective mitral valve area is reduced. It can rarely lead to the development of significant MS. Even Impella, a temporary ventricular support device, can cause functional MS if the shaft of the device lies on the anterior mitral leaflet.[19]

SUMMARY

RHD is the most common cause of mitral stenosis; other causes are relatively uncommon.

Congenital MS is seen in the pediatric age group. Mitral annular calcification causing degenerated MS is a rare disease of the elderly. In this, valve thickening and calcification predominantly involves the base of the leaflets without any commissural fusion. This contrasts with rheumatic MS, where thickening and calcification predominates at the tips of valve leaflets, and there is commissural fusion. Radiation exposure is a definite risk factor for the development of clinically significant valvular heart disease. Usually it involves the aortic valve; the development of hemodynamic significant MS is rare. Findings of restrictive motion of posterior mitral leaflet and commissural fusion, which are hallmarks of rheumatic MS, are usually absent in radiation-induced MS. Iatrogenic causes are increasingly being recognized and clinicians should be aware of this possible complication.

REFERENCES

1. Horstkotte D, Niehues R, Strauer BE. Pathomorphological aspects, aetiology and natural history of acquired mitral valve stenosis. *Eur Heart J* 1991 Jul;12 Suppl B: 55–60.
2. Gordon SP, Douglas PS, Come PC, Manning WJ. Two-dimensional and Doppler echocardiographic determinants of the natural history of mitral valve narrowing in patients with rheumatic mitral stenosis: Implications for follow-up. *J Am Coll Cardiol* 1992 Apr;19(5):968–73.
3. Collins-Nakai RL, Rosenthal A, Castaneda AR, Bernhard WF, Nadas AS. Congenital mitral stenosis. A review of 20 years' experience. *Circulation* 1977 Dec;56(6):1039–47.
4. Iung B, Baron G, Butchart EG et al. A prospective survey of patients with valvular heart disease in Europe: The Euro Heart Survey on Valvular Heart Disease. *Eur Heart J* 2003 Jul;24(13):1231–43.
5. Aronow WS, Kronzon I. Correlation of prevalence and severity of mitral regurgitation and mitral stenosis determined by Doppler echocardiography with physical signs of mitral regurgitation and mitral stenosis in 100 patients aged 62 to 100 years with mitral anular calcium. *Am J Cardiol* 1987 Nov 15;60(14):1189–90.

6. Gujral DM, Lloyd G, Bhattacharyya S. Radiation-induced valvular heart disease. *Heart Br Card Soc* 2016 Feb 15;102(4):269–76.

7. Cutter DJ, Schaapveld M, Darby SC et al. Risk of valvular heart disease after treatment for Hodgkin lymphoma. *J Natl Cancer Inst* 2015 Apr;107(4).

8. Malanca M, Cimadevilla C, Brochet E, Iung B, Vahanian A, Messika-Zeitoun D. Radiotherapy-induced mitral stenosis: A three-dimensional perspective. *J Am Soc Echocardiogr* 2010 Jan;23(1):108.e1–2.

9. Pohjola-Sintonen S, Tötterman KJ, Salmo M, Siltanen P. Late cardiac effects of mediastinal radiotherapy in patients with Hodgkin's disease. *Cancer* 1987 Jul 1;60(1):31–7.

10. Misch KA. Development of heart valve lesions during methysergide therapy. *Br Med J* 1974 May 18;2(5915):365–6.

11. Leder AA, Bosworth WC. Angiokeratoma corporis diffusum universale (Fabry's disease) with mitral stenosis. *Am J Med* 1965 May 1;38(5):814–9.

12. Hasegawa R, Kitahara H, Watanabe K, Kuroda H, Amano J. Mitral stenosis and regurgitation with systemic lupus erythematosus and antiphospholipid antibody syndrome. *Jpn J Thorac Cardiovasc Surg* 2001 Dec;49(12):711–3.

13. Dave B, Godkar D, Niranjan S, Lin K. Mitral stenosis as a rare presentation of carcinoid syndrome. *J Investig Med* 2007 Jan;55(1):S113. Accessed June 12, 2017. Retrieved from http://jim.bmj.com/content/55/1/S113.6.

14. Rose AG. Mitral stenosis in Whipple's disease. *Thorax* 1978 Aug;33(4):500–3.

15. Fischer TA, Lehr HA, Nixdorff U, Meyer J. Combined aortic and mitral stenosis in mucopolysaccharidosis type I-S (Ullrich-Scheie syndrome). *Heart Br Card Soc* 1999 Jan;81(1):97–9.

16. Harries I, Chandrasekaran B, Barnes E, Ramcharitar S. Iatrogenic mitral stenosis following transcatheter aortic valve replacement (TAVR). *Indian Heart J* 2015;67(1):60–1.

17. Pope NH, Lim S, Ailawadi G. Late calcific mitral stenosis after MitraClip procedure in a dialysis-dependent patient. *Ann Thorac Surg* 2013 May;95(5):e113–4.

18. Cockburn J, Fragkou P, Hildick-Smith D. Development of mitral stenosis after single MitraClip insertion for severe mitral regurgitation. *Catheter Cardiovasc Interv* 2014 Feb;83(2):297–302.

19. Toggweiler S, Jamshidi P, Erne P. Functional mitral stenosis: A rare complication of the Impella assist device. *Eur J Echocardiogr* 2008 May;9(3):412–3.

4

The pathophysiology of mitral stenosis

SUDHEER ARAVA, KUSUMA HARISHA, AND RUMA RAY

ANATOMY OF THE MITRAL VALVE

The mitral (bicuspid/left-atrioventricular) valve is a complex structure that resembles the pointed headdress of Bishop's miter.[1] It is obliquely situated in the immediate vicinity of the aortic valve. The normal area of the mitral valve orifice is 4–6 cm^2, which is sufficient to allow the flow of blood from the left atrium to the left ventricle. In the open state, the valve looks like a funnel extending from the hinge line of the atrioventricular junction to the free margins.[2] The main function of mitral valve is to prevent the backflow of blood from the left ventricle during active ventricular systole. For its proper function, the mitral valve requires all its structural components along with part of the adjacent left-atrial and left-ventricular musculature.[1] Structurally, the mitral valve complex consists of four components, namely: 1) the mitral valve annulus; 2) the mitral valve leaflets; 3) tendinous chords; and 4) the papillary muscles (Figure 4.1a and b).[1]

The mitral valve annulus

The mitral valve annulus is a solid, strong, fibrous, "D"-shaped hinge-like structure that separates the left atrium from the left ventricle and gives attachment to the mitral leaflets. The straight border of the "D" is in very close proximity to the aortic valve.[1] The remaining curvilinear portion of the mitral valve annulus covers the rest of the atrioventricular area. The area of fibrous expansion on either side of the aortic and mitral valve continuity are known as the right and left fibrous trigones.[1,3] The right fibrous trigone, along with the fibrous portion of the septum, is called the central fibrous body. The atrioventricular bundle (bundle of His) usually passes through the right fibrous trigone. The annulus near the attachment of the mitral valve fibrous continuity is weak when compared to the other parts of the mitral valve annulus. This is the area commonly affected in annular dilatation.[1,2] It is also the area involved in the annular calcification of the mitral valve.

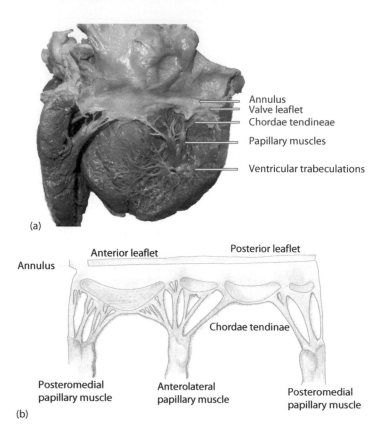

Figure 4.1 (**a** and **b**) Components of normal mitral valve.

The mitral valve leaflets

The mitral valve leaflets are two obliquely placed, thin, translucent, and shiny fibrous cusps with varying shape and circumferential length, termed the "aortic (anterior) leaflet" and the "mural (posterior) leaflet."[1] The septal leaflet, which is a characteristic feature of the tricuspid valve, is not present in the mitral valve. Each of the leaflets has two surfaces, i.e., the atrial and ventricular surfaces.[2] The aortic leaflet is a round structure and occupies one-third of the valve circumference, whereas the mural leaflet is long and narrow and occupies the remaining two-thirds of the circumference. The aortic leaflet is in fibrous continuity with the aortic valve. When a closed valve is viewed from the atrial side, it resembles a "smile" (Figure 4.2). The free lining end of the closure or the junction between two leaflets is known as a "commissure." The free edge of the mural commissure is again divided into scallops or segments, as lateral (P1), middle (P2), and medial (P3).[1–3]

These three scallops are those most commonly observed and are not of equal size. However, the middle scallop is found to be larger in the majority of hearts. The free edge of the aortic leaflet has A1, A2, and A3 segments.[3] Indentations on the valve leaflets do not reach the mitral annulus and end approximately 5 mm short of the annular attachment in an adult heart. In a floppy valve, it is the middle leaflet that is commonly prolapsed. Both leaflets show two zones known as the clear zone and the rough zone, which are divided by the attachment of the chordae tendineae.[1] The clear zone does not have any chordal attachment, whereas the rough zone (irregular and nodular) near the free edge in the atrial surface has the tendinous chord attachment.[3] The prominent ridge that separates these two zones is the line of leaflet closure. (Also see "Surgical Anatomy of the Mitral Valve" in Chapter 14.)

Line of coaptation: When both the valve leaflets close, the line of closure lies below the plane of atrioventricular junction rising towards the

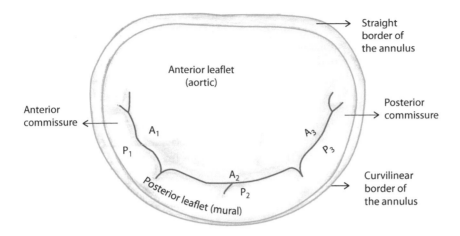

Figure 4.2 Normal mitral valve.

commissures at the periphery. The line of coaptation usually does not extend above the junction level in the ventricular systole. Occasionally, the leaflets may form a hooded appearance with a pocket-like doming towards the atrium. This should not be considered as an indicator of valve prolapse.

Commissures: Aortic and mural leaflets form an arc-shaped closure line (zone of apposition) when they approximate with each other. This line is obliquely situated when compared to the body plane. Each end of the closure line is known as a commissure. Hence, the two commissures in the mitral valve are known as the 1) anterolateral and 2) posteromedial commissure.

Subvalvular apparatus

Tendinous chords: These are string-like fibrous structures that attach to the ventricular surface of the mitral valve leaflet on one end and to the papillary muscles on the other end (true chordae tendineae). Sometimes, chords may also attach directly to the posteroinferior aspect of the left ventricular wall to form the tensor apparatus of the valve (false chordae tendineae).[1] Chords arising from the tip of the papillary muscle usually attach to both the atrial and mural leaflets. They are anatomically grouped as primary, secondary, and tertiary chords depending on their attachment.[3] As the tendinous chords branch distally, the number of chords is approximately five times closer to the

valve attachment than on the papillary muscles.[4] First-order chords are numerous and delicate and insert into the free edge of the valve. Second-order chords insert into the ventricular aspect of the leaflet and form the rough zone of the valve cusps. These are thicker than first-order chords. Third-order chords attach directly to the mitral valve leaflets. They arise directly from the ventricular wall and form small trabeculations. They insert into the basal portion of the valve and are shorter.[1,4]

Papillary muscles: These are the muscular components of the mitral valve apparatus. They commonly arise from the apical and midportion of the left ventricular wall.[1] For normal valvular function, papillary muscles require part of the left-ventricular musculature. They are present in two close groups located beneath the commissures, anterolateral and posteromedial.[3] The anterolateral papillary muscle is larger and is supplied by the circumflex or anterior descending branch of the left coronary artery. The posteromedial papillary muscle is supplied by the right coronary artery. At their base, they sometimes fuse or form muscular/fibrous continuity before attaching to the left ventricular wall. Extensive fusion results in parachute malformation leading to mitral stenosis (MS). Any alteration in the left-ventricular structure distorts the position of the papillary muscle, leading to abnormality in mitral valve function. Rupture of the papillary muscle, which is one of the complications of left-ventricular infarction, usually results in mitral valve regurgitation.[1]

Left atrial wall

The left atrial wall forms an important functional unit of mitral valvular performance.[1] The atrial myocardial fibers are in continuity with the atrial side of the posterior mitral valve leaflet. Due to this, any increase in the atrial diameter subsequently leads to mitral valve dysfunction (left-atrial dilatation causing mitral regurgitation). The degree of muscular extension may vary from heart to heart.[1]

DEVELOPMENTAL EMBRYOLOGY

The development of the mitral valve is a complex process with the involvement of tightly regulated genes. The heart develops from a primitive heart tube. Later, the heart tube forms the atrioventricular canal, which then divides into the right and left atrioventricular junctions. Atrioventricular valves begin to form between the fifth and eighth week of gestation. The first evidence of valvulogenesis is the formation of endocardial cushions in the atrioventricular canal by highly proliferative progenitor cells. Endocardial cushion formation is induced by myocardial production of signaling molecules that inhibit the expression of chamber-specific genes in the atrioventricular canal. The primordial valve formed continues to grow and elongate into a thin fibrous leaflet with the gradual accumulation of extracellular matrix (ECM) proteoglycans, which cause the valve tissue to protrude into the interior lumen of the heart. During late gestation and soon after birth the valve leaflets become stratified into a highly organized collagen, proteoglycan, elastin-rich ECM compartment. The anterior leaflet is derived from the superior and inferior cushions while the posterior mitral leaflet is derived from the lateral cushion. Cell lineage studies from mouse models demonstrated that the majority of valve cells originate from the endothelial endocardial cushion. Myocytes are usually absent from the mature valve. Embryological hypothesis reveals the detachment and migration of endothelial cells into the mesenchyme, which then transdifferentiate into interstitial fibroblastic cells. This process is known as endothelial mesenchymal transition (EMT).[5] Around the tenth week of life, ventricular trabeculae become compact and the small papillary muscle is observed. During the eleventh to thirteenth week of gestation, papillary muscle becomes more distinct and the rudimentary chordae develop. By the fifteenth week, mitral valve leaflets, chordae, and papillary muscles develop completely.

NORMAL HISTOLOGY

A properly oriented section of the mitral valve leaflet consists of four layers (Figures 4.3 and 4.4).

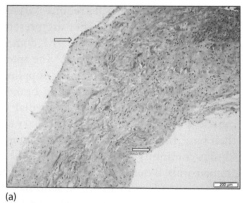

(a)

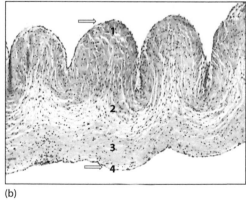

(b)

Figure 4.3 Histology of mitral valve: Properly oriented mitral valve specimen consists of four layers. From above downwards: **(a)** Hematoxylin and eosin section of the mitral valve and **(b)** Schematic diagram showing valve layers: 1) Lamina atrialis 2) Lamina spongiosa 3) Lamina fibrosa and 4) Lamina ventricularis. Arrow indicates the single layer of endothelial cell layer which continues with the atrial and ventricular endocardium.

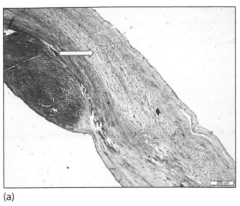
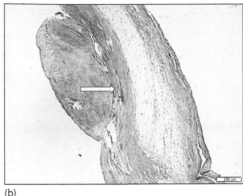

(a)   (b)

Figure 4.4 Special histochemical stain reveals the clear distinction of the mitral valve layers: **(a)** Alcian blue-Periodic acid Schiff stain (ABPAS) demonstrates the lamina spongiosa (arrow). **(b)** Lamina fibrosa is clearly highlighted by Masson trichrome stain (arrow).

The first layer is the *lamina atrialis*, composed of properly oriented elastic and collagen fibers. It is covered with a single layer of endothelium, which continues with the endocardial lining of the left atria. The *lamina spongiosa* lies beneath the atrialis and separates the lamina fibrosa. It contains abundant proteoglycans, which give it a spongy and loose appearance. This layer acts as a shock absorber. The *lamina fibrosa* is a dense full-length layer that contains collagen fibers, and it is continuous with the fibrous annulus. This layer gives structural support and strength to the mitral leaflets. The *lamina ventricularis* is similar to the *lamina atrialis* but is continuous with the endocardium of the ventricular surface.[3]

Normally all the valves are avascular except for a small area near the base of the valve attachment, which contains few capillaries and smooth muscle cells. Generally, valves are devoid of any inflammatory cells.

MITRAL STENOSIS

MS is characterized by the abnormal narrowing of the mitral valve orifice causing obstruction to the normal forward flow of blood. This disorder was first reported in 1668 by John Mayow, an Oxford physiologist, and, until recently, it was the most discussed valvular heart disease.[6–10] Rheumatic heart disease is still one of the most common etiological factor of MS worldwide, with varying incidence and distribution. Hence, the detailed

pathophysiological features of this condition will be mentioned later in this chapter. Other conditions causing MS are categorized below.

Mitral annular calcification

The pathophysiological process in mitral annular calcification (MAC) is similar to any other vascular calcification in the body (Figure 4.5). In MAC, calcification is mainly limited to the mitral annulus and leaflet base. Occasionally, it may extend to the leaflet resulting in restricted mobility. In fewer than 1% of cases, the calcified mass may contain a radiolucent core. This finding has been termed "caseous" calcification of the mitral valve annulus. Microscopic examination of this condition shows presence of dystrophic calcification, fibrosis, and sometimes osteoblastic differentiation in the region of mitral annulus. The amount and degree of calcification may vary from case to case. There is no grading system available to assess the degree of calcification. Calcification commonly affects the posterior portion of the valve annulus rather than the anterior portion.[11–13] MAC can serve as a nidus for secondary infective endocarditis. Younger patients may also develop MAC due to abnormal wear and tear of the annulus in conditions like rheumatic heart disease, chronic renal failure, and mitral valve prolapse, or in metabolic disorders. MAC is also associated with other conditions including increased left-ventricular afterload, systemic hypertension, hypertrophic obstructive

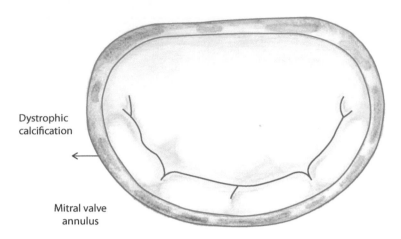

Dystrophic
calcification

Mitral valve
annulus

Figure 4.5 Mitral annular calcification.

cardiomyopathy, and valvular aortic stenosis. The pathophysiological mechanism behind the development of MAC is increased annular tension. Elevated mitral valve closing pressure results in excess annular tension and repetitive trauma. These sites of annular trauma undergo dystrophic calcification, leading to MAC. Any condition that causes an increase in left-ventricular pressure can result in increased mitral valve stress and accelerated progression of MAC.[13] In pure mitral annular calcification, fusion of the mitral valve commissures is not noted. If commissural fusion is noted, then an alternative diagnosis of rheumatic valvular heart disease should be considered.

Congenital mitral stenosis

Congenital MS is defined as a developmental anomaly of the mitral valve leaflets, commissures, interchordal spaces, papillary muscles, and the annulus causing obstruction to left-ventricular filling.[14-16] Congenital malformation of the mitral valve is very rare, with an estimated incidence of about 0.4% in patients with congenital heart disease.[17-19] When present, it usually involves other valves and multiple segments of the valve apparatus in several forms. Fusion and poor development of the commissures is one of the most frequently observed anatomic features of congenital MS.[15] Other common variants include hypoplasia of the mitral valve annulus,[19] supravalvular ring in the left atrium, abnormalities of the chordae tendineae, parachute mitral valve (chordal apparatus is inserted into a single-papillary muscle or a

muscle group),[16] and double mitral valve orifices. Unileaflet mitral valve,[17] and accessory mitral valve[18] (if present) is usually seen on the ventricular aspect. Ruckman and Van Praagh[20] have described four classical types of congenital MS. They are: (1) typical MS caused by short chordae tendineae with obliteration of the interchordal space and reduction of inter-papillary distance; (2) hypoplastic congenital MS; (3) supramitral ring; and (4) parachute mitral valve.

Infective endocarditis

Infective endocarditis causing mitral valve regurgitation is a well-recognized complication, but infective endocarditis leading to MS is very rare.[21] Rarely, only large valvular vegetations may cause MS. The anterior mitral leaflet is the most common site for infective vegetations in a patient of infective endocarditis. Vegetations are usually large in cases of fungal etiology as compared to those of a bacterial nature (see Figure 4.6).

Radiation-associated mitral valve stenosis

Radiation-induced valvular heart disease is uncommon and affects approximately 6%–15% of patients exposed to mediastinal radiotherapy.[22] The pericardium is the most commonly affected structure.[23] Mediastinal radiation is used in the treatment of a variety of diseases, such as Hodgkin's lymphoma, seminoma, breast cancer, and lung cancer.[24,25] The heart is now considered

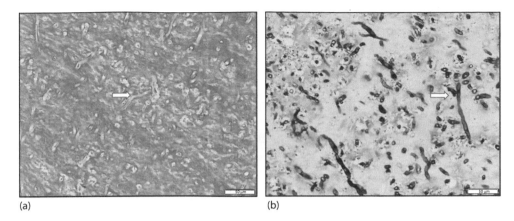

(a)   (b)

Figure 4.6 Infective fungal endocarditis: **(a)** Routine hematoxylin and eosin stain from the vegetation shows many negatively stained fungal profiles (arrow). **(b)** Grocott silver methenamine stain highlights and shows the acute angle branching septate fungal hyphae (arrow).

a radiosensitive organ that undergoes pathological changes as a result of radiation. The complication usually manifests after 15–20 years of therapy. Common cardiac disorders include premature coronary artery atherosclerotic disease, valvular disorders, pericardial fibrosis, conduction defects, and cardiomyopathy. Valvular dysfunction mainly results from chronic inflammation, fibrosis, and calcification.[24,25] The incidence of valvular abnormalities varies according to different studies. Regurgitant lesions tend to occur earlier than stenotic lesion. MS occurs late and is characterized by leaflet thickening, involving the base and midbody of the valve with the absence of commissural fusion. The mechanisms of radiation-induced cardiac disease are not clear. However, the disease progresses slowly and long-term follow-up is important.[24,25] Over time, cellular injury combined with pressure-related trauma leads to valvular thickening, chronic inflammation, fibrosis, and calcification.

Metabolic or enzymatic abnormalities

Some common metabolic diseases associated with MS are Fabry's disease, Whipple disease, mucopolysaccharidosis, and valvular involvement in carcinoid disease.[26] Endomyocardial fibrosis and autoimmune diseases like systemic lupus erythematosus (SLE) and rheumatoid arthritis may also present as MS.

RHEUMATIC MITRAL STENOSIS

Rheumatic mitral stenosis remains the most common cause of MS. Rheumatic MS is the sequelae of acute rheumatic fever.

Acute rheumatic fever

Rheumatic fever is an inflammatory disease that usually affects children and young adults aged between 1 and 19 years. It is a prototype of a postinfectious autoimmune disease caused by untreated oropharyngeal infection by group A β-hemolytic streptococcus (GAS).[27] Only 0.3%–3% of individuals affected by streptococcus develop rheumatic fever. Approximately two-thirds of rheumatic fever patients progress to rheumatic carditis and only a portion of them suffer from severe cardiac manifestations.[28,29] The exact mechanism leading to chronic inflammation of the heart valves is still unclear. However, studies have shown evidence of an epitope-spreading phenomenon (molecular mimicry) and the development of a long-lasting cellular immune response that are responsible for the cardiovascular damage.[27]

CAUSATIVE ORGANISM: GROUP A β-HEMOLYTIC STREPTOCOCCI

Group A streptococcus pyogenes is an important pathogenic bacterium that causes a wide variety of clinical conditions ranging from pharyngitis to severe invasive infections and necrotizing fasciitis. The most common mode of disease transmission is by direct contact of mucus droplets from an infected person. The organisms are gram-positive, non-motile, non-sporing, facultative anaerobes that grow in pairs and chains (Figure 4.7a). According to the Lancefield classification, they are categorized as group A because they display antigen A on their cell wall. They are called β-hemolytic because, on a blood culture agar plate, they typically produce a small zone of complete hemolysis (Figure 4.7b). The outer layer of *streptococcus pyogenes* is covered by a hyaluronic acid capsule that is chemically similar to the host connective tissue; therefore, it is non-antigenic. This is vital for these bacteria to survive in the host. The cytoplasmic membrane has antigens similar to human cardiac, skeletal, and smooth muscle cells. Some of the important surface antigens of streptococcus are as follows (Figure 4.8):

1. *C-Carbohydrates:* Protect the streptococcus from being dissolved by the lysosomal defense mechanisms of the host. One specific carbohydrate is N-acetyl glucosamine.
2. *Lipoteichoic acid:* Enables *streptococcus pyogenes* to adhere to the epithelial cells in the skin or respiratory mucosa.
3. *M-protein:* A fibrillary surface projection that contributes to the virulence of the organism by resisting phagocytosis and improving adherence.

4. *Hyaluronic acid:* Also found in human tissue; hence, it does not provoke an immune response from the host.
5. *C5a protease:* Catalyzes the cleavage of the C5a protein of the complement system.[29]

Streptococci express various fimbria-like structural proteins on their cell surfaces, which bind to human extracellular matrix proteins including fibronectin (Fn), laminin, and collagen. There are many known fibronectin-binding proteins, but each is expressed and distributed in a particular group of M-serotype organisms and is involved in adhesion and invasion. *Streptococci* express two major classes—M- and T-antigen—and two minor classes—R- and F-antigen. M-protein has a fibrillary coiled structure. It is strongly antiphagocytic and is a major virulent factor. It binds to serum H-factor, destroys C3 convertase, and prevents opsonization by C3. However, plasma B-cells can generate antibodies against M-protein, which further helps in opsonization and destruction of the organisms by macrophages and neutrophils. M-protein is type-specific and is resistant to heat and acid but sensitive to trypsin. T-antigens are the non-virulent factor and are resistant to heat, acid, and trypsin. Until now, over 220 M-protein and 20 T-serotypes are known.[29]

The genome of *streptococcus pyogenes* has 1,852,441 base pairs and contains 1752 predicted protein coding genes. Studies have identified more than 40 virulence-associated genes.

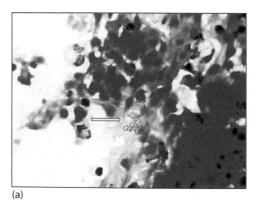

(a)

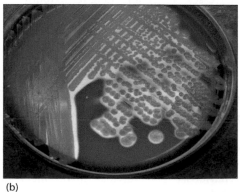

(b)

Figure 4.7 Streptococcus pyogenes: **(a)** Bacteria arranged in straight chains [arrow] and **(b)** beta hemolysis: Blood culture plate shows a small zone of hemolysis around the colonies of streptococcus.

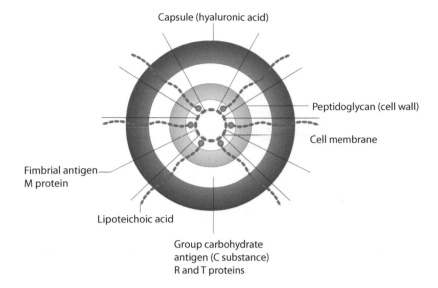

Figure 4.8 Schematic diagram showing the various surface antigens of Group A beta hemolytic streptococci.

CLINICAL FEATURES OF ACUTE RHEUMATIC FEVER

Rheumatic fever is diagnosed by the revised Jones criteria.[30] The common clinical findings[27,28] include: 1) carditis, the most severe presentation; 2) migratory polyarthritis, seen in almost 100% of individuals, with more severity in younger adults than in teenagers and children. Migratory polyarthritis occurs for between a few days and a few weeks and resolves completely; 3) Sydenham chorea, involuntary, purposeless, jerky movements of the hands and arms, shoulders, feet, legs, face, and trunk, along with hypotonia and weakness, which disappear during sleep; 4) subcutaneous nodules, commonly noticed over the occiput, elbows, knees, ankles, and Achilles tendons. These are firm, painless, and freely mobile with size varying from 0.5–2 cm. On microscopic examination, these nodules show central fibrinoid degeneration of the collagen surrounded by chronic mononuclear inflammatory cell infiltrate; 5) erythema marginatum, less commonly found, these present as a pink, non-pruritic skin rash present over the upper parts of the arms or trunk but not on the face. The rash generally occurs early or late in the course of the disease and extends centrifugally with a clear center.

Pathophysiology includes the deposition of immune complexes on joints causing non-destructive synovitis and non-destructive reactions in the basal ganglia, whereas the development of autoimmune cytotoxic reactions destroys the heart valves, causing a severe form of cardiac involvement. An accurate description is as follows: "rheumatic fever licks the joint, but bites the heart."[27,28]

The minimum latent period between throat infection and the development of antibody induced immunological damage to the heart valves and joints is approximately 1–3 weeks. The extra-cardiac manifestations are self-limiting with no residual injury.

Rheumatic heart disease

RHD is the chronic sequelae of recurrent bouts of acute rheumatic fever by GAS. The exact prevalence of RHD varies in different countries and regions, but it is a major public health problem in developing countries, with high morbidity and mortality. The mitral valve is the most commonly involved valve, seen in approximately 90% of cases, followed by the aortic and other valves in decreasing order of frequency.[28–31] In cases of multiple-valve involvement, a combination of mitral and aortic valves is the most common, as they are in close proximity. As RHD is a chronic condition, cardiac manifestations appear as late sequelae. The inflammatory process in the valve and the heart is mainly due to the cross-reactivity of streptococcal cell wall proteins and enzymes against the heart valve tissue. The main protein involved in this cross-reactivity is the streptococcal M-protein with the cardiac myosin. Valve leaflets will not show any evidence of active infection. Many studies have supported this mechanism and the culture report studied in all these valves was negative for any pathogens unless if there was any superadded secondary infection. Chronic RHD after decades causes many pathological changes in the mitral valve apparatus leading to mitral valve stenosis. The mean period of RHD and the symptomatic phase is usually found to be around 10–20 years.[27,28,31] Hence, it is a slow, progressive disease with a valve-narrowing speed of approximately 0.1 cm^2/year. Patients with RHD do not have a significant elevation of troponins.

PATHOGENESIS

Genetic susceptibility:[28] Only a small percentage of individuals with untreated streptococcal sore throat develop rheumatic fever and only a subset of these proceed with persistent inflammation and chronic RHD, suggesting a genetic susceptibility (see Flowchart 4.1). Studies have shown that the risk of acute rheumatic fever is six times higher in monozygotic twins when compared with that of dizygotic twins. Different Human leucocyte antigen (HLA) class II antigens have been found to be associated with several populations and HLA-DR 7 is the antigen most frequently associated with RHD. This may indicate the association of different strains of streptococcus in different regions of the world. This evidence has led researchers to study various susceptible gene associations in RHD patients. Some authors have documented that the majority of these genes were found to be involved in the regulation of the immune system. Major proteins involved in the innate immunity protection response are mannose-binding lectin protein (MBL), the family of toll-like receptors (TLR), and ficolins. MBL and ficolins are pattern recognizing proteins that are helpful in identifying the surface proteins of the pathogens for further processing. MBL binds to N-acetylglucosamine (GlcNAc), the major immune-epitope of GAS cell wall carbohydrates. This protein has immunological similarities to the cardiac valve laminin. Ficolin-2 has shown to bind selectively to lipoteichoic acid, a cell wall constituent of GAS. TLRs play a key role in host immunity by

mediating inflammatory mediators. TLR 2 interacts with bacterial lipoprotein, peptidoglycans, and lipoteichoic acid, which are the constituents of GAS cell wall. Polymorphisms are known to be associated with RHD. Some of the important known polymorphisms are cytotoxic T-lymphocyte-associated antigen-4 (CTLA-4) gene polymorphism, signal transducer and activation of transcription (STAT) 3, STAT5b, IL-10, and IL-6. Transforming growth factor (TGF) beta is the key regulator of fibrosis and calcification.[31]

Cytokines in RHD:[28,31] Tissue damage in RHD is mainly due to the persistence and maintenance of adaptive immunity that causes an increase in inflammatory cells and other cytokines. Some important cytokines include interleukin-1, tumor necrosis factor (TNF) alpha, and CTLA-4. Interleukins produced by inflammatory cells further activate other inflammatory cells and their adhesion molecules. They also heighten the immune response. Some studies showed that genetic variation in the IL-1RN allele 2 (A2) has an exacerbated immunological response when compared to IL-1RM allele 1 (A1). TGF beta is an important cytokine that is mainly responsible for immune cell proliferation and differentiation. Its levels in RHD patients were found to be elevated; hence, TGF beta could be responsible for the development of valve fibrosis and calcification in cases of RHD.

Autoimmunity: RHD has both an autoimmune and auto-inflammatory mechanism. Each mechanism is distinct with some overlap. Autoimmunity is a primarily adaptive immune response driven by T and B lymphocytes. Auto-inflammation is a primarily innate immune response driven by inflammasome-induced IL-1 beta and IL 8. The M-protein of the streptococcal antigen shares structural homology with cardiac myosin, tropomyosin, laminin, and vimentin. Hence, infection with streptococcal pyogenes triggers the autoimmunity responsible for pathological changes in the heart, joints, and central nervous system. This mechanism is called molecular mimicry. Antibodies produced against N-acetylglucosamine cross-react with laminin in the heart valves. Cardiac myosin and vimentin are the other target antigens. Streptococcal M5 and M6 proteins cross-react with cardiac myosin. Sydenham's chorea is mediated by antibodies against lysoganglioside GM1 of neuronal cells. Cunningham's group[33]

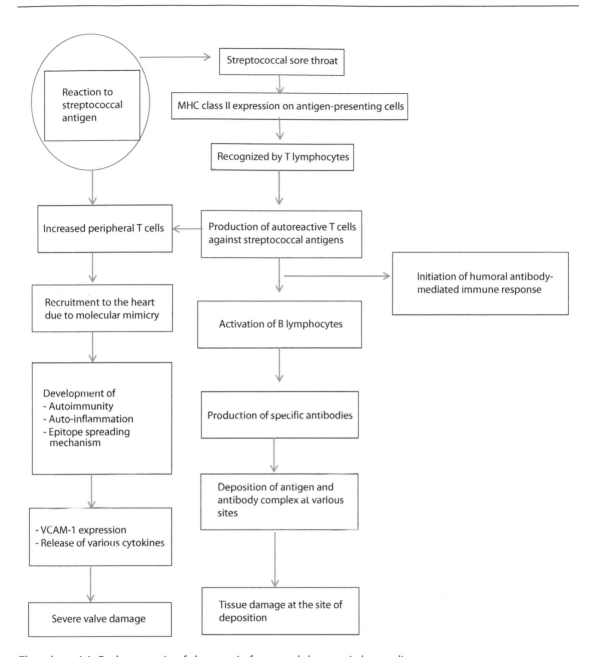

Flowchart 4.1 Pathogenesis of rheumatic fever and rheumatic heart disease.

showed that VCAM-1 is upregulated in cases of rheumatic fever, which leads to cellular infiltration, inflammation, and valve scarring. These mechanisms have been studied by many researchers who had demonstrated the presence of gamma globulin in the myocardium of rheumatic atrial appendage, valvulitis, and myocarditis. C-reactive protein (CRP) levels were known to correlate with the progression of MS. Endothelial injury is found to be the primary event in RHD. Galvin et al.[32]

demonstrated that antistreptococcal antibodies were cytotoxic for cultured human endothelial cells as well as human valvular endothelium and underlying basement membrane.

Pathogenesis of endothelial injury: Endothelial injury is an important mechanism in the pathogenesis of RHD. It has been demonstrated that antistreptococcal antibodies were cytotoxic for cultured endothelial cells, valvular endothelial cells, and the underlying basement membrane in humans.[31]

Role of cellular immune response: The increased cellular immune response is evident by the presence of CD 4-positive lymphocytes in rheumatic heart lesions. CD 4-positive T-lymphocytes are an important cellular component in RHD. Molecular mimicry of the T-cells is mainly mediated by the recognition of the self-antigens through HLA class II antigen presentation on antigen-presenting cells. These cells may include macrophages, dendritic cells, and B-lymphocytes.[27,28,31] Because of a molecular mimicry mechanism, autoreactive T-cells that are produced against GAS antigens escape immune tolerance. These autoreactive T-lymphocytes further activate the B-cells to produce more self-specific antibodies, further enhancing the inflammatory process. This is the mechanism of humoral-mediated antibody production in the initiation of cardiac inflammation via cellular immune response. Studies have also described the presence of peripheral and cardiac T-cells, which are capable of cross-reacting with streptococcal M5 protein and cardiac myosin, laminin, and tropomyosin. A final explanation for the mechanism is by an increased number of peripheral antigen-specific T-cells migrating to the heart because of antigenic mimicry. These cells expand locally and become capable of recognizing new self-antigens by the epitope spreading mechanism.[28,31]

HISTOPATHOLOGY

Acute rheumatic carditis: Rheumatic carditis involves all three layers of the heart (pancarditis):[27] 1) the pericardium shows thickening of both the parietal and visceral layers with serofibrinous exudate (bread-and-butter pericarditis) and chronic inflammatory cell infiltrates like lymphocytes, histiocytes, and plasma cells; 2) endocardium: inflammation involves either cardiac valves or the mural endocardium or both. All four cardiac valves may be involved. The frequency of valvular involvement in descending order is as follows: mitral valve, aortic valve, tricuspid valve, and pulmonary valve (pulmonary valve involvement is very rare). The mitral valve is commonly involved in cases of RHD. In the acute stage, the affected valves are edematous and opaque and lose their normal transparency. Gross examination of the affected valve may show tiny, uniformly sized thrombotic vegetations measuring approximately 1–3 mm in diameter that are present along the line of closure of the valve.

These are called rheumatic vegetations. They are firm in consistency and contain fibrinoid necrosis of the valve collagen surrounded by few histiocytic cells. These vegetations do not produce valve destruction. They are characteristically present on the atrial surface in case of mitral valves and ventricular surface in case of semilunar valves. Microscopic examination of the affected valves may also reveal Aschoff nodules. Rheumatic vegetations are formed mainly due to endothelial injury as a result of hemodynamic turbulence. Endothelial injury causes exposure of the subendothelial collagen and elastin to the flowing blood, which is highly thrombogenic and causes deposition of fibrin and platelets on the damaged site. These vegetations are sterile and do not yield any organisms on culture. Due to the change in the hemodynamic force, the endocardium of the posterior left atrial wall becomes irregular and thickened and is known as a MacCallum's patch, which can be easily visualized on gross inspection.[27] Microscopic examination of this area reveals edema and inflammation of the endocardium and subendocardial connective tissue deposits. The inflammatory infiltrate usually consists of lymphocytes, histiocytes, a few polymorphs, and eosinophils. Antischkow cells and Aschoff cells may also be seen; 3) myocardium: on gross examination, the heart becomes soft and flabby in acute myocarditis along with the dilatation of all chambers, especially the ventricles. Microscopic examination reveals presence of non-specific interstitial inflammation along with the presence of Aschoff bodies in the interstitium. Myocyte destruction is a rare phenomenon.

Chronic rheumatic heart disease

Gross findings (Figures 4.9 through 4.11): Post-inflammatory and postrheumatic valve disease is usually diagnosed at the time of surgery by gross inspection of the valve. In the chronic stage, heart valves show dense fibrosis, commissural fusion, calcification, and scarring of the valve components resulting in severe stenosis and other deformities. Fibrosis may involve the valve leaflets, chordae tendineae, and papillary muscles. This results in characterized morphological deformities like a "funnel shaped valve," "fish mouth," and "button hole," depending upon the severity. These changes occur due to the fusion of the commissures.

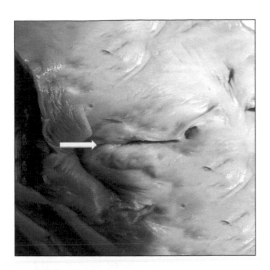

Figure 4.9 Severe mitral stenosis: Gross exami-nation of the mitral valve from the left atrial view shows severe narrowing of the mitral valve open-ing (arrow). Inner surface of the opening shows gray-white areas of fibrosis.

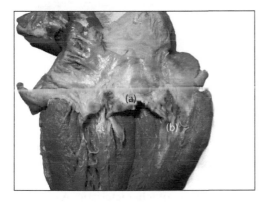

Figure 4.10 Rheumatic heart valve: Mitral valve is thickened, fibrosed and shows commissural fusion **(a)**. **(b)** Shows extension of the patchy gray-white fibrosis into the papillary muscles.

Pathological changes (Figure 4.12): Most com-monly observed microscopic findings in the surgi-cally excised rheumatic heart valve specimens are:

1. *Chronic inflammation.* The severity of inflamma-tion varies depending upon the disease status and activity. Commonly, chronic inflammation is focal and limited to the base of the valve. The inflam-matory infiltrate usually consists of lymphocytes, histiocytes, and plasma cells. Sometimes, when there is superadded infection/inflammation, polymorphonuclear neutrophils and eosinophils

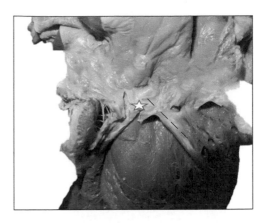

Figure 4.11 Rheumatic heart valve: The mitral valve complex is thickened, scarred and shows commissural fusion (star). Fibrosis is extending into the papillary muscles with fusion and short-ening of the chordae tendineae (dotted line).

may also be present. Immunohistochemical stain-ing reveals the CD 4 and CD 8 subsets of T-cells in acute rheumatic valvular involvement. Major histocompatibility complex class II (MHC-class II) antigens are commonly expressed on the vessel endothelium and valve fibroblasts.

2. *Fibrosis.* Fibrosis is mainly due to the deposi-tion of varying amounts of collagen in the valve substance, which is nothing but the sequelae of any chronic inflammation. Fibrosis of the valve leads to fusion of the valve commissures, leading to stenosis. This finding is a charac-teristic feature of chronic inflammatory/ rheumatic valve disease. The deposited col-lagen may show areas of hyalinization, at a later stage. Fibrosis involving the chordae tendineae and papillary muscles may cause shortening and thickening, leading to valve regurgitation.

3. *Aschoff body/nodules.*[34] These are the oval or elliptical nodules formed by the central area of fibrinoid degeneration/necrotic collagen of the valve substance surrounded by specialized cardiac histiocytes and lymphocytes. Macro-phages are the first cells to migrate and aggre-gate around the degenerated collagen and fibrinoid necrosis at the site of injury. These cells secrete various cytokines that will attract the T-lymphocytes followed by B-lymphocytes. Aschoff nodules may be present in various sites but they are most commonly located in the interstitium of the myocardium, often

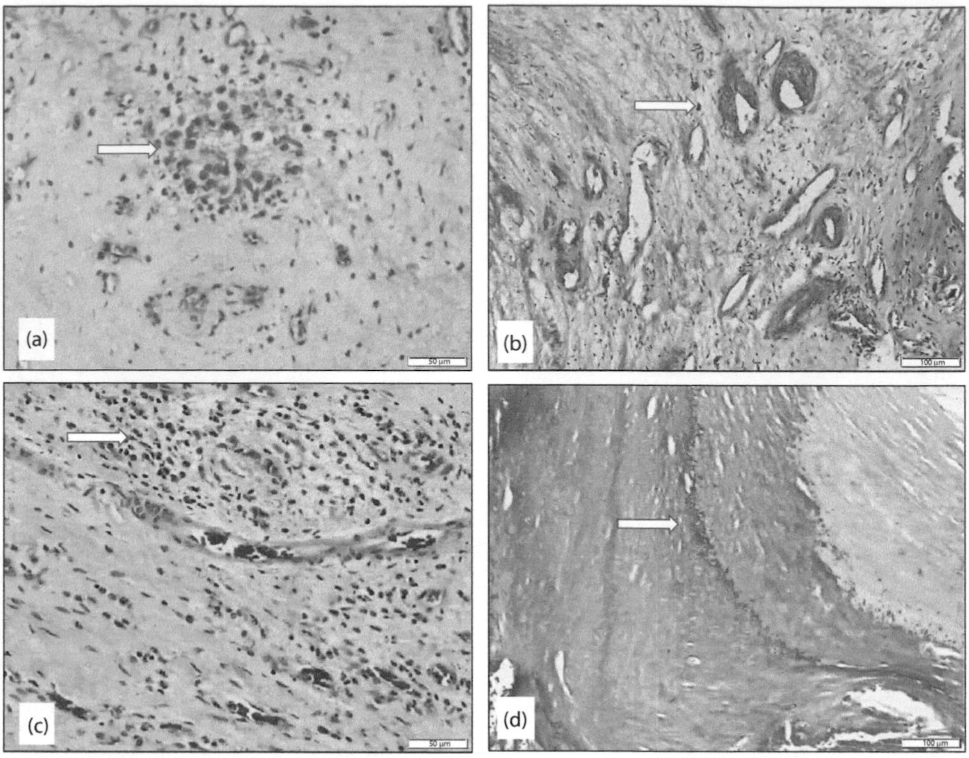

Figure 4.12 Histopathological changes seen in the Rheumatic mitral valve excision specimens - arrows; **(a)** Elliptical Aschoff nodule, **(b)** prominent neovascularization showing both thick and thin walled blood vessels, **(c)** chronic inflammatory cell infiltrate, and **(d)** dystrophic calcification.

adjacent to the intramyocardial blood vessels. These nodules may occasionally be encountered in the pericardium and adventitia of the aorta. A large number of Aschoff nodules are commonly present in the left-atrial appendageal specimens that are excised at the time of mitral valvotomy in cases of MS. The mononuclear cardiac histiocytes in the Aschoff nodule are called Antischkow cells. They are also known as caterpillar cells because of the wavy and serrated look of the chromatin, which resembles a caterpillar (Figure 4.13). The same cell in transverse section shows central chromatin with surrounding clear halo, which is also known as an "owl-eyed" nucleus. Sometimes, multinucleated giant cells are also present, known as Aschoff giant cells. The presence of Aschoff nodules in a histopathology section is a pathognomonic feature of RHD, but they are not always seen in all the suspected cases of rheumatic valve excision specimens. Silver and Stollerman defined three developmental stages of Aschoff nodules:

stage 1) central fibrinoid necrosis, edema, and infiltration by histiocytes, lymphocytes, and plasma cells (exudative and degenerative phase); stage 2) a specific granulomatous phase with accumulation of characteristic Aschoff giant cells and Antischkow cells; and stage 3) a late stage with diminution of the cellular infiltrate and replacement by scar tissue.[34] On immunohistochemistry, the Aschoff and Antischkow cells will show positivity for histiocytes/macrophage markers like CD 68 and MAC 387.

4. *Neovascularization.* Normally, valves are avascular and may show the presence of a few capillaries near their attachment at the base. In RHD and in all other inflammatory conditions, the mitral valve will show the presence of thick- and thin-walled proliferating blood vessels within the valve substance, known as neovascularization. Neovascularization is one of the most important and consistent features seen in resected specimens of mitral valve with a suspected history of RHD.

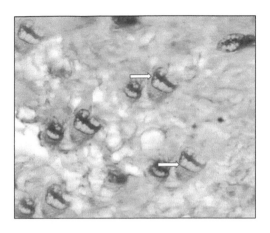

Figure 4.13 Antischkow cells: They are also called caterpillar cells because of their serrated chromatin pattern (arrow).

5. *Calcification.* Dystrophic calcification may be seen focally in the degenerated valve. Its amount and distribution vary in different cases and depend on the duration of the disease. Sometimes, the valve may show extensive calcification with surrounding foreign body giant cell reaction to the deposited calcium.

6. *Vegetation* (Figure 4.14). Repetitive trauma due to changes in hemodynamic stress and the chronic inflammatory process of the valve tissue leads to the formation of vegetations on the mitral valve surface near the line of closure. These are usually fibrin-rich vegetations without any organisms (aseptic vegetations). Sometimes, repetitive trauma may also be the precedent factor for superadded secondary infections, leading to secondary infective vegetations.

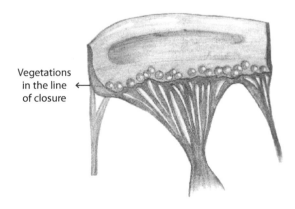

Vegetations in the line of closure ←

Figure 4.14 Rheumatic valve vegetations.

Hemodynamic changes in mitral stenosis

The normal cross-sectional area of the mitral valve is 4–6 cm². Clinical symptoms appear when the area becomes less than 2.0 cm².[9] The sequences of hemodynamic changes in MS patients are described below (and see Flowchart 4.2):

INCREASED HEMODYNAMIC PRESSURE IN THE LEFT ATRIUM

Due to the obstruction in the normal blood flow, there will be an increased transmitral pressure gradient in the left atrium. In severe MS, left-atrial pressure will be significantly elevated even at rest. This will lead to decreased filling in the left ventricle, which further causes a decrease in blood volume and decreased stroke volume resulting in a decrease in cardiac output.

LEFT-ATRIAL REMODELING

A constant increase in left-atrial pressure leads to pathological adaptive modifications in the left atrial wall. Commonly associated adaptive changes include hypertrophy of the atrial muscle fibers and interstitial fibrosis due to the deposition of collagen between the cardiac myocytes, which leads to geometric remodeling and dilatation of the left atrium. These changes are known to cause the development of atrial fibrillations and intra-atrial luminal thrombus.

INCREASED PULMONARY VASCULAR BED PRESSURE

Cases of chronic MS are always associated with secondary pulmonary vascular hypertension. This is mainly because of the transmission of back pressure from the left atrium to the pulmonary veins and subsequently to the pulmonary capillaries and arteries. Studies have shown that patients of MS with pulmonary hypertension can have a threefold increase of endothelin factor-1 as compared to that of normal healthy individuals. The level of endothelial factor-1 decreases and comes to near-normal after 6 months of correction of MS.[35]

REMODELING OF THE PULMONARY VASCULATURE

A constant increase in back pressure leads to histopathological alterations in the pulmonary vasculature.[36,37] Variable degrees of changes are observed in muscular branches of pulmonary

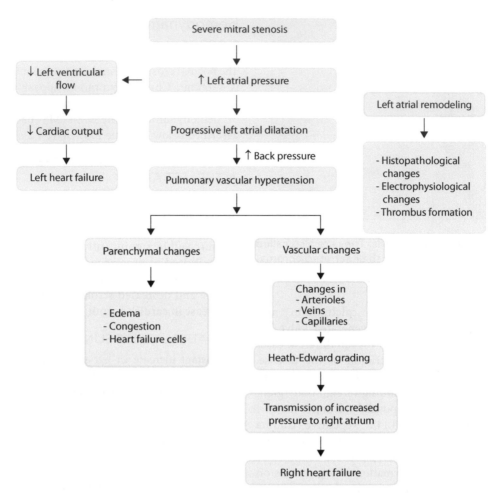

Flowchart 4.2 Pathophysiological sequelae in mitral stenosis.

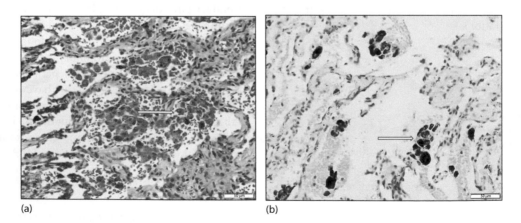

Figure 4.15 **(a)** Numerous hemosiderin-laden macrophages in the alveolar lumen (arrow). They are also called heart failure cells. **(b)** Perl's Prussian blue stain imparts blue color to the iron present in the cytoplasm of these cells.

arteries, pulmonary arterioles, veins, and lymphatics. Quantitative pulmonary parenchymal and vascular changes are usually seen consistently in almost all cases, with more severity in younger individuals. The most consistent finding is muscularization of arterioles. There will be narrowing of the lumen due to the proliferation of intimal cells. Vascular changes are graded according to the Heath-Edwards grading system.

CHANGES IN THE PULMONARY PARENCHYMA

Lung parenchyma may show accumulation of proteinaceous fluid and red blood cells in the alveolar interstitium and lumen due to pulmonary edema. The interstitial space may show congestion of the septal capillaries and areas of hemorrhage because of the rupture of small-caliber vessels due to increased luminal pressure. In chronic stages, the extravasated red blood cells will be degraded by the alveolar macrophages, which in turn form hemosiderin-laden macrophages. These cells are also known as heart failure cells (see Figure 4.15).

RIGHT-HEART CHANGES

If the chronic stage persists for a longer duration, back pressure will be transmitted to the right atria, leading to similar histopathological changes as seen in left atria that ultimately result in right-heart failure.

SUMMARY

MS is one of the major global causes of morbidity and mortality, with rheumatic heart disease still being the most common cause worldwide. Etiopathogenesis includes the chronic inflammatory disease process affecting the heart valves due to cross-reactivity of streptococcal antigens with the cardiac myosin. Valve neovascularization, fibrosis, and chronic inflammatory infiltrate are consistently present in most of the resected mitral valve specimens with a suspected history of RHD. Although Aschoff nodules are rarely seen in histopathological specimens, they are a pathognomonic feature of rheumatic valvular heart disease. The number of Aschoff nodules may vary but their presence does not indicate the activity of the disease process. The presence of "bread-and-butter" fibrinous pericarditis and acute rheumatic vegetations denote activity in cases with RHD.

REFERENCES

1. Ho SY. Anatomy of the mitral valve. *Heart* 2002;88(Suppl IV):5–10.
2. Yacoub M. Anatomy of the mitral valve, chordae and cusps. In: Kalmanson D (ed.). The Mitral valve. London: Edward Arnold; 1976:15–20.
3. McCarthy KP, Ring L, Rana BS. Anatomy of the mitral valve: Understanding the mitral valve complex in mitral regurgitation. *Eur J Echocardiogr* 2010;11:3–9.
4. Lam JH, Ranganathan N, Wigle ED, Silver MD. Morphology of the human mitral valve. I. Chordae tendineae: A new classification. *Circulation* 1970;41(3):449–58.
5. Combs MD, Yutzey KE. Heart valve development: Regulatory networks in development and disease. *Circ Res* 2009;105(5):408–21.
6. Turi ZG. Mitral valve disease. *Circulation* 2004;109:38–41.
7. Waller BF, Howard J, Fess S. Pathology of Mitral Valve stenosis and pure Mitral Regurgitation-Part I. *Clin Cardiol* 1994;17:330–6.
8. Harb SC, Griffin BP. Mitral valve disease: A comprehensive review. *Curr Cardiol Rep* 2017;19(8):73.
9. Arı H, Arı S, Karakuş A et al. The impact of cardiac rhythm on the mitral valve area and gradient in patients with MS. *Anatol J Cardiol* 2017;18(2):90–8.
10. Sorajja P, Goss M, Bae R et al. Severe mitral annular calcification. First experience with transcatheter therapy using a dedicated mitral prosthesis. *JACC Cardiovasc Interv* 2017;10:1178–9.
11. Lyle MA, Snipelisky DF, Aggarwal NR, Miller FA, Anavekar NS. Exuberant mitral annular calcification. *Int J Cardiovasc Imaging* 2017;33:615–21.
12. Mallisho M, Hwang I, Alsafwah SF. Liquefaction necrosis of mitral annuluscalcification. *J Clin Ultrasound* 2014;42(6):382–3.
13. Floria M, Baroi LG, Georgescu CA. Mitral annular calcification: Left atrial size and left ventricular dysfunction. *Anatol J Cardiol* 2016;16:548.
14. Seguela PE, Houyel L, Acar P. Congenital malformations of the mitral valve. *Arch Cardiovasc Dis* 2011;104:465–79.

15. Collins-Nakai RL, Rosenthal A, Castaneda AR, Bernhard WF, Nadas AS. Congenital MS. A review of 20 years' experience. *Circulation* 1977;56:1039–47.

16. Mohan JC, Shukla M, Mohan V, Sethi A. Spectrum of congenital mitral valve abnormalities associated with solitary undifferentiated papillary muscle in adults. *Indian Heart J* 2016;68(5):639–45.

17. Zhang W, Wang Y, Ma C, Zhang Z, Yang J. Congenital uni-leaflet mitral valve with severe stenosis: A case report with literature review. *Echocardiography* 2017;34(3):468–71.

18. Wilkes JK, Fraser CD, Seery TJ. Accessory mitral valve leaflet causing severe left ventricular outflow tract obstruction in a preterm neonate with a partial atrioventricular septal defect. *Tex Heart Inst J* 2016;43(6):543–5.

19. Plymale JM, Frommelt PC, Nugent M, Simpson P, Tweddell JS, Shillingford AJ. The infant with aortic arch hypoplasia and small left heart structures: Echocardiographic indices of mitral and aortic hypoplasia predicting successful biventricular repair. *Pediatr Cardiol* 2017;38(6):1296–1304.

20. Ruckman RN, Van Praagh R. Anatomic types of congenital MS: Report of 49 autopsy cases with consideration of diagnosis and surgical implications. *Am J Cardiol* 1978; 42(4):592–601.

21. Roberts WC, Ewy GA, Glancy DL, Marcus FI. Valvular stenosis produced by active infective endocarditis. *Circulation* 1967;36(3):449–51.

22. Malanca M, Cimadevilla C, Brochet E, Iung B, Vahanian A, Messika-Zeitoun D. Radiotherapy-induced MS: A three-dimensional perspective. *J Am Soc Echocardiogr* 2010;23(1):108.

23. Bose AS, Shetty V, Sadiq A, Shani J, Jacobowitz I. Radiation induced cardiac valve disease in a man from Chernobyl. *J Am Soc Echocardiogr* 2009;22(8):973.

24. Tamura A, Takahara Y, Mogi K, Katsumata M. Radiation-induced valvular disease is the logical consequence of irradiation. *Gen Thorac Cardiovasc Surg* 2007;55(2):53–6.

25. Raghunathan D, Khilji MI, Hassan SA, Yusuf SW. Radiation-induced cardiovascular disease. *Curr Atheroscler Rep* 2017;19(5):22.

26. Afshar M, Luk K, Do R et al. CHARGE Extracoronary Calcium Working Group. Association of triglyceride-related genetic variants with mitral annular calcification. *J Am Coll Cardiol* 2017;69(24):2941–8.

27. Chopra P. Rheumatic heart disease. In: Chopra P. *Illustrated Textbook of Cardiovascular Pathology.* First edition. New Delhi: Jay Pee Brothers; 2003: 28–42.

28. Azevedo PM, Pereira RR, Guilherme L. Understanding rheumatic fever. *Rheumatol Int* 2012;32(5):1113–20.

29. Mangold M, Siller M, Roppenser B, Vlaminckx BJ, Penfound TA, Klein R, Novak R, Novick RP, Charpentier E. Synthesis of group A streptococcal virulence factors is controlled by a regulatory RNA molecule. *Mol Microbiol* 2004;53(5):1515–27.

30. Guidelines for the diagnosis of rheumatic fever. Jones Criteria, 1992 update. Special Writing Group of the Committee on Rheumatic Fever, Endocarditis, and Kawasaki Disease of the Council on Cardiovascular Disease in the Young of the American Heart Association. *JAMA* 1992;268(15):2069–73.

31. Yanagawa B, Butany J, Verma S. Update on rheumatic heart disease. *Curr Opin Cardiol* 2016;31(2):162–8.

32. Galvin JE, Hemric ME, Ward K, Cunningham MW. Cytotoxic mAb from rheumatic carditis recognizes heart valves and laminin. *J Clin Invest* 2000;106(2):217–24.

33. Roberts S, Kosanke S, Terrence Dunn S, Jankelow D, Duran CM, Cunningham MW. Pathogenic mechanisms in rheumatic carditis: Focus on valvular endothelium. *J Infect Dis* 2001;183(3):507–11.

34. Fraser WJ, Haffejee Z, Jankelow D, Wadee A, Cooper K. Rheumatic Aschoff nodules revisited. II: Cytokine expression corroborates recently proposed sequential stages. *Histopathology* 1997;31(5):460–4.

35. Chen MC, Wu CJ, Yip HK et al. Increased circulating endothelin-1 in rheumatic MS: Irrelevance to left atrial and pulmonary artery pressures. *Chest* 2004;125(2):390–6.

36. Tandon HD, Kasturi J. Pulmonary vascular changes associated with isolated MS in India. *Br Heart J* 1975;37(1):26–36.

37. Heath D, Edwards JE. The pathology of hypertensive pulmonary vascular disease. A description of six grades of structural changes in the pulmonary arteries with special reference to congenital cardiac septal defects. *Circulation* 1958;18:533–47.

5

Clinical features of mitral stenosis

JAGANMOHAN A. THARAKAN

INTRODUCTION

Isolated mitral stenosis (MS) comprises 25% of all patients with rheumatic valvular heart disease. Approximately 35% have MS with incompetence, another 35% have concomitant aortic valve disease, and 5% have organic tricuspid valve disease. In combined valve diseases, the clinical features are often modified by the severity of other associated valvular lesions.

EPIDEMIOLOGY AND THE NATURAL HISTORY OF RHEUMATIC MITRAL STENOSIS

In the natural history of rheumatic fever, MS develops over a period of time, often extending over decades. Typically, there is a latent period from the occurrence of rheumatic fever to the onset of symptoms. This latent period lasts an average of 16.3 ± 5.2 years. Once symptoms of MS develop, progression to severe disability takes an average of 9.2 ± 4.3 years. A significant minority do not recall an episode of past rheumatic fever and hence the temporal progression of MS is often speculative. However, there is a geographical variation in the age at presentation with MS. In the developed world, with rheumatic fever incidence as low as 1/100,000, patients present with symptoms attributable to MS, typically in the fifth decade of life or beyond. In less developed countries, where incidence of rheumatic fever is as high as 50/100,000, patients may present with symptoms as early as the second, and the vast majority present in the third to fourth, decade of life. Once symptoms develop, it may take almost a decade before they become disabling. Whether this difference is explained by a more aggressive form of disease progression after an episode of rheumatic carditis, or due to repeated subclinical carditis in highly endemic areas with rheumatic fever, is debatable. Rheumatic MS is found more frequently in females, with a ratio of between 2:1 and 3:1.[1]

A study from India[2] included 108 patients with isolated/predominant MS <20 years with a male:female ratio of 1.7:1. Of these, 67% had a history of rheumatic fever (RF) in the past and more than two-thirds of those with a history of rheumatic fever presented within 5 years of their first episode of acute rheumatic fever. This is at odds with the present data, where mitral regurgitation (MR) is overwhelmingly more common and MS is rarely detected as an isolated lesion post-RF, during an intermediate-term follow-up. This may be attributed to better awareness and early medical attention and treatment of all acute rheumatic fever cases, resulting in the survival of all patients with acute rheumatic fever—mitral incompetence being the major residual lesion in almost all of them.

PATHOPHYSIOLOGY AND HEMODYNAMICS

The anatomic substrate in MS is the reduction in mitral valve orifice area from a normal value of 4–6 cm² to less than 2 cm² over a period of time. This happens due to the fusion of the anterior and posterior mitral leaflets along the closure line extending from the mitral annulus, along the posteromedial and anterolateral commissures towards the center, resulting in a central oval stenotic orifice. Degenerative changes like fibrosis and

calcification of leaflets possibly accelerated by the turbulent transmitral flow (hemodynamic theory) can further accelerate and accentuate the valve stenosis, as well as chordal shortening and chordal fusion (second distal stenosis). The net result is a progressive increase in the transmitral diastolic flow gradient, causing elevation of left-atrial (LA) pressure, in an attempt to propel the same amount of stroke volume into the left ventricle (LV) to maintain adequate cardiac output. The diastolic transvalvular pressure gradient for any given valve area is a function of the square of the transvalvular flow rate. Similarly, to maintain the same forward stroke output, the transmitral gradient increases proportionately, as a function of the square of decrease in cross-sectional valve area. Doubling the transmitral flow quadruples the transmitral gradient; reducing cross-sectional area (CSA) by half will quadruple the transmitral gradient.

$$Flow = CSA \times Velocity \text{ and gradient} = 4 \times Velocity^2$$

Hence,

$$Flow = CSA \times \sqrt{Gradient}, \text{ so gradient} = Flow^2/CSA^2$$

$$(5.1)$$

Example. If flow is 5 L/min and CSA is 2 cm² then gradient = 5 × 5/2 × 2 = 6.25 mmHg. Keeping the flow constant, if the valve area is halved to 1 cm², then gradient = 5 × 5/1 × 1 = 25 mmHg. Similarly, keeping the CSA constant, if the transmitral flow is doubled then gradient = 10 × 10/2 × 2 = 100/4 = 25 mmHg. Stated simply, doubling transmitral flow quadruples the gradient; halving the valve area quadruples the gradient. As symptoms attributable to MS are dependent on an increase in absolute LA pressure, contributed entirely by the transmitral gradient (in the absence of LV systolic or diastolic dysfunction or aortic incompetence), changes in cross-sectional area and the quantum of transmitral flow have a profound influence on symptoms.

As the mitral valve orifice narrows, the pressure gradient across the valve increases, leading to an increase in LA pressure and volume. This triggers a vicious cycle of increased pulmonary venous and pulmonary capillary wedge pressure (PCWP), which eventually causes pulmonary artery hypertension (PAH). Over time, PAH causes right-heart failure, tricuspid regurgitation (TR), and pulmonary regurgitation. Right-heart failure leads to hepatic congestion, elevated jugular venous pressure, ascites, and bilateral pedal edema.

With the increase in LA pressure, transudation of fluid occurs into the lung interstitium leading to dyspnea on mild exertion, which can progress to dyspnea at rest. Rupture of the pulmonary veins from elevated hydrostatic pressure can result in hemoptysis. In addition, increased LA chamber size is a risk factor for atrial fibrillation (AF), which further elevates the LA pressure, and also predisposes the patient to thromboembolism and embolic complications such as stroke. Although left-ventricular end-diastolic pressure and cardiac output remains within the normal range in the early stages of the disease, cardiac output falls over time, leading to a state of low cardiac output.

PROGNOSTIC FACTORS AND SURVIVAL

Prognostic factors in MS include age, degree of mitral valve stenosis, presence of PAH, and the clinical status New York Heart Association functional class of the patient. PAH and AF are markers of poor prognosis with high risk of morbidity and mortality. Cardiac failure and cerebrovascular or pulmonary embolism are the major causes of morbidity and mortality in these patients. Associated cardiovascular morbidities as well as intercurrent illness can adversely affect the natural history.

Before recent advances in interventional and surgical practice, the prognosis of patients with MS was poor. Those having NYHA class III had a five-year survival rate of 62%, whereas in class IV it was only 15%. In individuals having been offered mitral valve surgery but who refused, survival with medical therapy alone was $44 \pm 6\%$ at 5 years, and $32 \pm 8\%$ at 10 years after they were offered correction. In the asymptomatic or minimally symptomatic patient, survival is greater than 80% at 10 years. When limiting symptoms occur, ten-year survival is less than 15% in the patient with untreated MS. When severe PAH develops, mean survival is less than 3 years. Most (60%) patients with severe untreated MS die of progressive pulmonary or systemic congestion, but others may suffer systemic embolism (20%–30%), pulmonary embolism (10%), or pulmonary infection (1%–5%). Generally, the prognosis is good in patients who undergo surgical

repair of the valve. However, the life expectancy of such patients is still low as expected for the age due to the related complications of the disease.

SYMPTOM PROGRESSION

The normal area of the mitral orifice is about 4–6 cm². In MS, this is significantly reduced; however, MS remains asymptomatic until the valve area reduces to 2–2.5 cm². At this point the patient may start experiencing exertional dyspnea with moderate exercise due to the increased LA pressure and transmitral gradient. Severe symptoms occur when the area becomes less than 1 cm². The course of MS varies between patients. The latent phase after an episode of rheumatic fever can last anywhere between a few years to a few decades, during which the mitral valve area (MVA) progressively reduces from about 4 cm² to less than 2 cm². Mild symptoms on accustomed effort will be present once the valve area falls below 2 cm². However, this may not be forthcoming from the history, as most patients will scale down their physical activity to avoid the unpleasant sensation of dyspnea. Following the onset of mild effort limitation and dyspnea, it takes around 7 to 9 years to develop severe complications. However, factors such as severe anemia, fever, thyrotoxicosis, exercise, pregnancy, or excitement may trigger an attack of dyspnea. Pregnant women with mild MS can develop symptoms in their second trimester due to increased cardiac output and blood volume.

The presentation depends on the severity of the disease. Patients may be totally asymptomatic in mild cases. As the stenosis worsens, symptoms of dyspnea on exertion, paroxysmal nocturnal dyspnea, or orthopnea develop. Several compensatory mechanisms triggered by elevated pulmonary venous and PCWP can ameliorate symptoms of dyspnea, including more efficient lymphatic drainage of the lungs that prevents development of interstitial edema, pulmonary congestion, and other associated symptoms.

More severe symptoms occur as the stenosis worsens and LA pressure and size increase. Coughing may occur due to bronchial compression by the enlarged LA. Rupture of the bronchial veins may result in hemoptysis. In an occasional patient, compression of the left recurrent laryngeal nerve by an enlarged hypertensive pulmonary artery (PA) results in hoarseness of voice (Ortner's syndrome).

NATURAL HISTORY AND CLINICAL FEATURES MODIFIED BY INTERVENTION

It is important to appreciate the influence of therapeutic interventions, especially percutaneous transvenous mitral commissurotomy (PTMC), on the clinical course of MS. After successful PTMC, there is a steady and progressive recurrence of MS over intermediate-term follow-up. In a series of 310 patients, of whom 206 (66%) had successful PTMC, restenosis (a loss of >50% of valve area) was noted in 40% at a six-year follow-up. Morphological characteristics with a Wilkins score of >8 predicted restenosis.[3] In a follow-up study of 561 patients undergoing PTMC, there was a gradual loss of MVA over time, and a reduction in valve area of up to 0.3 cm^2 was noted in 12%, 22%, and 27% of patients at 3, 5, and 7 years, respectively. Very few patients had progression of mitral regurgitation by more than one grade at follow-up and 67% of patients were functionally improved at 6 years.[4] During the follow-up period of 103 patients with significant MS, MVA decreased at a mean rate of 0.09 cm^2/year. In 28 patients there was no decrease, in 40 there was only relatively little change (<0.1 cm^2/year), and in 35 the rate of progression of mitral valve narrowing was more rapid (>0.1 cm^2/year). The rate of progression was significantly greater among patients with a larger initial MVA and milder MS (0.12 vs. 0.06 vs. 0.03 cm^2/year for mild, moderate, and severe stenosis, $p < 0.01$). The rate of mitral valve narrowing in individual patients is variable and cannot be predicted by initial MVA, mitral valve score, or transmitral gradient, alone or in combination. Right-heart disease can progress independent of mitral valve narrowing.[5]

DETERMINANTS OF SYMPTOMS AND CLINICAL SIGNS

Important factors contributing to symptoms and signs of MS are LA pressure and transmitral flow (effective stroke output/effective systemic blood flow).

Left-atrial pressure

LA pressure rises proportional to the degree of valve obstruction, to ensure adequate effective forward cardiac output. In effect, this increases the pulmonary venous and PCWP, and, in due course the pulmonary artery (PA), right-ventricular (RV), and right-atrial (RA) pressure, while the LV is not directly affected. However, chronic underfilling of the LV in severe MS with reduced forward stroke volume can result in reduced LV ejection fraction (EF) and stroke work. Up to 5% of patients with isolated MS have significant LV dysfunction in the absence of other secondary causes like coronary artery disease. Whether the chronic rheumatic process, by itself—in the setting of the longstanding natural history of chronic MS and a chronically underfilled (preload-starved) LV—can result in LV dysfunction is debatable (see Chapter 23).

Clinical conditions resulting in increased stroke output like anemia, fever, hyperthyroidism, pregnancy, and exercise can increase the LA pressure and the pulmonary venous and PCWP, precipitating acute dyspnea. Conditions leading to sinus tachycardia, such as exercise, thyrotoxicosis, pregnancy, and fever, also reduce the diastolic filling period, increasing the quantum of transmitral flow in respect to filling time, aggravating dyspnea. AF with a fast ventricular rate also causes increase in LA pressure due to shortened diastolic filling time. In AF, additionally, the loss of atrial contribution to ventricular filling requires that LA pressure increases proportionately to maintain identical forward stroke output.

FEATURES WITH A DIRECT BEARING ON LA PRESSURE

Severity of MS. This is determined by effective mitral valve orifice area contributed by commissural fusion (primary stenosis) and chordal thickening, shortening, and fusion (distal/second stenosis). LA pressure rises proportionate to the severity of mitral valve obstruction, in an attempt to maintain adequate stroke volume and cardiac output.

LA compliance. This is altered by a chronic inflammatory process with fibrosis and scarring (noncompliant LA/stiff LA syndrome). This causes LA pressures to be higher for the same LA volume and stroke volume. LA compliance is also altered by the acuteness and severity of LA dilatation as determined by hemodynamic factors. Acute myocardial stretch decreases LA compliance and raises the LA pressure disproportionate to volume load.

This is typically seen in situations of acute LA volume overload, such as in acute MR/chordal rupture/infective endocarditis. This is less important in MS, which is typically a slowly progressive chronic valve disease. However, acute fluid overload as seen with parenteral fluid resuscitation, blood transfusion, and the second and third stages of labor can precipitate acute pulmonary edema in MS, as LA pressure rises disproportionately to the additional LA volume increase.

Diastolic filling time. As the forward stroke volume has to be propelled to LV in the limited diastolic filling period, any compromise on diastolic filling time, typically tachycardia, will increase the transmitral gradient and LA pressure.

Venous inflow into LA (increased systemic cardiac output). Any physiological condition (pregnancy, exercise) that increases stroke volume and cardiac output will increase the transmitral gradient. So, too, will pathological states like fever, anemia, thyrotoxicosis, and other states of high cardiac output. All post-tricuspid left-to-right shunts like VSD and PDA will increase the transmitral gradient in the presence of MS.

LV diastolic filling characteristics (LV relaxation abnormality [lusitropy]/LV wall stiffness [LV hypertrophy]). Any impairment in LV relaxation in early diastole (negative lusitropy) compromising active LV suction (hampering early diastolic LV filling) as well as LV hypertrophy-related increase in LV stiffness (especially in mid- and late diastole) will result in an increase in mean LA pressure, to maintain the same forward stroke volume.

LA remodeling. Physiological chamber dilation (e.g., LV in chronic mitral incompetence) tends to normalize the chamber compliance and chamber pressure for the same chamber volume. Physiological LA hypertrophy normalizes LA wall tension for the same intra-atrial volume, and the LA pressure will tend to return to baseline.

Atrial contribution to diastolic ventricular filling. This is crucial in any condition leading to impairment to diastolic filling. An optimal PR interval is also a critical factor for optimizing left-atrial contribution to ventricular filling. A lack of atrial contraction typical in AF is an important cause for functional deterioration in MS. Any rhythm with atrioventricular dys-synchrony will increase the transmitral gradient and functional deterioration in MS.

Mechanical impedence to LV filling. In MS, ball valve thrombus/aortic incompetence jet are the two common mechanical hindrances to LV diastolic filling.

A chain of compensatory mechanisms in the pulmonary vascular bed. In the setting of elevated LA, pulmonary vein (PV), and PCWP pressures, several compensatory changes occur in the pulmonary vascular bed. Elevated LA pressure is directly transmitted to the pulmonary veins and the pulmonary capillaries, stressing the alveolo-capillary membrane permitting exudation of fluid into the alveoli. When the pulmonary alveolo-capillary membrane reserve is stressed, compensatory structural changes occur in the alveolo-capillary membrane with thickening, which helps prevent transudation of fluid into the alveoli and pulmonary edema. This helps the patient tolerate a higher chronically elevated PCWP than seen with an acute rise in PCWP. The efficiency of lymphatic drainage from the pulmonary interstitium improves in the setting of chronically elevated PCWP and this in turn relieves symptoms of interstitial edema of chronic pulmonary venous hypertension. Patients tolerate much higher levels of chronically elevated pulmonary venous pressures, unlike acute pulmonary venous hypertension.

Pulmonary arteriolar vasoconstriction Precapillary pulmonary arteriolar vasoconstriction results in the redistribution of pulmonary blood flow from lung bases to lung apices, especially marked in the upright position. Progressive pulmonary arteriolar vasoconstriction and muscularization of the arteriolar wall increases pre-capillary pulmonary vascular resistance, PAH and resultant RV hypertrophy, and RV decompensation. An increase in pre-capillary pulmonary vascular resistance prevents acute flooding of the pulmonary capillary bed, preventing acute pulmonary edema. RV dysfunction leads to TR, further hampering forward cardiac output. PA dilation and PAH lead to high-pressure pulmonary regurgitation (Graham Steell murmur). The changes described upstream to the PVs protect the pulmonary capillary bed from surges of increased blood flow flooding the pulmonary capillary bed and resultant pulmonary venous hypertension and pulmonary edema. More efficient pulmonary lymphatic drainage and thickening of the alveolo capillary membrane also prevents alveolar exudation and pulmonary edema even at very high chronically elevated PV pressure.

Patients of MS get relief of paroxysmal nocturnal dyspnea over the years, and the trade-off is fatigue due to reduced forward cardiac output.

Bronchial vein pressure elevation, bronchial vein dilation and bronchial vein drainage to systemic veins may permit decompression of the bronchial veins. However, these dilated thin-walled bronchial veins are susceptible to rupture leading to hemoptysis. As these dilated veins drain PV blood to systemic veins at high pressure, their rupture leads to hemoptysis with bright-red blood (oxygenated blood). Under high pressure, pulmonary veins also dilate, resulting in PV to bronchial vein flow reversal. These dilated venous channels are prone to rupture under high pressure, resulting in hemoptysis and, rarely, pulmonary apoplexy.

FACTORS AFFECTING THE EFFECTIVE FORWARD CARDIAC OUTPUT (EFFECTIVE SYSTEMIC BLOOD FLOW)

As discussed above, most compensatory mechanisms—including pulmonary arteriolar vasoconstriction leading to an increase in pre-capillary pulmonary vascular resistance, pulmonary thromboembolism, pulmonary incompetence, RV systolic dysfunction, and TR—contribute to a reduction in forward stroke output. Associated organic tricuspid valve disease with organic TR and/or TS will further aggravate the situation. Similarly, associated mitral incompetence and aortic valve disease (AS and/or AR) also contribute to reduced forward stroke output, especially when LV systolic and or diastolic dysfunction sets in. An occasional patient will have primary LV systolic dysfunction that aggravates the already-compromised stroke output. In the elderly, hypertension and coronary artery disease are common risk factors for diastolic and systolic LV dysfunction.

SYMPTOMS[6]

Symptoms pertain to MS per se, its cardio pulmonary consequences, other associated valvular lesions due to the rheumatic process, and complications related to MS (Table 5.1). As age advances, other common acquired heart diseases like hypertensive heart disease and coronary artery disease can influence the clinical presentation of MS.

MS results in back pressure in the LA, PV, and pulmonary capillary bed resulting in interstitial edema and decreased lung compliance resulting in

Table 5.1 Symptoms attributable to MS

Effort dyspnea
Paroxysmal nocturnal dyspnea/acute pulmonary edema
Orthopnea
Low output state
Hemoptysis
RV angina
Right-sided heart failure: acute/chronic/very chronic
Hepatic fibrosisà hepatic cirrhosis
Stroke, systemic, and pulmonary thromboembolism
Non-regression of PAH on relief of MS

effort dyspnea. An acute rise in LA pressure due to sinus tachycardia, exercise, tachyarrhythmia, and especially AF with fast ventricular response results in alveolar fluid exudation, which consequently results in tachypnea, basal crackles and wheeze/rhonchi, and frank pulmonary edema. More severe MS results in orthopnea due to chronic interstitial edema. With a reduction in forward stroke output and cardiac output, the pulse volume is low with peripheral vasoconstriction and occasionally peripheral cyanosis. Typical mitral facies may be appreciated, described in fair-skinned individuals with acrocyanosis of the nose and facial skin contrasting with purplish cheeks.

What causes symptoms of dyspnea in mitral stenosis?

Elevated LA pressure transmitted to the pulmonary capillary bed is the basic reason for dyspnea in MS. As discussed earlier, several factors influence the LA pressure as well as symptoms, depending on the acuteness of LA pressure elevation or chronicity of LA pressure elevation permitting several compensatory mechanisms to alleviate the catastrophic consequences of LA pressure elevation.

Normally, most of the transmitral forward flow occurs passively in early diastole across a widely patent mitral valve orifice, facilitated by a normally relaxing LV (positive lucitropy) with a suction effect. Obstruction to the MV orifice in diastole as in MS, as well as negative lucitropy of LV with relaxation abnormality, can affect transmitral forward flow in early diastole. Normally, atrial contribution to ventricular filling in late diastole is less than 25% of the forward stroke volume. However, atrial contribution to ventricular filling can be high in conditions causing an increase in LV wall stiffness, as seen with ventricular hypertrophy that hampers late diastolic LV filling. Atrial contribution to ventricular filling is also important when passive LV filling is hampered by MS. Atrial contraction contributes to LV filling with a minimal increase in LA mean pressure as atrial systole is short (less than 200 ms). The hemodynamic advantage of active LA contribution to LV filling is a larger transmitral flow with a marginal increase in LA pressure as the atrial contraction is of relatively short duration. Conversely, a lack of active atrial contribution to LV filling will result in a higher LA mean pressure to maintain the same forward stroke volume, as typically seen in AF. The transmitral gradient is very sensitive to the diastolic filling period. A compromise in the diastolic filling period, as seen in sinus tachycardia or a fast ventricular rate in AF, results in an increase in the transmitral flow rate during the curtailed diastolic filling time, resulting in an increased transmitral gradient to maintain the same forward stroke volume.

Associated mitral incompetence will increase the transmitral gradient and LA pressure as regurgitation fraction increases the transmitral flow for an equivalent effective forward stroke output. An aortic incompetence jet can compromise the functional MV orifice area, causing partial closure of the anterior mitral leaflet in diastole, increasing the transmitral gradient.

Paroxysmal nocturnal dyspnea

An acute paroxysmal episode of sudden-onset dyspnea paroxysmal nocturnal dyspnea (PND) is characteristic of left-sided heart failure. It can be life-threatening and is usually precipitated by an acute event. PND responds positively to a propped-up position, oxygen, mild sedation, and preload-reducing agents (venodilators and diuretics). With bed rest, fluid shifts from extracellular to intravascular compartment, and blood from splanchnic bed also moves to systemic circulation increasing intravascular volume and pulmonary blood flow. Sympathetic stimulation during REM sleep and resultant tachycardia and a less responsive respiratory center, precipitates acute pulmonary edema. In MS, PND is not due to LV dysfunction and hence, once treated, prognosis is better than when PND occurs in the setting of LV

dysfunction. AF with uncontrolled ventricular rate is an important cause of PND in MS.

Orthopnea

With chronically elevated pulmonary venous and PCWP there is interstitial fluid exudation, interstitial edema, peribronchial edema, and decreased lung compliance and increased work of breathing; the patient feels comfortable in a semi-upright position, using multiple pillows. This improves the diaphragmatic contribution of breathing while preventing the upward shift of the diaphragm by the enlarged liver. Orthopnea points to a more advanced and chronic stage of heart failure with a poorer long-term outcome, even in the absence of LV dysfunction as in MS.

Right-heart failure

Right-heart failure in isolated MS is due to PAH and secondary RV dysfunction and RV failure, and usually has a rapid downhill course. The patient presents with right hypochondriac pain, pedal edema, and occasionally orthopnea due to pulmonary congestion and bilateral/right-sided pleural fusion. Acute hepatic dysfunction with marked hepatic enzyme elevation can occur, as well as pre-renal azotemia contributed to by elevated renal vein pressure and the activation of the Renin angiotensin aldosterone system (RAAS) system.

Low-cardiac-output state with renal and hepatic dysfunction

Both the renal tubular system with its blood supply through the efferent glomerular arterioles and the hepatic portal system through the portal veins (portal circulation) are particularly susceptible to systemic hypotension and a state of low cardiac output, and both of these organs can be affected, resulting in renal and hepatic dysfunction.

Ortner's syndrome (cardio-vocal syndrome)

Ortner's syndrome, a clinical entity manifested by hoarseness of voice, caused by an impaired ability of the left recurrent laryngeal nerve to transmit impulse to the laryngeal musculature because of stretching or impingement of the nerve from the disease-induced changes in cardiac or greater vessel anatomy. Hoarseness of voice due to paralysis of the left recurrent laryngeal nerve postulated as caused by a dilated LA in MS was first discussed by Nobert Ortner in 1897. A variety of conditions can lead to paralysis of the left recurrent laryngeal nerve; these include thoracic aortic aneurysm, patent ductus arteriosus, primary pulmonary hypertension, atrial and ventricular septal defect, Eisenmenger's syndrome, and recurrent pulmonary embolism. In MS, its incidence ranges from 0.6% to 5%. Currently, it is believed that dilated hypertensive pulmonary arteries impinge on the recurrent laryngeal nerve. The most common cardiovascular cause—other than aortic aneurysm—is compression of the left recurrent laryngeal nerve by a hypertensive dilated PA, and this seems the most plausible reason in MS, as LA does not come in close proximity to the left recurrent laryngeal nerve, even with aneurysmal dilation.

Ascites precox

Gradual-onset, chronic longstanding right-heart failure can present with ascites as a more prominent feature than pedal edema and tender hepatomegaly, as is often seen in acute rapid-onset heart failure. MS is a slowly progressive disease even after symptom onset (MV area <1.5 cm^2) and many compensatory mechanisms take place proximal to the stenosis that tend to protect the pulmonary vascular bed from surges of increased pulmonary venous pressure and mitigating symptoms that can result in long-term survival and chronicity of the disease. This also allows for slow-onset RV systolic dysfunction to set in with TR and chronic right-heart failure, which favor ascites precox and hepatomegaly. This can lead to centrilobular necrosis, peri-centrilobular fibrosis, and hepatic cirrhosis in the long run. Organic tricuspid valve disease with tricuspid stenosis (TS) and/or TR also favors slow progression of the disease and chronicity, favoring ascites precox. More commonly, organic tricuspid valve disease with TR and or TS favor a slow, gradually progressive right-heart failure with preserved RV function, allowing longer survival but with chronic right-heart failure. Cardiac cirrhosis should be suspected in patients with prolonged decompensated mitral valve disease with TR associated organic tricuspid valve disease. Incidence has fallen because of early definitive therapy for rheumatic MS.

Hemoptysis

Hemoptysis can be the presenting symptom in MS and is often distressing to the patient and is occasionally life-threatening. The more life-threatening causes are acute pulmonary edema presenting with orthopnea, coughing and pink frothy sputum, requiring immediate management with oxygen, a propped-up position, morphine, diuretics, and ventilator support. Pulmonary venous and bronchial venous bleed results in hemoptysis with bright-red blood (oxygenated). In severe MS, there is a reversal of blood flow from pulmonary veins into bronchial veins with bronchial vein dilation and rupture, causing bright-red blood hemoptysis. Bronchitis can cause streaky hemoptysis with mucoid expectoration and is due to bleeding from distended submucosal bronchial veins under high pressure due to pulmonary venous hypertension. Pulmonary infarct leads to pleuritic chest pain with rusty/altered blood hemoptysis. Pulmonary hemosiderosis has also been mentioned as a cause for hemoptysis. Paul Wood found sudden massive hemoptysis ("pulmonary apoplexy") in 18.3% of his patients, and in close to 12.7% it was the presenting symptom even before effort dyspnea. This appears to be distinctly uncommon in the present clinical scenario. Shunting of blood from congested pulmonary veins to bronchial veins, which tend to bleed easily, is the likely cause of profuse haemorrhage. Hemoptysis of a lesser degree, blood-stained sputum accompanying congestion ("congestive hemoptysis"), was found in 16.5% of his series. The pleurohilar veins, which connect the pulmonary and azygos venous beds, have also been proposed as a source of bleeding.

Angina

RV hypertrophy with supply-demand mismatch can present as anginal pain. PAH per se can cause chest pain. Pleuritic pain of pulmonary infarction should be excluded in all patients complaining of chest pain.

Palpitation (atrial fibrillation)

Patients with MS typically experience palpitation with the onset of atrial fibrillation (AF). It may be described as a fast heartbeat or, less often, as an irregular heartbeat. Patients often claim a worsening of symptoms of dyspnea during such paroxysmal episodes. Paroxysmal episodes gradually become persistent. AF is an important complication of MS, resulting in clinical deterioration as well as a substrate for systemic and pulmonary thromboembolic complications. AF is a frequent complication of MS due to LA electrical remodeling because of LA dilation from chronic inflammatory process as well as hemodynamic stress. Age is another important contributing factor. AF is seen in less than 10% of patients with severe MS below 30 years of age, and AF incidence increases with the age of the patient. Left-atrial diameter, and age have been shown to be the most important risk factors in the occurrence of AF in patients with RHD. The highest frequency of AF in RHD occurs in patients with mixed MV lesion: MS with MR, and TR in combination. AF, while occurring in 29% of patients with isolated MS and in 16% with isolated mitral regurgitation, is an infrequent finding (1%) in patients with isolated aortic valve disease.

Acute stroke can be the presenting symptom of MS, especially beyond the third decade of life. Paroxysmal as well as persistent AF are at equal risk for thromboembolic complications.[7]

Embolic complications

Stroke is the most devastating complication. AF and age are important risk factors in the setting of significant MS. Peripheral embolism, especially saddle embolism at the aorto-iliac bifurcation, can be life-threatening and is a surgical emergency. Recurrent pulmonary embolism and pulmonary infarction may lead to PAH disproportionate to severity of MS and can be a cause for non-regression of PAH despite relief of MS. Emboli from the heart are distributed evenly throughout the body according to cardiac output, but more than 80% of symptomatic or clinically recognized emboli involve the brain. Of emboli to the brain, approximately 80% involve the anterior circulation (i.e., carotid artery territory), whereas 20% involve the vertebra-basilar distribution, proportional to the distribution of cerebral blood flow.

Age, severity of MS, reduced cardiac output, and associated valvular lesions like AR, LA size, spontaneous echo contrast in LA, and presence of LA thrombus are significant risk factors for thromboembolism. Needless to say, more than 80% of patients with thromboembolism and MS are in AF. AF is seen in less than 10% of patients with MS below 30 years of age, but the presence of AF can be as high as 50% in the sixth and seventh decade.

PHYSICAL EXAMINATION

General physical examination

In the setting of longstanding severe MS with low output and right-heart failure, cardiac cachexia, mitral facies, acrocyanosis, and peripheral edema may be present.

Arterial pulse

A low-volume pulse suggests low stroke volume and decreased cardiac output as a consequence of severe MS. Pulse irregularity points to AF. Pulse asymmetry should alert one to past or acute peripheral embolism.

Jugular venous pressure (JVP) and waveforms

JVP and waveforms are normal in MS with sinus rhythm. However, JVP waveform and pressure are altered by the onset of PAH, functional TR, and associated organic tricuspid valve disease with TS, TR, or a combination of both. Loss of an "a" wave in JVP suggests AF. With the onset of functional TR or organic TR, the "v" becomes prominent and the upstroke occurs earlier and earlier to obliterate the "x" descent, described as a "cv" wave. Typically, the "vy" descent is rapid, indicating unobstructive early diastolic transtricuspid flow. Any delay in the "vy" descent should alert to coexisting TS (organic obstruction to RV filling). An unusually tall and sharp flicking "a" wave in JVP is often seen with organic TS, especially in the absence of TR. Severe RV hypertrophy secondary to PAH can result in a prominent "a" wave in JVP due to RV diastolic dysfunction. The hepatic pulsations closely mimic the JVP and findings of hepatic pulsation should be recorded.

Inspection and palpation of precordium

MS per se does not result in clinically detectable cardiomegaly, as LA is a posterior structure.

LV apex is not displaced and the palpable S1 gives it a tapping character, superadded on a relatively underfilled LV. Apical diastolic thrill is often palpable in the left lateral decubitus at end expiration with a palpable S1 and points to organic MS. Other physical findings on precordial examination are typically determined by the presence of PAH, secondary RV hypertrophy, RV dysfunction, and functional TR. Other associated valvular lesions, especially organic TV disease, should be looked for.

With PAH, the pulmonary component of S2 may be palpable in the pulmonary area, as well as an RV heave in the left parasternal region. With onset of RV dysfunction and RV dilation, the cardiac apex gets displaced leftward, more laterally than downward. RA enlargement to the right of the sternum in the presence of severe TR or organic TV disease with TR and or TS may be elicited by percussion. Percussion, a rarely performed clinical tool, helps identify right-atrial enlargement, PA dilation, and associated significant pericardial effusion.

Auscultation

This discussion on heart sounds and murmurs in MS is only a primer, in order to understand the influence of various hemodynamic variables that can alter the auscultation findings. These basics will help a reader to understand, discuss, and unravel the protean auscultation features of MS.

FIRST HEART SOUND

First heart sound (S1) intensity is increased from the early stages of the disease and indicates the presence of end diastolic transmitral gradient, keeping the mitral valve in a wide-open position and allowing for a large excursion to closure with the onset of LV systole. S1 can become softer in later stages of the disease, with the calcification and scarring of the valve restricting its mobility. With onset of AF, the intensity of S1 will depend on the end diastolic transmitral gradient of each cardiac cycle. A constant and loud S1, regardless of length or duration of diastole, points to critical MS due to a persistent end-diastolic gradient even in long diastole, whereas a variable intensity of S1 with a varying duration of diastole points to a less critical MS. Important determinants of the intensity of S1 (mitral valve closure sound) are:

i. The mobility of the mitral valve leaflets (sail-like function)
ii. The position of the MV leaflets at the time of onset of ventricular contraction
iii. The adequacy of coaptation of leaflets at the time of onset of isovolumic contraction
iv. LV contractility and dp/dt at time of mitral valve closure

Mitral valve mobility and excursion are restricted by valve fibrosis and calcification, which occurs to a variable extent in the natural history of rheumatic MS. Heavily calcific immobile mitral leaflets result in attenuation of the mitral closure sound.

In hemodynamically significant MS, LA to LV gradients of varying degree persist to the end of diastole, before the onset of LV contraction, keeping the MV leaflets in a wide-open position, permitting large excursion and a loud S1 with the onset of LV contraction. Factors that can alter this situation are very prolonged diastole as in AF and long cardiac cycle or post ventricular ectopy pause—situations when the end diastolic gradient may diminish considerably especially in milder form of MS and S1 can be less intense after long diastole compared to normal/shorter cardiac cycles. A higher preload in the longer diastole will increase the force of contraction (Starling's law) and may partly offset the above feature as MV closes at a higher dp/dt. A prolonged PR interval causes S1 to be soft in normal hearts, but its influence in MS is debatable. Normal LV contractility will ensure that the MV closure and coaptation occur at a higher dp/dt, further accentuating the S1. Depressed LV contractility has the opposite effect.

A less recognized factor is that with increasing severity of MS, the mitral closure sound moves away from the QRS (the Q-S1 interval lengthens) and fuses with the TV closure sound (MC-TC fusion), resulting in the accentuation of S1.

The constancy of S1 in the setting of a variable diastolic filling period is considered an indicator of significant MS, and S1 variability excludes critical MS, on the premise that mitral leaflets are in the wide-open position at the end of even longer diastole, if MS is severe. Whether varying LV contractility with varying preload can influence this has not been well studied.

The lack of coaptation of mitral leaflets is seen invariably with associated mitral incompetence, which may attenuate S1 of MS even when the valve is bellowing well. It is important to appreciate various factors that oppose or complement each other in contributing to the physical findings.

SECOND HEART SOUND

The pulmonary component of the second heart sound (S2) is normal in the absence of PAH. The pulmonary component of S2 (P2) increases in intensity with the progression of PAH and the split of S2 becomes narrow due to reduced hang-out interval, though respiratory variation is still appreciable. With the onset of RV dysfunction, P2 may move away from the aortic component (A2), widening the split. It is debatable what happens to the splitting of S2 with significant TR, as RV ejection time may shorten. One must take note that, simultaneously, the forward stroke output across the aortic valve is also diminished.

THIRD AND FOURTH HEART SOUNDS

The third (S3) and fourth (S4) heart sounds should be carefully looked for as indicators of RV systolic and RV diastolic dysfunction, respectively. RV S3 can be present with either functional or organic TR.

OPENING SNAP

Opening snap (OS) is a sharp, short, high-pitched early diastolic sound that occurs 0.04 to 0.12 seconds after A2 and coincides with the sudden deceleration of the rapid early diastolic opening movement of the mitral leaflets due to the restraint caused by commissural fusion and resultant doming. The audibility of OS also depends on mobility of the mitral leaflets and can become soft when leaflets are fibrotic and calcific, lacking inherent leaflet mobility.

Differentiating opening snap from other early diastolic heart sounds

Differentiating P2 of S2 from OS can be challenging. Respiratory variation is far more pronounced in the A2-P2 interval with marked shortening of the A2-P2 interval in inspiration. The A2-OS interval remains the same or may increase with reduced pulmonary venous return and a reduction in LA pressure in inspiration. Prompt standing can reduce the A2-P2 interval (reduced RV stroke volume) and OS may move away from

A2, due to reduced pulmonary venous return. A change in heart rate due to sinus tachycardia can further complicate the hemodynamics, especially of MS.

Early LV filling sounds like S3 or pericardial knock are low-frequency sounds that occur later (beyond 160 ms of A2) at the end of peak early diastolic filling. Occasionally, tumor plop or a pericardial knock can be difficult to differentiate from the opening snap of MS, as these occur relatively early compared to the pathological LV S3 of LV dysfunction or increased flow. Clinically, the tumor plop is the most likely to be confused with OS in timing as well as character.

The A2-OS interval in mitral stenosis

The A2-OS interval is the time lapsed from the time the aortic valve closes to the opening of the mitral valve. In the cardiac cycle, this represents the isovolumic relaxation time as both the valves are in a closed position during this interval. A2 represents the closure of the aortic valve, which occurs a short time after the crossover of the LV and aortic pressure due to the hang-out interval. The hang-out interval is short on the left side because of the high-impedance characteristics of the systemic circulation as compared to the pulmonary circulation. The LV pressure can be considerably lower than the pressure in the aorta at the time of aortic valve closure if the hang-out interval on the left side is prolonged as in aortic stenosis. The mitral valve opens at the crossover of the LV and LA pressure. Thus, the A2-OS interval does not represent exactly the time taken for the LV pressure, at the LV-aorta pressure crossover, to drop below the LA pressure as A2 occurs a short time after the pressure crosses over due to the hang-out interval. (A2-OS interval = LV-AO pressure crossover to LV-LA pressure crossover time – left-sided hangout interval.)

What are the factors influencing the A2-OS interval?

As the A2-OS interval approximates the time for the LV pressure at the LV-aorta crossover to drop below the LA pressure (isovolumic relaxation period), conditions leading to a higher aortic pressure at the pressure crossover point (incisura on the central aortic pressure wave form), as in systemic hypertension, will increase the A2-OS interval, whereas elevation of the LA pressure, as in MS, will shorten the A2-OS interval. With increasing severity of MS, transmitral gradient increases and the LA pressure will rise, resulting in progressive shortening of the A2-OS interval. If the patient has systemic hypertension, the A2-OS interval will lengthen for the same degree of LA pressure. With normal LV function, the hangout interval may reduce with systemic hypertension and counter this effect. In MS, any maneuver which increases the transmitral gradient will reduce the A2-OS interval (e.g., exercise) and factors which reduce the gradient (e.g., inspiration, standing, hypovolemia) will lengthen the A2-OS interval. Increased LV contractility along with increased lusitropy will reduce the isovolumic relaxation time and thus reduce A2-OS interval and vice versa. Valvular AS increases the hangout interval and can shorten the A2-OS interval. If there is diastolic relaxation abnormality of the LV (LV hypertrophy, LV ischemia), the A2-OS interval can be prolonged due to prolonged isovolumic relaxation. The LV end diastolic pressure will also affect the LA pressure. The LA pressure will be higher for a higher LVEDP, for the same degree of MS and forward stroke volume. In summary, factors which alter the A2-OS interval are severity of MS, the cardiac output, the preload, the afterload, LV contractility, the aortic hangout interval, the diastolic relaxation abnormality of LV, impaired diastolic filling, and elevated end diastolic pressure. Any impairment to ventricular filling will increase the LA pressure and shorten the A2-OS interval. A reduction in preload will reduce the LA pressure and increase the A2-OS interval. An increase in after-load will elevate the aortic pressure at which the aortic valve closes and can increase the A2-OS interval. An increase in LV contractility shortens the isovolumic relaxation time while diastolic relaxation abnormality increases the isovolumic relaxation time. Though several factors influence the A2-OS interval in a complex way, A2-OS interval is a fairly reliable measure of the severity of isolated MS. An A2-OS interval of less than 60 ms indicates severe MS, and more than 100 ms indicates mild MS.

MURMURS

The only murmur attributable directly to MS is the mid-diastolic to presystolic murmur of turbulent transmitral flow, heard best at the cardiac apex. As discussed earlier, the hallmark of significant MS is an end-diastolic transmitral gradient, which should translate into an audible murmur reaching S1 (presystolic murmur). Mid-diastolic murmur results from rapid passive flow from LA to LV in mid-diastole with opening of the MV and active LV relaxation. The murmur tends to wane in later diastole with progressive reduction in LA to LV gradient (better appreciated with sinus bradycardia and in long diastole) and again accentuates during atrial systole (presystolic accentuation) due to active atrial contraction resulting in ventricular filling. Opening snap preceding a long mid-diastolic murmur points to MS. The transmitral mid-diastolic murmur of MS starts with the OS and extends beyond the rapid filling phase for variable length into diastasis depending on severity of MS and amount of transmitral flow. It may be noted that hemodynamically significant MS does not have a true diastasis period, as the LA pressure is continuously elevated above the LV diastolic pressure with a continuous downward trend in LA pressure and the LA and LV pressure moving towards each other, while, by definition, the diastasis period has a minimal recordable gradient between LA and LV and the two pressures move upwards in parallel, with reduced transmitral flow.

The mid-diastolic rumble of MS is a localized, low-pitched murmur best heard with the bell of the stethoscope, with the patient in the left-lateral decubitus position with breath held in end expiration. The duration of the rumble closely corresponds to the duration of the diastolic pressure gradient across the mitral valve. In mild MS, there are two phases of diastolic pressure gradient across the valve (during early diastolic rapid ventricular filling and again during presystole with atrial contraction), resulting in a rumble that can occur during mid- and late diastole with a distinct gap. When MS becomes severe, the diastolic rumble persists throughout diastole due to persistent pressure gradient across the valve. The intensity of murmur corresponds to both the severity of the obstruction and the forward flow across the stenotic valve and hence does not have a direct bearing on the severity of MS. This is evident from maneuvers like exercise, which increase murmur intensity by increasing transmitral flow in a given case of MS.

Presystolic accentuation of the diastolic rumble of mitral stenosis

Presystolic accentuation is attributed to atrial contraction accelerating transmitral flow and hence absent in AF. Factors like annular contraction with onset of ventricular systole in the preisovolumic phase (onset of LV contraction to S1) may play a minor role, as well as the auscultatory cadence of the murmur ending with a loud S1. Persistence of the diastolic murmur up to S1 in long diastole in AF is a clinical clue to severe MS as it indicates persisting gradient across the MV up to late diastole.

Differential diagnosis of a diastolic heart murmur

Differential diagnosis of a diastolic heart murmur that may mimic MS includes conditions with increased cardiac output states that produce high flow across the mitral valve, which include anemia and pregnancy, post-tricuspid left-to-right shunts like persistent ductus arteriosus and ventricular septal defect and mitral incompetence. Flow murmurs result in mid-diastolic rumble that does not extend beyond mid-diastole and is typically preceded by a third heart sound (S3). Though it can be difficult to differentiate the S3 from an opening snap, S3 is a low-frequency sound, occurring 160 ms or later after A2, whereas OS is a sharp, high-frequency sound occurring less than 120 ms after A2. Severe aortic insufficiency causes functional mitral valve obstruction, compromising the effective mitral orifice as the AR jet impinges on the anterior mitral leaflet (reverse doming of MV in diastole) leading to the Austin-Flint murmur, which can extend into presystole. A simple maneuver like isometric handgrip, which increases the aortic incompetence, accentuates the Austin Flint murmur, while MS murmur is not appreciably altered by this maneuver.

LA ball valve thrombus and LA myxoma must be kept in mind, especially if symptoms are episodic and the murmur is variable and intermittent and changes with posture or over time. Organic tricuspid stenosis can occasionally be confused with MS, but location of murmur and characteristic inspiratory augmentation points to TS (beware of a pseudo-Carvallo sign where MS murmur can increase in inspiration due to sinus tachycardia). Congenital parachute mitral valve and supramitral ring mimics rheumatic MS but is rarely associated with OS. Other causes of non-rheumatic MS are extremely uncommon.

In AF, the presystolic accentuation of the diastolic murmur contributed by the atrial contraction is absent, though the murmur can extend to S1 depending upon the severity of MS (i.e., presystolic component of murmur persists but there is no accentuation of murmur). AF also provides an opportunity to assess severity of MS, as presence of a diastolic murmur reaching to S1 in long diastole indicates critical MS, whereas the diastolic murmur stopping well short of S1 in longer diastole suggests less severe MS. Constant intensity of SI regardless of cycle length indicates critical MS.

Intuitively, a third heart sound that results from rapid flow into a normal LV or usual flow at high pressure into a noncompliant LV excludes MS; however, bedside differentiation of OS (sharp and early) from an S3 (low-frequency, soft, and late), can be difficult. It is not uncommon to hear a loud, widely audible thudding third heart sound in severe rheumatic MR. Mid-diastolic murmur extending to presystole (reaching to S1) points to hemodynamically significant MS. However, Austin Flint murmur of severe aortic incompetence can mimic MS. Isometric handgrip accentuates Austin Flint murmur but has no effect on murmur of MS. Austin Flint murmur may be preceded by S3 but not an OS. In the presence of severe AR, other features of MS like symptoms of PVH, hemoptysis, loud S1, features of PAH, and AF often points to underlying MS.

Murmurs arising secondary to complications of mitral stenosis

Severe PAH with RV dysfunction results in murmur of TR, heard typically at the left lower sternal edge, and may be heard up to the cardiac apex formed by the hypertrophied and dilated RV. The TR murmur is a high-frequency pansystolic murmur that increases in intensity with inspiration or, occasionally, appreciated only on careful auscultation during inspiration. RV S3 may be heard, as well as a soft mid-diastolic rumble due to excess flow across the TV due to significant TR. However, a long mid-diastolic murmur without preceding RV S3 should alert one to the possibility of organic TS.

Severe MS, if uncorrected, invariably results in PAH, which can result in PA annular dilation and pulmonary incompetence. Pulmonary incompetence results in high-frequency early diastolic murmur (Graham Steell murmur) best heard over the upper left sternal edge, increasing with inspiration. As aortic valve disease is a more common accompaniment of rheumatic MS, care should be taken not to mistake AR for pulmonary hypertensive PR.

Common valvular lesions associated with significant mitral stenosis[8]

MIXED MITRAL VALVE DISEASE

Detailed discussion of the physical findings of combination multivalvular disease is beyond the scope of this chapter. Though 25% of RHD patients have isolated/dominant MS, 35%–40% have MS with MR in varying combination of severity. The presence of mitral incompetence results in LV enlargement, accentuation of murmur of MS with additional flow across the mitral valve due to MR for the same effective forward output, earlier onset of PVH and PAH, and AF. Associated MR is suspected, in the presence of a high-frequency pansystolic murmur at the cardiac apex often directed to the mid-axilla and the back. LV cardiomegaly (cardiac apex shifted down and out with a well-localized hyperdynamic apical impulse) and intensity of apical pansystolic murmur are surrogate markers of severity of MR. Presence of S3 sound should caution against diagnosis of significant MS. As discussed earlier, mid-diastolic murmur at the cardiac apex can be entirely due to mitral incompetence and associated LV type cardiomegaly and LV S3 supports this assumption. However, mixed mitral valve disease with significant MS and significant mitral incompetence is a common clinical scenario and assessing the severity of each can be challenging.

TRICUSPID VALVE DISEASE

Organic tricuspid valve disease is present in up to 5%–10% of patients with MS. Clinical organic TS is distinctly uncommon, but when present, provides very classical physical findings. The JVP shows a flicking prominent "a" wave, well above the mean jugular venous pressure. RA enlargement can be demonstrated by percussion and presystolic hepatic pulsation is occasionally seen.

Mid-diastolic murmur at the lower sternal edge, increasing with inspiration, is typical of organic tricuspid stenosis, especially in the absence of significant TR. One must be aware of a pseudo-Carvallo sign of MS, wherein, due to sinus tachycardia associated with inspiration, MS murmur can get accentuated. More commonly, organic tricuspid valve disease presents with TS and TR. TR murmur of organic tricuspid valve disease is typically described as early systolic murmur, increasing with inspiration and best audible at the left sternal edge. JVP will reflect TR as a large "vy" wave. The rapidity of "y" descent will indicate presence or absence of TS as tricuspid valve inflow obstruction blunts the "vy" descent. Systolic hepatic pulsation can be seen and felt when TR is significant. It is not uncommon to have coexisting MS with PAH and organic TV disease. In this situation, TR results in pansystolic murmur. Book picture description of murmurs due to isolated valvular heart disease is often modified by coexistent hemodynamic alterations and other valve lesions.

AORTIC VALVE DISEASE

The presence of aortic incompetence can further complicate the physical signs of MS. An aortic incompetence jet can partially close the anterior mitral valve (reverse doming) and result in mechanical hindrance to forward flow, causing flow turbulence and murmur: Austin Flint murmur closely mimics MS murmur and it is not uncommon to mistakenly diagnose MS in the presence of free aortic incompetence. Maneuvers that increase aortic incompetence, like handgrip, will accentuate Austin Flint murmur. Lack of OS and peripheral signs of significant AR favor an Austin Flint murmur. When present, LVS3 is a useful sign to exclude significant MS. Severe AR elevates the LVEDP as well as causes preclosure of MV attenuating S1 intensity. Mild AR does not interfere with the assessment of MS. However, severe AR can mask findings of MS. The presence of PAH and AF should caution one to MS in the presence of severe AR.

LEFT-VENTRICULAR DYSFUNCTION

MS with LV dysfunction is a complex clinical scenario. A palpable LV apical thrust/impulse in the absence of aortic valve disease or mitral incompetence must caution one to suspect LV muscle disease. LV dysfunction in the absence of any identifiable causes is seen in up to 5% of patients with MS. Management of these patients is difficult, as symptoms are partly contributed to by LV dysfunction. Relief of MS, when significant, is an automatic choice if the valve is suited for PTMC at low risk. LV function may improve after successful relief of MS (preload-starved LV). Drugs like ACEI, which are generally not indicated in valvular obstructions like critical MS and AS, may be administered cautiously in patients with MS and LV dysfunction, especially if symptoms are attributable to LV systolic dysfunction in the presence of moderate MS.

SILENT MITRAL STENOSIS

Understanding the causation of murmurs and factors influencing audibility and loudness of murmurs is important. Reynold's number is an arbitrary dimensionless, "unitless" number related to fluid mechanics, as a determinant of laminar against turbulent flow. When the number exceeds approximately 4000, turbulent flow results—which is the cause of cardiac murmur. Reynold's number is directly related to the quantum of flow, velocity of flow, and effective flow orifice. However, in turbulent flow, Reynold's number increases as a function of the square root of gradient, which means gradient is a less important factor in raising the Reynold's number. Hence, it is conceivable that large gradients with markedly diminished flow through a very small orifice (e.g., critical MS with low cardiac output) may not cause as much turbulence and an audible murmur (silent MS) as against a large flow through a relatively larger orifice with increased velocity.

When the mitral diastolic murmur is not audible despite the presence of severe MS, it is called silent MS. RV hypertrophy causes clockwise rotation of the heart so that the left ventricle lies more posteriorly and the apex is formed by the RV. Hence the mitral diastolic murmur may not have been heard at the apex. Another reason is the decreased flow across the mitral valve in very severe MS, diminishing the intensity of the murmur. The decreased mobility of the thick and calcified mitral leaflets in severe calcific MS may contribute to the decrease in intensity of the mitral diastolic murmur. Lutembacher's syndrome, pulmonary emphysema, and obesity are other possible causes for silent MS. Severe tricuspid stenosis is another cause of silent MS. In this scenario, the transmitral gradient can be low,

despite having severe MS, because of markedly reduced forward cardiac output. Silent MS can present as PAH with right-heart failure or with Ortner's syndrome due to compression of the left recurrent laryngeal nerve by massively dilated hypertensive pulmonary artery.

In 1965, Ueda et al.[9] studied patients with silent MS and described severe valve fibrosis with immobile cusps, chordal thickening and shortening, and a second distal stenosis due to subvalvular chordal shortening and fusion, with a postero-medially oriented deformed mitral orifice and often with left-atrial thrombus. These features were more common in patients of silent MS.

CONCLUSION

MS is not an uncommon valvular disease in regions and population with a high incidence of rheumatic fever. The majority of patients present in the third and fourth decade of life and women may present for the first time during pregnancy. Diagnosis and assessment for definitive therapeutic intervention, such as balloon mitral valvotomy, in moderate to severe MS early in the course of the disease in symptomatic patients, is the key to favorably altering the natural history of the disease and its progression, preventing complications and in turn morbidity and mortality.

REFERENCES

1. Selzer A, Cohn KE. Natural history of mitral stenosis: A review. *MD Circulation* 1972; XLV.
2. Roy SB, Bhatia ML, Lazaro EJ et al. Juvenile mitral stenosis in India. *The Lancet* 1963;2:1193–6.
3. Wang A, Krasuski RA, Warner JJ, Pieper K, Kisslo KB, Bashore TM, Harrison JK. Serial echocardiographic evaluation of restenosis after successful percutaneous mitral commissurotomy. *J Am Coll Cardiol* 2002;39:328–34.
4. Hernandez R, Bañuelos C, Alfonso F, Goicolea J, Fernández-Ortiz A, Escaned J, Azcona L, Almeria C, Macaya C. Long-term clinical and echocardiographic follow-up after percutaneous mitral valvuloplasty with the Inoue balloon. *Circulation* 1999;99:1580–6.

5. Sagie A, Freitas N, Padial LR, Leavitt M, Morris E, Weyman AE, Levine RA. Doppler echocardiographic assessment of long-term progression of MS in 103 patients: Valve area and right heart disease. *J Am Coll Cardiol* 1996;28:472–9.

6. Wood P. An appreciation of mitral stenosis. *Br Med J* 1954;1(4870):1051–83.

7. Diker E, Aydogdu S, Ozdemir M, Kural T, Polat K, Cehreli S, Erdogan A, Göksel S. Prevalence and predictors of AF in rheumatic valvular heart disease. *Am J Cardiol* 1996;77(1):96.

8. Carabello BA. Modern management of mitral stenosis. *Circulation* 2005;112:432–7.

9. Ueda H, Sakamoto T, Kawai N, Watanabe H, Uozumi Z, Okada R, Kobayashi T, Kaito G. Silent MS: Patho-anatomical basis of the absence of diastolic rumble. *Jap Heart J* 1965.

6

Complications of mitral stenosis

SENGUTTUVAN NAGENDRA BOOPATHY AND AMBUJ ROY

INTRODUCTION

The incidence of rheumatic fever (RF) and rheumatic heart disease (RHD) has started decreasing, but it remains a major public health problem in low- and middle-income countries. Mitral stenosis (MS), the most common sequela of rheumatic fever, leads to many complications, especially if not treated in time. Though valve replacements and percutaneous transvenous mitral commissurotomy (PTMC) have improved outcomes, their longevity remains shortened by the disease process, primarily due to the complication associated with the disease. They include acute pulmonary edema, atrial fibrillation, systemic embolism, pulmonary hypertension, infective endocarditis, and (rarely) dysphagia and dysphonia. In this review, we elucidate the various complications of mitral stenosis, except for atrial fibrillation, which has been discussed elsewhere.

THE NATURAL HISTORY OF MITRAL STENOSIS

Mitral stenosis develops after an initial episode of acute rheumatic fever. It occurs a few decades earlier after acute rheumatic fever in developing countries as compared to developed countries.[1] This might be due to initial severity of disease and ongoing rheumatic activity, which might be occult. One prospectively conducted study identified the severity of carditis, recurrences of rheumatic fever, and low educational level of the mother as three risk factors determining the progression of disease.[2] According to their rate of progression, patients have been classified into three categories. Almost one-third had their valve area stable, another third had a progression of 0.01 cm²/year, and a third category had rapid progression with decrease in valve area between 0.1 to 0.3 cm²/year.[3,4] A Wilkins score ≥8 and a peak mitral gradient of 10 mmHg or more are predictors of rapid progression.[5] The natural history of MS depends on the symptomatic status of patients and pulmonary artery hypertension (PAH).[6] Asymptomatic patients had a 20-year survival of more than 80%. Nearly half of such patients develop symptoms after 10 years. Sudden deterioration happened in 50% of individuals. More than 60% of patients died of heart failure, while 20% of patients died of thromboembolic complications.[5]

ACUTE PULMONARY EDEMA

Mitral stenosis causes increase in pulmonary venous hypertension (PVH). As PVH increases, it causes exudation of fluid from the pulmonary capillaries into the interstitium. Interstitial fluid leads to a decrease in lung compliance that increases the effort of breathing. If not effectively drained by lymphatics, this leads to acute pulmonary edema. It is important to note that a sudden increase in PVH can lead to pulmonary edema at lower pulmonary venous pressure as compared to gradual chronic increase in PVH. Common precipitants of acute pulmonary edema include fever, anemia, intercurrent infections, atrial fibrillation with fast ventricular rate and pregnancy.[7]

SYSTEMIC EMBOLISM

Mitral stenosis provides the perfect milieu for the formation of clots inside the left atrium (LA). Among the three criteria predisposing to the formation of clots as per Virchow's triad, patients with mitral stenosis have two. This includes stasis of blood due to obstruction and AF. Another possible factor is endothelial dysfunction inside the LA due to rheumatic activity. This leads to the formation of clots inside LA, usually in the left-atrial appendage (LAA). Though systemic embolism seems to be unrelated to the severity of MS,[8] it is logical that more stasis will happen in severe stenosis and thus there would be greater probability of thromboembolism as the severity of MS increases. Liu et al. have shown that treatment of MS with PTMC could significantly decrease the incidence of embolic stroke in patients with MS.[9] This again is indirect evidence for the association of severity of MS and thromboembolism. The exact prevalence of embolism in patients with MS is difficult to assess as some of these episodes might be asymptomatic. In general, about 20% of patients with MS have had a history of systemic embolism in the past. Embolism to cerebral circulation leading to stroke is very common, accounting for 60%–70% of episodes of systemic embolism.[8] The presence of atrial fibrillation increases the risk of stroke. In patients who are in sinus rhythm, the presence of spontaneous echo contrast was found in 50% of individuals with embolism. The presence of LAA dysfunction has also been correlated to the formation of LAA clots.[10] The presence of subclinical atrial fibrillation has also been associated with increased cardiac embolism in patients of MS. In a 24-hour Holter study of patients in sinus rhythm, the presence of subclinical atrial fibrillation on Holter resulted in five times higher chances of systemic embolism as compared to patients who did not have atrial fibrillation on Holter monitoring.[11] Global fibrinolytic index (GFI) was assessed in patients with rheumatic MS with atrial fibrillation, non-rheumatic atrial fibrillation, patients with MS in sinus rhythm, and normal controls.[12] GFI was significantly lower in patients with MS with AF, as compared to the rest of the groups. Similarly, patients with MS in sinus rhythm were found to have lower GFI as compared to controls. This emphasizes that the fibrinolytic activity was lower in patients with MS. It was concluded that hypofibrinolysis, as measured by GFI, could be one of the important reasons for elevated risk of thromboembolism in such patients. Murugesan et al. have shown that patients with severe MS with left-atrial clot had raised fibrinogen, homocysteine, and platelet aggregation with lower level of homocysteine-vitamin determinants (vitamin B12 and folate).[13] In summary, the potential reasons for clot formation in LA in patients with MS are stasis of blood due to MS, atrial standstill due to atrial fibrillation, increased thrombogenicity along with decreased fibrinolytic activity, endothelial dysfunction due to possible rheumatic activity, and dysfunctional LAA.

Though there are no significant differences in the management of patients with cardioembolic and atheroembolic stroke, cardioembolic stroke has been shown to have the worst prognosis, which might be due to the tendency of occlusion of major cerebral arteries in patients with stroke due to cardioembolism. Arboix et al. reported that the in-hospital mortality of cardioembolic stroke (that included all possible cardiac causes) was 27%. They found it to be the highest in their series. They also found a recurrence of 77% within a week.[14] This underscores the importance of identifying the potential cardiac cause and treating it so as to decrease the complication. Other than symptomatic stroke, silent infarction is frequently diagnosed in patients with mitral stenosis. It is defined as any brain infarction that is identified by brain imaging in an asymptomatic patient (without prior clinical history of transient ischemic attack or stroke). Akedemir et al.[15] studied patients with mitral valve disease to assess the risk of silent brain infarction. They excluded patients with carotid artery disease, diabetes, hypertension, left-atrial thrombus, left-ventricular dysfunction and other valve disease. They found that the incidence of silent brain infarction was 24.5% in patients with MS (47% cortical, 53% lacunar). LA dimension >4 cm or atrial fibrillation or both were associated with significantly increased silent brain infarction. They also found presence of moderate to severe mitral regurgitation to be negatively associated with silent brain infarction. There was no significant difference between calcific and non-calcific MS. Similarly, Wood et al. found that amongst patients with stroke, rheumatic mitral valve disease is associated with the worst clinical outcomes, including increased risk of mortality, infections, arrhythmias, and sepsis after stroke.[16] This might be related to coexisting diseases like atrial fibrillation, ongoing endothelial dysfunction due to recurrent infections and their poor cardiovascular adaptability. Identifying patients who are at risk of developing systemic embolism is helpful in formulating preventive strategies in this subgroup. Chaing et al. prospectively studied 534 consecutive patients with mitral valve areas of <2 cm². Seventy-five percent of these patients were in atrial fibrillation. They found that 11.4% of patients with atrial fibrillation and 9.1% of patients with sinus rhythm developed systemic embolism on follow-up. The presence of left-atrial thrombus, higher age, lower mitral valve area, and moderate aortic regurgitation were found to be associated with an increased risk of systemic embolism in patients with MS and sinus rhythm. In patients with atrial fibrillation, prior embolism was associated with an increased risk of recurrent embolism, while PTMC was associated with a lower risk of embolism. They concluded that it might be appropriate to give anticoagulation to patients with prior embolism, left-atrial thrombi, or significant aortic regurgitation. It is also prudent to do early PTMC in symptomatic patients to prevent such complications.[17]

PULMONARY ARTERY HYPERTENSION

The passive obstruction of the mitral valve leads to elevated left-atrial pressure that gets transmitted into pulmonary capillaries, leading to elevated pulmonary capillary wedge pressure. There exists a normal mean pulmonary artery (PA) to LA gradient that forces the blood to flow from PA to LA, which is usually 10–12 mmHg. When LA pressure and pulmonary capillary wedge pressure (PCWP) elevates in MS, it also elevates the mean PA pressure accordingly. This is called passive PAH. Hence, there is a proportional increase in PA pressure according to the increase in LA pressure. Once the obstruction is relieved by either mitral valve replacement or PTMC, PA pressure drops down to the normal range. However, persistently elevated pulmonary venous hypertension may lead to significant changes in the alveolo-capillary membrane, along with pulmonary arterioles and pulmonary arteries (Figure 6.1). Possible mechanisms include endothelial dysfunction, vasoconstriction, an increase in endothelin 1 and its receptors, a decrease in nitric oxide, and a decrease in response to BNP. In order to differentiate between passive PAH and disproportionately elevated PAH, Vachiery et al.[18] proposed newer terminologies like isolated post-capillary PAH and combined post-capillary and pre-capillary PAH in patients with left-heart disease. They proposed that when the difference between diastolic pressure and mean LA pressure is >6 mmHg, combined pre-capillary and post-capillary PAH should be suspected.[18] The presence of PAH in patients with MS is closely related with symptoms and associated with markedly worse outcomes. However, limited data are available from modern series. Maoqin et al. found that patients with severe PAH and severe MS had higher New York Heart Association (NYHA) class symptoms, both before and after intervention, respectively.[19] They also found a higher cardiovascular event rate in such patients during follow-up. Similarly, from a cohort of 531 patients referred for PTMC, 15% had severe PAH (systolic PAP >60 mmHg), and these patients exhibited a significantly reduced long-term cardiac event-free survival compared with those

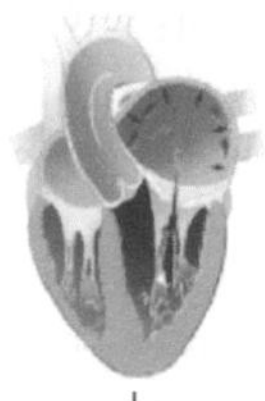

Increase in left atrial pressure

↓

Passive backward increase in pulmonary venous pressure (PVH)

↓

Passive backward increase in pulmonary arterial pressure (PAH)

↓

Persistent increase in PVH leads to alteration in anatomy of alveolar capillary membrane (ACM) and pulmonary arteries
Increased deposition of type IV collagen in ACM
Muscularization of arterioles
Hypertrophy of media
Formation of neointimal layer in distal PA

↓

Out of proportional raise in PA pressure (reactive with or without irreversible PAH)

↓

Right ventricle dysfunction

↓

Decline in stroke volume leading to fall in PA pressure
Right heart failure

Figure 6.1 Mitral stenosis and pulmonary artery hypertension.

with normal systolic PAP.[19] Overall, once symptomatic patients develop severe PAH, their mean survival drops down significantly.

The treatment of MS leads to regression of the PA pressure. Fawzy et al. reported that all patients with mild, moderate, and severe PAH had similar PA pressure 6–12 months after PTMC, though the regression in PA pressure was slower in patients with severe PAH.[20,21] However, persistent PAH (PA systolic pressure >40 mmHg) after PTMC has been reported in patients at one year in up to 40% of patients. These patients were older, sicker, and had advanced rheumatic mitral valve disease. On follow-up, these patients had higher incidence of restenosis, new-onset heart failure, and need for re-interventions.[22]

HEMOPTYSIS

Another well-known complication of MS is hemoptysis. The etiology of hemoptysis in MS may be diverse. It includes: (1) pulmonary apoplexy due to raised pulmonary venous hypertension; (2) acute pulmonary edema resulting in pink frothy sputum; (3) bronchitis; (4) co-existent lung infection due to tuberculosis; (5) pulmonary thromboembolism causing pulmonary infarct and hemoptysis.

The bronchial arterial circulation forms the bronchial venous plexus, which is connected to the pulmonary venous circulation. Approximately two-thirds of the blood from this venous plexus drains to the pulmonary veins and thus to the LA.[23,24] An increase in pulmonary venous pressure due to MS leads to a reverse flow of blood from the pulmonary veins to the bronchial venous plexus, visible as engorged bronchial vasculature. When there is a sudden increase in LA pressure, these veins are prone to rupture, leading to hemoptysis, which can be massive and require blood transfusion and surgery.[25] In rare cases, this may be the only presenting feature of MS. This complication occurs more commonly early in the course of the disease when the bronchial veins are more prone to rupture. Long-standing PVH leads to thickening of these veins and thus they are able to withstand greater pressure. Susceptibility to tuberculosis in patients with MS is much debated. Rokitansky, in 1846, enunciated the theory that chronic passive congestion of the lungs excludes probability of tuberculosis of the lungs.[26] However, this concept has been argued against and patients of MS in endemic areas are as susceptible to it. Pulmonary thromboembolism may also occur in these patients especially in untreated cases with PAH and right-heart failure. The resulting pulmonary infarct can be a cause of hemoptysis.

INFECTIVE ENDOCARDITIS

The deformity of the mitral valve in patients of MS makes the patient susceptible to infective endocarditis. This complication is more common with mild MS when the valve is stiff and fibrotic and becomes less likely once it is calcified and very rigid. However, overall infective endocarditis is uncommon in isolated MS. Rowe et al., in their ten-year follow-up of medically treated patients of MS, reported 5% of all deaths as being due to infective endocarditis.[27] The presence of associated mitral regurgitation or aortic regurgitation increases the probability of infective endocarditis. When endocarditis does occur, it may cause mitral regurgitation or may lead to an increase in the degree of stenosis due to mechanical obstruction of the valve by the vegetation. Current guidelines do not recommend antibiotic prophylaxis in uncomplicated cases of MS.

RARE COMPLICATIONS

Other complications of MS may include ball valve thrombus formation. This is most often due to a cleavage of a clot from the left-atrial wall, which is then free-moving within the LA. This is a potentially fatal complication if not treated in time due to mechanical obstruction of systemic embolism.[28] Other rare complications of MS include Ortner's syndrome or cardiovocal syndrome due to left recurrent laryngeal nerve palsy leading to hoarseness of voice. Ortner's syndrome was first described by Nobert Ortner, a Viennese

physician, in 1897, in a case of mitral stenosis with dilated LA. Initially, enlarged LA was thought to be the main culprit; however, the current understanding favors pressure in the pulmonary artery playing the most important role in causing the nerve compression in a majority of the cases. The incidence of Ortner's syndrome in MS ranges from 0.6% to 5%.[29] MS with enlarged LA is also associated with dysphagia, the mechanism of which has been attributed to mechanical compression of the esophagus or to the compression of the autonomic plexus, which coordinates the peristaltic movement of the esophagus. The latter is the more likely mechanism since the pressure generated within the LA is unlikely to be higher than the pressure within the esophagus lumen, which reaches a peak of 40–80 mmHg.[30] Ortner's syndrome and dyshagia are not unique to MS as any condition that can increase LA or PA pressure can produce such complications.

REFERENCES

1. Roy SB, Bhatia ML, Lazaro EJ, Ramalingaswami V. Juvenile mitral stenosis in India 1963. *Natl Med J India* 2011 Jul-Aug;24(4):248–53.
2. Meira ZM, Goulart EM, Colosimo EA et al. Long-term follow-up of rheumatic fever and predictors of severe rheumatic valvar disease in Brazilian children and adolescents. *Heart* 2005; 91:1019–22.
3. Dubin AA, March HW, Cohn K et al. Longitudinal hemodynamic and clinical study of mitral stenosis. *Circulation* 1971; 44:381–9.
4. Gordon SP, Douglas PS, Come PC et al. Two-dimensional and Doppler echocardiographic determinants of the natural history of mitral valve narrowing in patients with rheumatic mitral stenosis: Implications for follow-up. *J Am Coll Cardiol* 992 Apr;19(5):968–73.
5. Lung B, Vahanian A. Rheumatic mitral valve disease, Chapter 14. In: Otto Cm, Bonow RO Eds. *Valvular Heart Disease: A Companion to Braunwald's Heart Disease.* 3rd Edition. Saunders 221.
6. Olesen KH. The natural history of 271 patients with mitral stenosis under medical treatment. *Br Heart J* 1962 May;24:349–57.

7. Bader RA, Bader ME, Rose DJ et al. Hemodynamics at rest and during exercise in normal pregnancy as studied by cardiac catheterization. *J Clin Invest* 1955;34:1524.

8. Alpert JS, Rahimtoola SH, Dalen JE. Valvular Heart Diseases, 3rd edition; Lippincott Williams & Williams; 75–112.

9. Liu TJ, Lai HC, Lee WL et al. Percutaneous balloon commissurotomy reduces incidence of ischemic cerebral stroke in patients with symptomatic rheumatic mitral stenosis. *Int J Cardiol* 2008 Jan 11;123(2):189–90.

10. Goswami KC, Yadav R, Bahl VK. Predictors of left atrial appendage clot: A trans-esophageal echocardiographic study of left atrial appendage function in patients with severe mitral stenosis. *Indian Heart J* 2004 Nov-Dec;56(6):628–35.

11. Karthikeyan G, Ananthakrishna R, Devasenapathy N et al. Transient, subclinical atrial fibrillation and risk of systemic embolism in patients with rheumatic mitral stenosis in sinus rhythm. *Am J Cardiol* 2014 Sep 15;114(6):869–74.

12. Atalar E, Ozmen F, Haznedaroroglu I et al. Impaired fibrinolytic capacity in rheumatic mitral stenosis with or without atrial fibrillation and nonrheumatic atrial fibrillation. *Int J Hematol* 2002 Aug;76(2):192–5.

13. Murugesan V, Pulimamidi, VK, Rajappa M et al. Elevated fibrinogen and lowered homocysteine-vitamin determinants and their association with left atrial thrombus in patients with rheumatic mitral stenosis. *Br J Biomed Sci* 2015;72(3):102–6.

14. Arboix A, Alio J. Cardioembolic stroke: Clinical features, specific cardiac disorders and prognosis. *Curr Cardiol Rev* 2010 Aug;6(3):150–6.

15. Akdemir I, Dagdelen S, Yuce M et al. Silent brain infarction in patients with rheumatic mitral stenosis. *Jpn Heart J* 2002 Mar;43(2):137–44.

16. Wood AD, Mannu GS, Clark AB et al. Rheumatic mitral valve disease is associated with worse outcomes in stroke: A Thailand national database study stroke. 2016 Nov;47(11):2695–701.

17. Chiang CW, Lo SK, Ko YS et al. Predictors of systemic embolism in patients with mitral stenosis. A prospective study. *Ann Intern Med* 1998 Jun 1;128(11):885–9.

18. Vachiéry JL, Adir Y, Barberà JA et al. Pulmonary hypertension due to left heart diseases. *J Am Coll Cardiol* 2013;62:D100–8.

19. Maoqin S, Guoxiang H, Zhiyuan S et al. The clinical and hemodynamic results of mitral balloon valvuloplasty for patients with mitral stenosis complicated by severe pulmonary hypertension. *Eur J Intern Med* 2005;16:413–8.

20. Fawzy ME, Osman A, Nambiar V et al. Immediate and long-term results of mitral balloon valvuloplasty in patients with severe pulmonary hypertension. *J Heart Valve Dis* 2008;17:485–91.

21. Fawzy ME, Hassan W, Stefadouros M et al. Prevalence and fate of severe pulmonary hypertension in 559 consecutive patients with severe rheumatic mitral stenosis undergoing mitral balloon valvotomy. *J Heart Valve Dis* 2004 Nov;13(6):942–7; discussion 947–8.

22. Nair KKM, Pillai HS, Titus T et al. Persistent pulmonary artery hypertension in patients undergoing balloon mitral valvotomy. *Pulm Circ* 2013 Apr–Jun;3(2):426–31.

23. Ashour MH, Jain SK, Kattan KM. Massive haemoptysis caused by congenital absence of a segment of inferior vena cava. *Thorax* 1993 Oct;48(10):1044–5.

24. Baile EM. The anatomy and physiology of the bronchial circulation. *J of Aerosol Med* Mar 2009;9(1):1–6.

25. Wood P. An appreciation of mitral stenosis. Part 1. Clinical features. *Br Med J* 1954;1:1051.

26. Tileston W. Passive hyperemia of the lungs and tuberculosis. *JAMA* 1908;l(15):1179–82.

27. Rowe JC, Bland EF, Sprague HB et al. The course of mitral stenosis without surgery: Ten- and twenty-year perspectives. *Ann Intern Med* 1960 Apr;52:741–9.

28. Roy A, Naik N, Nagesh CM et al. Fatal freely mobile left atrial thrombus: Fallout of anti-coagulation? *J Am Soc Echocardiogr* 2009 Jul;22(7):863.e5–6.

29. Solanki SV, Yajnik VH. Ortner's syndrome. *Indian Heart J* 1972;24:43–6.

30. Daley R. Massive dilatation of the LA. *Br Heart J* 1980 Dec;44(6):724.

PART 2

Investigations

7

Electrocardiogram, chest radiograph, and ancillary investigations

ARUN SHARMA, KANIKA BHAMBRI, GURPREET S. GULATI, AND NEERAJ PARAKH

ELECTROCARDIOGRAM

Electrocardiogram (ECG) changes in rheumatic mitral stenosis (MS) are a reflection of hemodynamic consequences of the left-atrial outflow obstruction. Pressure overload of the left atrium (LA) due to MS results in a variable degree of LA enlargement, depending upon the severity and duration of mitral valve disease. Associated mitral regurgitation may further increase the insult on LA. A variable degree of scarring and conduction abnormalities in the LA also exist because of hemodynamic insult and underlying rheumatic heart disease. Back pressure from LA results in pulmonary venous hypertension followed by pulmonary arterial hypertension. This results in right-ventricular hypertrophy and later on right-atrial (RA) enlargement. In many cases, accompanying tricuspid valve disease augments the RA abnormalities. Pressure and volume overload of atria results in various rhythm abnormalities ranging from atrial premature beats to atrial tachycardia, atrial flutter, and atrial fibrillation (AF). Since mitral valve per se has no ECG contribution, there are few or no ECG abnormalities in hemodynamically insignificant MS.[1] The presence of concomitant abnormalities of other valves will have a variable effect on the ECG changes due to MS. Thomas Lewis, credited for the first textbook of electrocardiography in 1913, described extensively various ECG changes in MS. He described these ECG changes as characteristic for MS, though it was later realized that these changes may be present in many other conditions affecting the heart.[2]

Left-atrial abnormality

Left-atrial depolarization contributes to the middle and terminal part of the surface P-wave. The LA P-wave vector is directed leftwards and posteriorly as per the anatomical orientation of the LA in the thoracic cavity. A combination of LA enlargement, scarring, and pressure overload results in the delayed depolarization of the LA along with increased P-terminal force. A conduction delay in Bachman's bundle also contributes to prolonged LA depolarization. Electrophysiological studies in MS have shown an LA activation delay of 35 ms in coronary sinus electrodes as compared to a normal P-wave.[3,4] Various ECG changes resulting from abnormal LA activation in MS are set out below.

P-WAVE DURATION, AREA, AND DISPERSION

A P-wave duration of 0.12 sec or more in limb lead II or any other limb lead is a marker of LA enlargement. The degree of P-wave widening correlates well with LA enlargement. P-wave widening correlates better with LA volume than LA pressure.[5,6] The overall sensitivity of P-wave duration in diagnosing LA enlargement in MS is around 50%, while specificity is 95%.[7] A P-wave area of ≥4.0 ms.mV in lead II as a marker of LA enlargement has been found to be more sensitive than P-wave duration (85% vs. 45%–60%); however, specificity of both criteria is similar (~94%).[8] P-wave dispersion is defined as the difference between maximum and minimum P-wave duration. Increased P-wave dispersion is a marker of discontinuous and inhomogeneous conduction of sinus impulse in the atria. Increased sympathetic activity in MS may also contribute to increased P-wave dispersion. An increased P-wave dispersion has been identified as a marker of increased risk for future AF.[9] P-wave dispersion is increased in MS. Mitral valvotomy and β-blocker therapy has shown to decrease the P-wave dispersion in some studies but their effect on the prevention of future AF is not established.[10–12]

NOTCHED OR BIFID P-WAVE

Some notching in the P-wave may be seen in normal ECG due to differential activation of right and left atria. A definite notch with interpeak distance of greater than 0.04 sec and depth of 0.1 mV or more is indicative of LA enlargement. A bifid and wide P-wave has classically been described as a P-mitrale, as it is commonly associated with mitral valve disease.[13] However, a P-mitrale is not specific for mitral valve disease and occurs in many other conditions, such as left-ventricular hypertrophy, constrictive pericarditis, etc. These changes are most prominent in lead II as this lead is maximally aligned with the P-wave axis. Limb lead I and other limb leads may also show a notched P-wave (Figure 7.1). In patients with significant MS who were undergoing valve surgery, P-mitrale was present in one-third of cases.[14]

MORRIS INDEX

The product of the amplitude and duration of the terminal negative component of the P-wave in lead

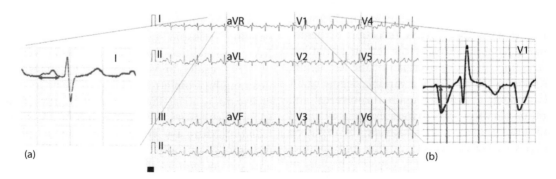

(a)

(b)

Figure 7.1 ECG from a patient of longstanding MS. Inset (a) shows P mitrale in lead I with P-wave duration of 3 mm and interpeak distance of more than 1 mm. Inset (b) shows a big negative component of P-wave in lead V1 with a Morris index of 0.032 mV.sec.

V1 is less than 0.003 mV.sec in the normal population (less than one small square in width and depth at standard ECG paper speed). Morris et al. termed this as P-terminal force at V1 (TFP-V1), also known as the Morris index.[15] A value of more than 0.003 mV.sec has sensitivity of 75%–85% and specificity of more than 90% for LA enlargement (Figure 7.1). The Morris index is one of the most accurate indicators of LA enlargement in MS with overall accuracy in the range of 90%.[7,16] Cor pulmonale, chest deformities, and a markedly enlarged right atrium may result in false-positive Morris index for LA enlargement. Alteration of the atrial activation axis is responsible for this pattern.[17]

MACRUZ INDEX

The ratio between the P-wave duration and PR segment (P/PR segment) is termed the Macruz index. Normally, this is between 1.0 and 1.6, and a value of more than 1.6 is indicative of LA enlargement.[18] The Macruz index requires accurate measurement of P-wave and PR segment as even minor errors will substantially change the value. Besides this, its utility is also limited in the presence of biatrial enlargement.[19] The Macruz index can accurately diagnose LA enlargement in two-thirds of patients with MS.[7]

LEFTWARD P-WAVE AXIS

A leftward shift in P-wave axis (less than +30°) is manifested by a negative terminal P-wave deflection in III and a VF and positive terminal P-wave deflection in lead aVL. This is an uncommon finding and present in only 10% of patients.[20]

Left-atrial abnormality regresses after successful percutaneous transvenous mitral commissurotomy (PTMC). A mitral valve area of ≥1.7 cm² at follow-up is an independent predictor of P-wave normalization.[21]

Bi-atrial abnormality

Right-atrial enlargement in MS occurs due to pulmonary hypertension or coexistent tricuspid valve disease. ECG manifestations of biatrial abnormality are[22]:

1. An increase in both duration and amplitude of P-wave (>0.12 ms and 0.25 mV, respectively)
2. Tall peaked P-wave (>0.15 mV in V1 and wide, notched P-wave in lead II)
3. A large initial positive P-wave deflection in V1 with area of >0.006 ms.mV along with a positive Morris index (Figure 7.2)

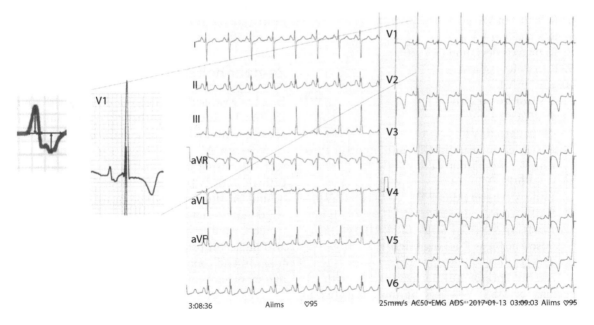

Figure 7.2 ECG of a 15-year-old girl with severe MS and pulmonary artery hypertension. There are features of biatrial enlargement with right-ventricular hypertrophy. R >7 with T inversion and right axis deviation are other features of RVH. P-wave duration and amplitude is also increased in II. Inset shows enlarged V1 and magnified P-wave of V1 showing large initial positive and later negative P-wave.

Right-ventricular hypertrophy

Right-ventricular hypertrophy (RVH) indicates pulmonary artery hypertension (PAH) in MS, although the degree of PAH varies from patient to patient and is not always proportional to the severity and duration of disease. Younger patients and poor LA compliance also predisposes to the development of PAH. Standard ECG criteria of RVH also apply in MS.[21-24] These criteria have low sensitivity (~10%) and high specificity (85–99%),[25] except for the Lewis criteria, which have high sensitivity (80.4%) and low specificity (16.8%).[26] Butler's criteria have a sensitivity of 66% and specificity of 94%.[27] A combination of various criteria (three or more) has better accuracy in predicting RVH.[28,29] R/S >1 in V1 is one of the most common ECG findings of RVH in MS, while presence of qR pattern in V1 is one of the most specific findings for RVH.[30] Various ECG features of RVH are as follows:

1. R/S of more than 1 in V1
2. An increase in the intrinsicoid deflection of onset of QRS in V1 (>35 ms)
3. A sum of R in V1 and S in V5 or V6 of more than 1.05 mV
4. S V1 <0.2 mV
5. R V1 >0.7 mV
6. R/S <0.4 in V6
7. R/S <0.75 in V5
8. Right axis deviation (> + 110°)
9. R in aVR >0.4 mV
10. rSR' in V1
11. S V5 or V6 >0.7 mV
12. R V5/6 <0.5 mV
13. qR pattern in V1
14. A sudden increase in QRS amplitude of three times or more from V1 to V2
15. R:S V5/R:S V1 <0.4
16. Butler's criteria (Max R V1,2 + Max S I, aVL) – S V1 >0.6mV
17. Lewis criteria (R1 + SIII) – (S1 + RIII) <0.15 mV (also known as Einthoven sign)

The presence of RBBB may correlate with the severity of MS.[31] V4R may be more sensitive in predicting LA enlargement and right-ventricular hypertrophy.[32] Vectorcardiographic studies suggest transition from type B RVH to type C and then type A as pulmonary hypertension progresses.[33] The presence of RVH in ECG has 93% sensitivity and 92% specificity for predicting systolic pulmonary artery pressure of 60 mmHg or more, although the absence of RVH in ECG does not exclude RVH or PAH.[34] As a rule, left-ventricular hypertrophy is absent in pure MS. Its presence indicates significant MR or aortic valve disease.

ST-T changes

ST-T changes in right precordial leads are indicative of right-ventricular strain. Patients on digoxin, especially those with AF, may show an inverted tick sign of the ST segment in precordial leads. QT dispersion is significantly prolonged in the presence of MS and is directly related to the severity of MS and plasma NT pro BNP levels.[35]

Arrhythmias

Atrial fibrillation is the most significant rhythm abnormality seen in MS. Various arrhythmias are discussed separately in Chapter 18.

Stress ECG

A false-positive treadmill test may be seen in MS. Digitalis therapy, AF, and a higher maximum heart rate are predictors for ST changes without any significant coronary artery disease.[36]

24-hour holter

Heart rate variability is decreased in MS with sinus rhythm. Increased sympathetic activity is the likely cause for this and may be a marker for future AF. In MS with AF a markedly increased heart rate variability denotes the effect of increased parasympathetic activity on the AV node.[37] Holter is also helpful in detecting asymptomatic or paroxysmal AF, otherwise not documented of routine ECG. The incidence and severity of ventricular arrhythmia is also higher in patients with MS. The presence of frequent and complex ventricular ectopy may be a marker of left-ventricular dysfunction.[38]

CHEST RADIOGRAPH

Chest radiograph is the initial imaging tool in the evaluation of MS and is frequently diagnostic. Moreover, the radiographic findings also provide

Table 7.1 Radiographic findings in mitral stenosis

- Normal to slightly enlarged cardiac size in isolated MS. Moderate to severe cardiomegaly in cases of associated mitral regurgitation.
- Elevation of left main bronchus, double-density sign-LA enlargement.
- Enlargement of the LA appendage (suggestive of rheumatic etiology).
- Pulmonary venous hypertension or edema, hilar haze, or pleural effusion.
- Enlargement of the pulmonary arterial segment, indicative of associated pulmonary arterial hypertension.
- Right-ventricular enlargement, indicative of pulmonary arterial hypertension or associated tricuspid regurgitation.
- Right-ventricular enlargement in the absence of prominence of the main pulmonary artery suggests associated tricuspid regurgitation. The right atrium may also be enlarged with tricuspid regurgitation.
- Inconspicuous ascending aorta and aortic arch. Even slight enlargement of the thoracic aorta raises the possibility of associated aortic valve disease.
- Loss of parallelism of ipsilateral ribs, hypertranslucent ipsilateral lung, loss of LA appendage prominence-post thoracotomy status for MS.

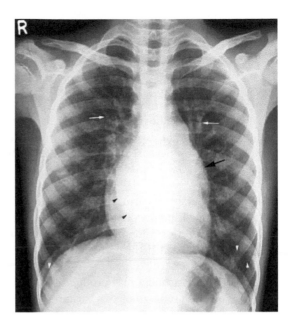

Figure 7.3 Chest radiograph showing normal-sized heart in a patient with MS. Note is made of retrocardiac double density (black arrowheads), left-atrial appendage enlargement (third mogul-black arrow) with presence of cephalization (white arrows), and interstitial edema in the form of Kerley B lines (white arrowheads) in this patient.

considerable insight into the severity of MS and are useful in documenting the progression of disease (Table 7.1).

Heart size

Heart size is usually normal or mildly enlarged in isolated MS (Figure 7.3). This occurs due to posteriorly directed enlargement of the LA. Moderate to severe cardiomegaly may, however, be seen in cases of MS associated with mitral regurgitation.

Left atrium

Left-atrial enlargement usually causes retrocardiac double density (double density sign) with splaying of the carina and/or elevation of the left main bronchus (Figures 7.3 and 7.4). In normal subjects,

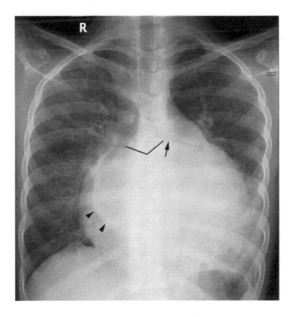

Figure 7.4 Chest radiograph showing cardiomegaly with retrocardiac double density (arrowheads), uplifting of left mainstem bronchus (arrow), and splaying of carina in a patient with MS.

subcarinal and interbronchial angle measurements (Figure 7.5) vary widely, as below.[39,40]

- Interbronchial angle: normal mean 67°–77° (range 34°–109°) (angle between the central axis of right and left main bronchi)
- Subcarinal angle: normal mean 62°–73° (range 34°–90°) (angle of divergence of right and left main bronchi measured along their inferior margins)

On chest radiograph, a carinal angle of more than 90° is an acceptable predictor of LA enlargement.[41,42] Moreover, an LA dimension more than 50 mm can be correctly predicted if the carinal angle is more obtuse (100° or greater).

Left-atrial enlargement may produce characteristic signs on chest radiograph or a barium swallow:

- Superior displacement of the left mainstem bronchus on frontal view (Figure 7.4)
- Posterior displacement of a barium-filled esophagus or nasogastric tube

The size of the LA can be measured as the distance from the middle of the right lateral border of the LA to the middle of the inner margin of the left main bronchus. This distance is usually less than 7 cm in the majority of normal subjects and is generally 7 cm or greater in 90% of MS patients.[43–45] Massive LA enlargement can result in the LA becoming border-forming on the right side, a condition also known as atrial escape (Figure 7.6). The LA can approach within a few centimeters of the chest wall on one or both sides, as seen in longstanding mitral regurgitation with AF.

On a lateral chest radiograph, an enlarged LA may cause posterior displacement of the left upper or lower lobe bronchi relative to the right bronchi, creating right and left legs, giving the appearance of the "walking man sign".[43] However, this sign is not pathognomonic of an enlarged LA, and may occur in cases of mediastinal mass, subcarinal lymphadenopathy, and thoraco-lumbar scoliosis.

Rheumatic MS results in characteristic enlargement of the LA appendage. It can appear as straightening of the left heart border or as a convexity along the left cardiac border, just below the pulmonary artery segment—the "bump" is often referred to as the "third mogul"[46] (Figures 7.3 and 7.6). (Moguls are mounds of snow formed on a ski slope. The first and second moguls on the left

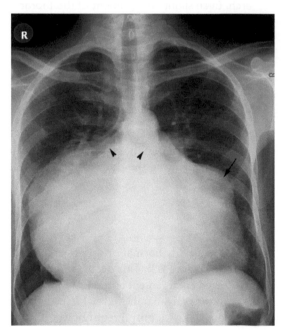

Figure 7.6 Chest radiograph in a patient with severe MS showing gross LA enlargement forming right-heart border ("atrial escape sign") with splaying of carina (arrowheads). Note is made of LA appendage enlargement (third mogul) in this patient (arrow).

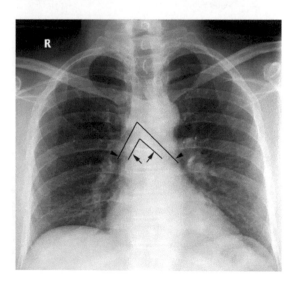

Figure 7.5 Chest radiograph demonstrating measurement of carinal (arrows) and interbronchial (arrowheads) angles in a normal subject.

mediastinal contour are the aortic knob and main pulmonary artery respectively. The fourth mogul is the cardiac apex.)

Mitral valve calcification

Calcification of the mitral apparatus may be seen in MS of rheumatic etiology (Figure 7.7). This generally involves valve leaflets or tips and is more commonly associated with valvular stenosis. This is distinct from mitral annular calcification (MAC), which appears as C-shaped calcification. MAC is a degenerative process seen with aging in up to 35% of elderly patients, and is usually not symptomatic.[47] Posterior mitral annulus is more commonly involved than anterior mitral annulus in annular calcification and there is a lack of mitral leaflet commissural fusion, as compared to MS due to rheumatic etiology.

In order to differentiate between aortic and mitral valve calcification, a lateral chest radiograph can often be helpful. A line drawn from the anterior costophrenic sulcus to the carina helps in differentiating valvular involvement. Aortic valve calcification would lie above this line, while mitral valve calcification would be seen below this line. A fluoroscopy can also be used to detect and identify the location of valvular calcification.

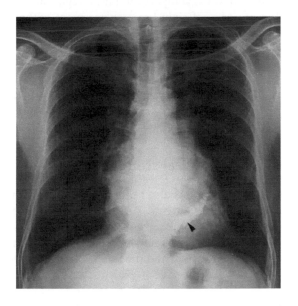

Figure 7.7 Chest radiograph showing extensive calcification (arrowhead) of mitral valve in a patient of MS.

Pulmonary vasculature in mitral stenosis

The severity and chronicity of MS, as well as monitoring the effect of treatment on the pulmonary vasculature, can be assessed on a chest radiograph. The degree of pulmonary venous hypertension (PVH) acts as a rough guide for assessing the severity of MS.

Mild PVH. In mild disease, there is equalization or reversal of the diameter of upper and lower lobe pulmonary veins (cephalization). This is the earliest sign of pulmonary venous hypertension, and the prominence of upper lobe pulmonary veins is thought to resemble the antler of a stag ("stag's antler sign" or "inverted moustache sign") (Figure 7.3). This correlates with a pulmonary capillary wedge pressure (PCWP) of 13–18 mmHg.[48] This sign occurs due to recruitment of resting upper lobe vessels that become more prominent as compared to lower lobe vessels. The compression of lower lobe vessels due to an increase in hydrostatic pressure at the lung bases also contributes to this finding. On a radiograph, this comparison between the upper and lower lobe vessels should be made at an equal distance from the hilar point/angle, which is formed by junction between the superior pulmonary vein and the descending pulmonary artery.

Moderate PVH. With increasing LA pressures, interstitial pulmonary edema develops.[47] This is typically seen as interlobular septal thickening (Kerley B lines), and is frequently visible on a chest radiograph. Typical Kerley B lines appear as short (1–2 cm), horizontal white lines perpendicular to the pleural surface at lung bases (Figure 7.3). These findings are seen in moderate PVH and correlate with PCWP of 18–25 mmHg.[48] Less frequently identified signs of interstitial edema include Kerley A and C lines. Kerley A lines represent distension of lymphatic channels between peri-venous and peri-bronchovascular lymphatics, and can be seen as larger lines (larger than B lines, 2–6 cm in length) extending obliquely from the hilum to the upper lobes. Kerley C lines represent reticular opacities in the lung bases and may represent Kerley B lines en face.

Severe PVH. With increasing LA pressures (PCWP >25 mmHg), alveolar pulmonary edema develops with fluid seepage into the alveoli.[48]

On chest radiograph, it appears as diffuse, confluent areas of ground-glass opacity with peripheral sparing ("bat-wing appearance"). With the institution of decongestant therapy, the clearing generally takes three days or less. Resolution usually starts from the periphery and moves centrally. This is useful to differentiate it from other acute conditions that can present with perihilar opacification, such as hypersensitivity pneumonitis, infection, pulmonary hemorrhage, etc. Associated cardiomegaly is helpful in the differential diagnosis of cardiogenic pulmonary edema. Moreover, sequential progression of changes, signs of infection, bleeding diathesis, or occupational history should be kept in mind while evaluating chest radiograph, as these are helpful clues in arriving at the exact diagnosis.

Hemosiderosis and ossification

There may be diffuse pulmonary hemorrhage in patients of hemosiderosis and ossification. In the early phase of the disease, hemorrhage may be due to rupture of microvasculature; however, in the later course of the disease it may relate to abnormally engorged submucosal bronchial veins exposed to raised pressures through anastomoses with the pulmonary veins.[49] There may be deposition of hemosiderin or fibrosis following repeated episodes of pulmonary edema or hemorrhage. Hemosiderosis is frequently seen in autopsy specimens of these patients; however, it may be visible radiographically in 10%–25% of chronic MS cases.[50] It is characterized by small, 1–3-mm-diameter, ill-defined nodules, or by coarse reticular areas of increased opacity with preference for the middle and lower lobes. Pulmonary parenchymal ossification can also be seen in 3%–13% of the cases and is usually pathognomonic for chronic MS.[51] Radiographically, it appears as densely calcified, 1–5-mm nodules, mainly in the middle and lower lobes, with a tendency for the occasional presence of trabeculae and confluence.

Assessment of etiology and associated conditions

Chest radiograph can give a clue to the etiology of the disease. Enlargement of the LA appendage is invariably associated with rheumatic etiology, as described earlier. A coexisting ASD may be present in 0.6% of the cases, which may relieve the

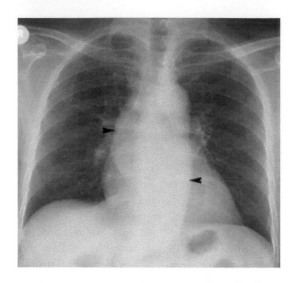

Figure 7.8 Chest radiograph showing dilated ascending and descending aorta (arrowheads) in a patient with MS with aortic regurgitation.

LA hypertension—also known as Lutembacher syndrome.[52]

Enlargement of the right ventricle and convexity of the pulmonary arterial segment usually indicate the development of pulmonary artery hypertension. However, pulmonary arterial and venous hypertension is much more commonly seen with MS as compared to mitral regurgitation. The presence of right-heart enlargement without pulmonary arterial hypertension is usually due to concomitant rheumatic tricuspid regurgitation.

In isolated mitral valve disease, the ascending aorta and aortic arch are characteristically small. However, coexisting aortic valve disease should be suspected (Figure 7.8) even if there is slight prominence of the thoracic aorta.[53]

Operated mitral stenosis

Chest radiograph is also helpful in the assessment of operated MS patients. Postoperative changes of lateral thoracotomy can be seen in the form of loss of parallelism of ribs on the same side, hyperlucent ipsilateral lung, and the loss of LA appendage prominence. Moreover, in patients with mechanical prosthetic heart valves, fluoroscopy plays an important role in functional assessment of valves (Figure 7.9) with early recognition of stuck valves (Figure 7.10), thereby helping the timely institution of thrombolytic therapy in these patients.

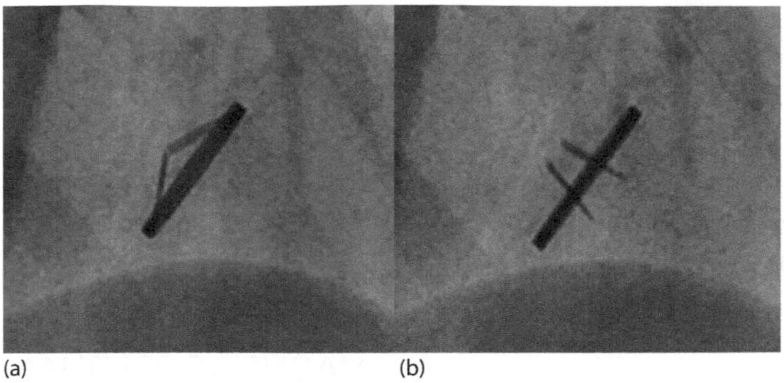

Figure 7.9 Fluoroscopic images show prosthetic mitral valve in systole **(a)** and diastole **(b)**.

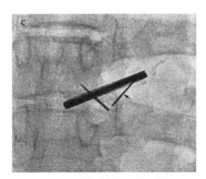

Figure 7.10 Fluoroscopic image shows stuck prosthetic mitral valve leaflet (arrow) that fails to open in diastole.

It is also helpful in follow-up of these patients with documentation of normal valve movement following thrombolysis. Knowledge of the opening and closing angles of the mechanical valves is essential. The normal opening and closing angles for the St. Jude bileaflet valve are 85° and 25°–30°, and for the carbomedics valve are 78°–80° and 15°, respectively. The normal opening and closing angles for the tilting-disc Medtronic Hall valve are 70° and 0°, and for the TTK Chitra valve are 70° and 0°, respectively.[54,55]

COMPUTED TOMOGRAPHY

Normal mitral valve anatomy on computed tomography

The mitral valve annulus is a D-shaped ring within the left atrioventricular groove and is the site of valve leaflet attachment (Figure 7.11). It is bordered

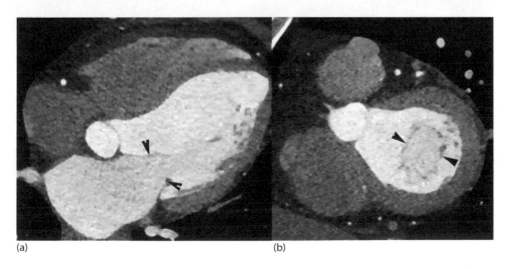

Figure 7.11 CT angiography: normal mitral apparatus in diastole (arrowheads) in four-chamber **(a)** and short axis **(b)** views.

by the left circumflex artery and the coronary sinus. Valve leaflets (normally of thickness <5 mm) are supported by chordae, which in turn attach to two papillary muscles that arise from the lateral wall of the left ventricle. This complex is referred to as the mitral apparatus.[56,57] The anterior leaflet is wider and attaches to nearly two-fifths of the annulus. The anterior leaflet covers more of the valve orifice than the narrower posterior leaflet and also forms part of the left ventricular outflow tract.[58]

Computed tomography in mitral stenosis

Cardiac computed tomography (CT) is particularly helpful in the detection of mitral valve leaflet, commissural and annulus calcification, valvular planimetry, and for detection of the presence of thrombus and calcification (Figure 7.12). For the evaluation of valve components, reconstructions at 5% and 65% of the R-R interval are usually recommended for closed and open mitral valves, respectively. The geometric orifice area is measured by direct planimetry and has been shown to correlate well (R = 0.88; $p < 0.001$) with TEE.[59] It also provides information regarding LA size/volume, the presence or absence of thrombus, right ventricular hypertrophy, and evidence of pulmonary edema or hypertension. It is extremely useful in preoperative coronary artery assessment,

the mapping of pulmonary venous anatomy (Figure 7.13), and in the detection of postoperative complications.[60–62] Dynamic CT images may also reveal restricted movement of valve leaflets or evidence of stuck prosthetic valves. However, it is not indicated for routine valve disease assessment owing to its inability to provide sufficient hemodynamic information and its inherent need for iodinated contrast and ionizing radiation.

MAGNETIC RESONANCE IMAGING

Cardiac magnetic resonance imaging (MRI) is valuable for its ability to provide hemodynamic data in those patients where echocardiographic assessment is inadequate. It remains the gold standard investigation for providing reproducible measurements of ventricular volumes, mass, and function. It also depicts LA size, volume, wall thickness, and presence or absence of mass lesion (Figures 7.14 and 7.15) or thrombus.[63,64] The differentiation and characterization of associated thrombus from the mass lesion are much better on MRI. Delayed enhanced imaging is the technique of choice for detecting and quantifying LA fibrosis or scar.

DIFFERENTIAL DIAGNOSIS

In the majority of cases, MS is most commonly due to rheumatic etiology. Congenital and acquired

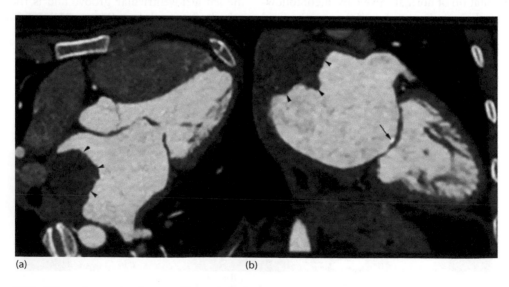

(a) (b)

Figure 7.12 CT angiography: large adherent thrombus [arrowheads in **(a)**] in LA with thickened mitral valve leaflets with hockey stick deformity of anterior mitral leaflet in a patient of MS. Note is made of presence of calcification [arrow in **(b)**] of valve leaflet.

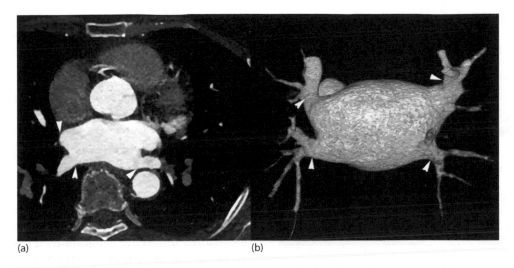

Figure 7.13 CT angiography: role of CT in pulmonary venous mapping (a and b). Arrowheads show drainage of pulmonary veins into LA.

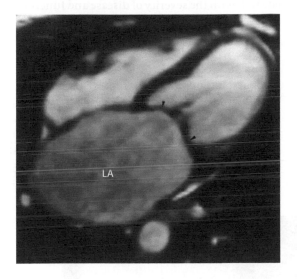

Figure 7.14 MRI image shows dilated LA with thickened mitral valve leaflets (arrowheads) in a patient with MS.

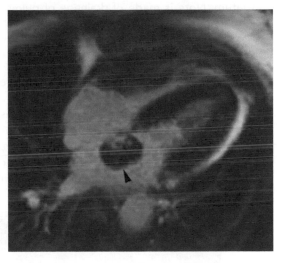

Figure 7.15 MRI of myxoma. Contrast-enhanced, delayed MRI in four-chamber view shows well-defined mass (arrowhead), attached to interatrial septum and projecting into LA.

(other than rheumatic etiology) forms occur less frequently; however, knowledge of these entities is helpful in differential diagnosis.

Congenital mitral stenosis

Causes of congenital MS may include association as a part of Shone's syndrome (supravalvar mitral ring, parachute mitral valve, subaortic stenosis, and coarctation of aorta), cor-triatriatum (Figure 7.16) or—rarely—pulmonary venous stenosis, which may present with similar findings as that

of MS. Computed tomography or MRI are useful modalities where echocardiography is inadequate to provide the diagnosis.

Acquired mitral stenosis (other than rheumatic etiology)

This may occur secondary to mitral annular calcification, LA thrombus, myxoma (Figure 7.17), vegetation, or inflammatory disorders like systemic lupus erythematosus, rheumatoid arthritis,

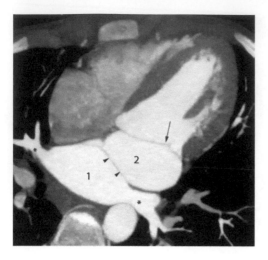

Figure 7.16 CT angiography: there is division of LA into the proximal (1) and distal (2) chamber by a membrane (arrowheads), in a patient of cortriatriatum. Note is made of drainage of pulmonary veins (*) into the proximal chamber, which drains into the distal chamber, and finally to the left ventricle across the mitral valve (arrow).

and mucopolysaccharidosis.[65,66] Thrombi are more commonly seen as compared to myxoma and are generally seen in the atrial appendage. Vegetations appear as a thickened valve or as irregular, homogeneous, hypodense masses attached to the valve or other endocardial structures. They are mobile during the cardiac cycle and develop frequently on the atrial side of the mitral valve.

BLOOD INVESTIGATIONS

Blood investigations are not required to establish the diagnosis of MS; however, they may be required for diagnosing associated complications or for monitoring anticoagulant therapy. Throat swab culture, total leucocyte count, ESR, Antistreptolysin O, antistreptococcal DNAse, antistreptococcal hyaluronidase antibodies, and C reactive protein need to be carried out if acute rheumatic fever is suspected. Those on oral anticoagulation therapy require regular INR for monitoring therapy. Digoxin levels are indicated for suspected digoxin toxicity. Blood cultures might be required if infective endocarditis is suspected. Work up for anemia and intercurrent infection may be required for the worsening of symptoms. NT pro-BNP levels are increased in MS and correlate well with the severity of disease and functional status. The presence of AF, large LA, and high pulmonary artery pressure also correlates with higher NT pro-BNP levels.[67] Successful PTMC leads to a significant decline in NT pro-BNP levels within 24 hours, although this decline is less marked in the presence of AF.[68] Plasma coagulant activity is increased in the form of increased platelet reactivity, higher fibrinopeptide A, thrombin-antithrombin III complex, and D-dimer levels. These abnormalities may arise from LA or hypertensive pulmonary vasculature but their clinical significance is unknown.[69]

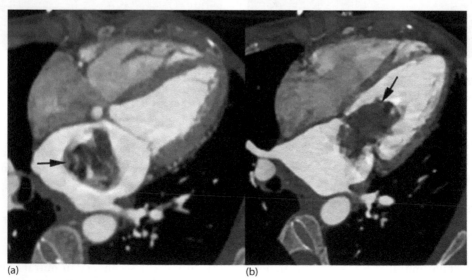

(a)   (b)

Figure 7.17 CT angiography images show LA mass (arrow in **a**), which is seen to prolapse across the mitral valve in diastole (arrow in **b**) in a patient of myxoma.

REFERENCES

1. Wood P. An appreciation of mitral stenosis: II. Investigations and results. *Br Med J* 1954; 1(4871):1113–24.

2. Lewis T. Clinical Electrocardiography. Shaw-Sons, 1913; chapter X, Special conditions: 105.

3. Yuce M, Davutoglu V, Akkoyun C et al. Interatrial block and P-terminal force: A reflection of mitral stenosis severity on electrocardiography. *J Heart Valve Dis* 2011; 20:619–23.

4. Josephson ME, Scharf DL, Kastor JA et al. Atrial endocardial activation in man. *Am J Cardiol* 1977;39:972–81.

5. Reynolds G. The atrial electrogram in mitral stenosis. *Br Heart J* 1953;15:250–8.

6. Gordon R, Neilson G, Silverstone H. Electrocardiographic P wave and atrial weights and volumes. *Br Heart J* 1965;27: 748–55.

7. Kasser I, Kennedy JW. The relationship of increased left atrial volume and pressure to abnormal P wave on the electrocardiogram. *Circulation* 1969;39:339–43.

8. Zeng C, Wei T, Zhao R, Wang C, Chen L, Wang L. Electrocardiographic diagnosis of left atrial enlargement in patients with mitral stenosis: The value of the p wave area. *Acta Cardiol* 2003;58:139–41.

9. Dilaveris PE, Gialafos EJ, Sideris S et al. Simple electrocardiographic markers for the prediction of paroxysmal idiopathic atrial fibrillation. *Am Heart J* 1998;135:733–8.

10. Turhan H, Yetkin E, Senen K et al. Effects of percutaneous mitral balloon valvuloplasty on P-wave dispersion in patients with mitral stenosis. *Am J Cardiol* 2002;89:607–9.

11. Erbay AR, Turhan H, Yasar AS et al. Effects of long-term beta-blocker therapy on P-wave duration and dispersion in patients with rheumatic mitral stenosis. *Int J Cardiol* 2005; 102:33–7.

12. Guntekin U, Gunes Y, Tuncer M, Gunes A, Sahin M, Simsek H. Long-term follow-up of P-wave duration and dispersion in patients with mitral stenosis. *Pacing Clin Electrophysiol* 2008;31:1620–4.

13. Thomas P, DeJong D. The P wave in the electrocardiogram in the diagnosis of heart disease. *Br Heart J* 1954;16:241–54.

14. Saunders JL, Calatayud JB, Schulz KJ et al. Evaluation of ECG criteria for P-wave abnormalities. *Am Heart J* 1967;74:757–65.

15. Morris JJ Jr, Estes EH Jr, Whalen RE et al. P-wave analysis in valvular heart disease. *Circulation* 1964;29:242–52.

16. Mishra A, Mishra C, Mohanty RR, Behera M. Study on the diagnostic accuracy of left atrial enlargement by resting electrocardiography and its echocardiographic correlation. *Indian J Physiol Pharmacol* 2008; 52:31–42.

17. DeOliveira JM, Sambhi MP, Zimmerman HA. The electrocardiogram in pectus excavatum. *Br Heart J* 1958;20:495–501.

18. Macruz R, Perloff JK, Case RB. Method for the electrocardiographic recognition of atrial enlargement. *Circulation* 1958;17: 882–9.

19. Hunman GP, Snyman HW. The value of the Macruz index in the diagnosis of atrial enlargement. *Circulation* 1963;27:935–8.

20. Saunders JL, Calatayud JB, Schulz KJ et al. Evaluation of ECG criteria for P-wave abnormalities. *Am Heart J* 1967;74:757–65.

21. Tarastchuk JC, Guérios EE, Perreto S et al. Changes in P-wave after percutaneous mitral valvuloplasty in patients with MS and left atrial enlargement. *Arq Bras Cardiol* 2006; 87:359–63.

22. Hancock EW, Deal BJ, Mirvis DM et al. AHA/ACCF/HRS recommendations for the standardization and interpretation of the electrocardiogram: Part V: Electrocardiogram changes associated with cardiac chamber hypertrophy: A scientific statement from the American Heart Association Electrocardiography and Arrhythmias Committee, Council on Clinical Cardiology; the American College of Cardiology Foundation; and the Heart Rhythm Society: Endorsed by the International Society for Computerized Electrocardiology. *J Am Coll Cardiol* 2009;53:992–1002.

23. Myers GB, Klein HA, Stofer BE. The electrocardiographic diagnosis of right ventricular hypertrophy. *Am Heart J* 1948;35:1–40.

24. Sokolow M, Lyon TP. The ventricular complex in right ventricular hypertrophy as obtained by unipolar precordial and limb leads. *Am Heart J* 1949;38:273–94.

25. Selzer A. Limitations of the electrocardiographic diagnosis of ventricular hypertrophy. *JAMA* 1966;195:1051.

26. Lewis T. Observations upon ventricular hypertrophy with special reference to preponderance of one or the other chamber. *Heart* 1914;5:367–402.

27. Butler PM, Leggett SI, Howe CM, Freye CJ, Hindman NB, Wagner GS. Identification of electrocardiographic criteria for diagnosis of right ventricular hypertrophy due to mitral stenosis. *Am J Cardiol* 1986;57:639–43.

28. Whitman IR, Patel VV, Soliman EZ et al. Validity of the surface electrocardiogram criteria for right ventricular hypertrophy: The MESA-RV Study (Multi-Ethnic Study of Atherosclerosis-Right Ventricle). *J Am Coll Cardiol* 2014;63:672–81.

29. Hiroki H, Arakawa K, Muramatsu J et al. New electrocardiographic criteria for diagnosing right ventricular hypertrophy in mitral stenosis—Comparison with the Bonner's and Mortara's criteria. *Jpn Circ J* 1988;52:1114–20.

30. Chou TC. *Electrocardiography in Clinical Practice. Adult and Pediatric.* 4th ed. Philadelphia, Saunders; 1996:63.

31. Ocal A, Yildirim N, Ozbakir C et al. Right bundle branch block: A new parameter revealing the progression rate of mitral stenosis. *Cardiology* 2006;105:219–22.

32. Mittal B, Mittal SR. Comparison of leads V4R and V1 in the electrocardiographic diagnosis of left atrial enlargement and right ventricular hypertrophy in mitral stenosis. *Indian Heart J* 1995;47:412.

33. Tseng CD, Tseng YZ, Lo HM, Hsu KL, Chiang FT, Wu TL. Hemodynamic significance of vectorcardiographic pattern in patients with mitral stenosis. *J Formos Med Assoc* 1990; 89:565–70.

34. Deniz A, Tüfenk M, Acartürk E. Electrocardiographic right ventricular hypertrophy predicts the severity of pulmonary hypertension in patients with mitral stenosis. *Turk Kardiyol Dern Ars* 2012;40:405–8.

35. Kılıçkesmez KO, Bulut G, Başkurt M, Coşkun U, Yıldız A, Küçükoğlu S. QT dispersion in patients with rheumatic MS and its relation with echocardiographic findings and serum NT-proBNP levels. *Turk Kardiyol Dern Ars* 2011;39:183–90.

36. Ueshima K, Chiba I, Saitoh M et al. Factors affecting ST depression during cardiopulmonary exercise testing in patients with mitral stenosis without significant coronary lesions. *Jpn Heart J* 2004;45:251–5.

37. Al-Hazimi A, Al-Ama N, Marouf M. Heart rate variability in patients with mitral stenosis: A study of 20 cases from King Abdulaziz University Hospital. *Ann Saudi Med* 2002; 22:143–8.

38. von Olshausen K, Treese N, Schwarz F, Kübler W, Meyer J. Ventricular arrhythmias in mitral valve disease: Incidence, severity and relations to hemodynamic parameters. *Z Kardiol* 1986;75:196–201.

39. Murray JG, Brown AL, Anagnostou EA et al. Widening of the tracheal bifurcation on chest radiographs: Value as a sign of left atrial enlargement. *Am J Roentgenol* 1995; 164(5):1089–92.

40. Karabulut N. CT assessment of tracheal carinal angle and its determinants. *Br J Radiol* 2005;78(933):787–90.

41. Taskin V, Bates MC, Chillag SA. Tracheal carinal angle and left atrial size. *Arch Intern Med* 1991;151:307–8.

42. Lin SC, Lee JH, Hsieh CM. The correlation between subcarinal angle and left atrial volume. *Acta Cardiol Sin* 2012;28:332–6.

43. Parker MS, Chasen MH, Paul N. Radiologic signs in thoracic imaging: Case based review and self-assessment module. 2009; 192(3 Suppl):S34–48.

44. Webb WR, Higgins CB. *Thoracic Imaging.* Lippincott Williams & Wilkins; 2010. ISBN:1605479764.

45. Brant WE, Helms C. *Fundamentals of Diagnostic Radiology.* Lippincott Williams & Wilkins; 2012. ISBN:1608319113.

46. A chest radiograph showing abnormal mediastinal contour. *Chest* 1996;109(5):1383–4.

47. Vijayvergiya R, Vaiphei K, Rana SS. Severe mitral annular calcification in rheumatic heart disease: A rare presentation. *World J Cardiol* 2012;4(3):87–9.

48. Cardinale L, Volpicelli G, Lamorte A, Martino J, Veltri A. Revisiting signs, strengths and weaknesses of standard chest radiography in patients of acute dyspnea in the emergency department. *J Thorac Dis* 2012; 4(4):398–407.

49. Fraser RG, Paré PD, Fraser RS, Genereux GP. *Diagnosis of diseases of the chest.* 3rd ed. Vol 2. Philadelphia, PA: Saunders; 1989:1863–79.

50. Steiner RE, Goodwin JF. Some observations on mitral valve disease. *J Fac Radiol* 1954; 5:167–77.

51. Galloway RW, Epstein EJ, Coulshed N. Pulmonary ossific nodules in mitral valve disease. *Br Heart J* 1961; 23:297–304.

52. Kulkarni SS, Sakaria AK, Mahajan SK, Shah KB. Lutembacher's syndrome. *J Cardiovasc Dis Res* 2012;3(2):179–81.

53. Higgins CB. *Essentials of cardiac radiology and imaging.* Philadelphia: JB Lippincot; 1992.

54. Lancellotti P, Pibarot P, Chambers J et al. Recommendations for the imaging assessment of prosthetic heart valves: A report from the European Association of Cardiovascular Imaging endorsed by the Chinese Society of Echocardiography, the Inter-American Society of Echocardiography, and the Brazilian Department of Cardiovascular Imaging. *Eur Heart J Cardiovasc Imaging* 2016;17:589–90.

55. Muralidharan S, Muthubaskeran V, Chandrasekar P. Ten years outcome of Chitra heart valves. *Indiana J Thorac Cardiovasc Surg* 2011;27:24–7.

56. Perloff JK, Roberts WC. The mitral apparatus: Functional anatomy of mitral regurgitation. *Circulation* 1972;46(2):227–39.

57. Fuster V. *Hurst's the Heart.* 12th ed. New York: McGraw-Hill Medical; 2008.

58. Morris MF, Maleszewski JJ, Suri RM et al. CT and MR imaging of the mitral valve: Radiologic-pathologic correlation. *Radiographics* 2010;30(6):1603–20.

59. Messika-Zeitoun D, Serfaty JM, Laissy JP et al. Assessment of the mitral valve area in patients with MS by multislice computed tomography. *J Am Coll Cardiol* 2006; 48:411–13.

60. Uçar O, Vural M, Cetfin Z et al. Assessment of planimetric mitral valve area using 16-row multidetector computed tomography in patients with rheumatic MS. *J Heart Valve Ds* 2011;20(1):13–17.

61. Lacomis JM, Wigginton W, Fuhrman C, Schwartzman D, Armfield DR, Pealer KM. Multi-detector row CT of the left atrium and pulmonary veins before radio-frequency catheter ablation for atrial fibrillation. *Radiographics* 2003;23 Spec No: S35–48; discussion S48–50.

62. Nasis A, Mottram PM, Cameron JD, Seneviratne SK. Current and evolving clinical applications of multidetector cardiac CT in assessment of structural heart disease. *Radiology* 2013;267(1):11–25.

63. Heidenreich PA, Steffens J, Fujita N et al. Valuation of MS with velocity-encoded cine-magnetic resonance imaging. *Am J Cardiol* 1995;75:365–9.

64. Didier D, Ratib O, Lerch R, Friedli B. Detection and quantification of valvular heart disease with dynamic cardiac MR imaging. *Radiographics* 2000;20(5):1279–99; discussion 1299–1301.

65. Horstkotte D, Niehues R, Strauer BE. Pathomorphological aspects, aetiology and natural history of acquired mitral valve stenosis. *Eur Heart J* 1991;12 Suppl B:55–60.

66. Chandrashekhar Y, Westaby S, Narula J. Mitral stenosis. *Lancet* 2009;374:1271–83.

67. Arat-Ozkan A, Kaya A, Yigit Z et al. Serum N-terminal pro BNP levels correlate with symptoms and echocardiographic findings in patients with MS. *Echocardiography* 2005;22:473–8.

68. Chadha DS, Karthikeyan G, Goel K et al. N-terminal pro-BNP plasma levels before and after percutaneous transvenous mitral commissurotomy for MS. *Int J Cardiol* 2010; 144:238–40.

69. Yamamoto K, Ikeda U, Seino Y et al. Coagulation activity is increased in the left atrium of patients with MS. *J Am Coll Cardiol* 1995;25:107–12.

8

Echocardiogram

VIVEK CHATURVEDI

INTRODUCTION

The diagnosis and management of mitral stenosis (MS) has been revolutionized by the advent of modern echocardiography. Echocardiography is an indispensable component in the assessment of mitral stenosis. While the mechanical obstruction of the left-ventricular inflow by thickened, restricted mitral leaflets is easily discerned on a two-dimensional (2D) scan, its functional consequences in terms of disturbed flow and elevated pressures are evident on doppler echocardiography. Other features influencing management and natural course of MS, like left-atrial (LA) thrombus, pulmonary arterial hypertension, left and right-ventricular (LV and RV) function, co-existing valvular lesions, anatomy of interatrial septum, etc., are also comprehensively evaluated on echocardiography. The backbone of a good echocardiographic evaluation of MS remains a thorough 2D scan and a careful doppler assessment, despite advances in echo-technology.

In this chapter, we will be discussing the various aspects of echocardiographic examination that are relevant to MS in day-to-day practice, as well as in special situations. Besides a targeted examination of the mitral valve, a thorough evaluation of cardiac structures and function is essential for the comprehensive management of MS; however, this would not be the emphasis or focus of this chapter. Several excellent general and valvular echocardiography references are available for the same. This work is also practice-oriented with an emphasis on practical situations and techniques. As such, it assumes a certain knowledge and familiarity of the clinician with echocardiographic examination. Further, as congenital MS and degenerative MS have been dealt elsewhere, this chapter focuses on MS due to rheumatic heart disease (RHD).

TWO-DIMENSIONAL ECHOCARDIOGRAPHY

Two-dimensional echocardiography (2D echo) in mitral stenosis reflects the morphology and severity of obstruction at the mitral valvular and subvalvular level. It is also used to evaluate the size and functions of cardiac chambers, presence of clot, pericardial effusion, and associated valvular abnormalities. All of these have a bearing on the management decisions related to MS.

Equipment and examination settings

While these are usually carried out as per the standard protocols described for echocardiographic examination,[1,2] the structural changes caused by MS require tweaking of conventional views for better visualization of the cardiac structures. A left recumbent position is the default approach for echocardiographic examination. Sometimes due to severe RV and atrial enlargement, the left-sided chambers are pushed posteriorly, such that to get a proper apical four-chamber view, one may need the patient to lie straight or only slightly left lateral. Further, with massive enlargement of the LA it becomes difficult to see the LV and even the LA in their entirety. In these cases, a better and more representative image may be obtained from epigastric area. Finally, patients with severe MS are thin-chested or emaciated, requiring necessary alterations in depth and gain settings. A high-gain setting may lead to underestimation of the cross-sectional valve area. Thus, while one must proceed with standard position and setting of the patient and equipment, one should be prepared to change them to better suit visualization of the mitral valve. It is desirable to have electrocardiographic (ECG) monitoring for defining cardiac timing events; however, a reasonably good examination, sufficient to guide management decisions, can be performed without the same. It is advisable to repeat an echocardiographic examination in the presence of uncontrolled atrial fibrillation (AF) after rate control, for an accurate assessment of valve morphology and area.

An assessment of mitral valve affected by the rheumatic process should focus on the morphology of pathologic changes in each component of the MV apparatus. These consist of the anterior and posterior mitral leaflet, medial and lateral commissures, and the submitral apparatus (the anteromedial and posterolateral papillary muscles and the chordae tendineae connecting papillary muscles to the leaflet surfaces) (Figure 8.1).

- Leaflets: Doming, asymmetric thickening, nodularity, restricted movement, calcification, prolapse
- Commissures: Thickened, fused, partially or fully calcified
- Chordae tendineae: Thickened, fused in chords, calcified
- Papillary muscles: Thickened, retracted

On echocardiography, the reduced leaflet motion manifests as "doming" of the anterior mitral leaflet (Video 8.1a and Video 8.1b). The leaflets typically show thickening at the tips, giving a hockey stick appearance to the anterior mitral leaflet (AML). The thickening is usually uneven with thin hinge points in midportion and thickened base and tips. The posterior mitral leaflet is thick, fused, and immobile (rather than moving anteriorly).[3] The leaflets may have bright echogenicity due to nodules (Video 8.14) or calcification (see below). Due to restricted mobility, the AML tip may prolapse below the coaptation point. The leaflet morphology is best seen in parasternal long-axis and apical views.

The commissures (medial and lateral) are best seen in parasternal short-axis view used in planimetry (Figure 8.2, Video 8.2). Sometimes varying views may be required as both commissures may not be seen simultaneously due to irregular subvalvular deformity (SVD). It should be noted whether they are split, fused, thickened, or calcified and if the pathologic process is asymmetric. Calcification can be focal, patchy, or the entire commissure may be calcified. All bright echogenic areas should not be labeled as calcified. Areas that remain bright even when the gain has been turned down sufficiently to hide most of the cardiac structures or those that are associated with shadowing should be labeled as calcific. This has implications for suitability for percutaneous transvenous mitral commissurotomy (PTMC), as complications (as well as success) are adversely impacted with increasing calcification. This has not, however, prevented operators from performing PTMC even with one commissure fully calcified.

The subvalvular apparatus, consisting of chordae tendineae and the two papillary muscles,

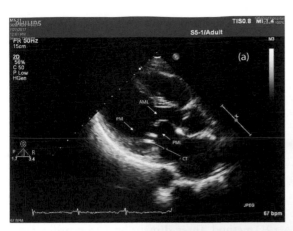
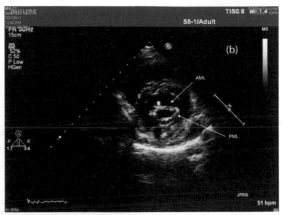
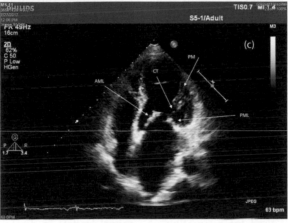

Figure 8.1 Effect of rheumatic mitral stenosis on different components of mitral annulus; doming and uneven thickening of leaflets, fusion of commissures, subvalvular thickening. (a) Parasternal long-axis view (PLAX); (b) parasternal short-axis view at valve level (PSAX); (c) apical four-chamber view (A4C). AML, anterior mitral leaflet; PML, posterior mitral leaflet; CT, chordae tendinae; PM, papillary muscle.

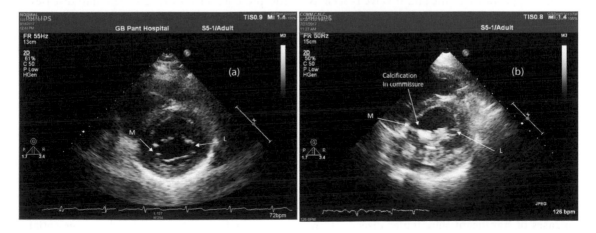

Figure 8.2 Parasternal short-axis view at valve level showing medial (M) and lateral (L) commissures. Normally these are thin and echofree (a), but are fused, asymmetric, and thickened in rheumatic MS (b).

is a complex structure. The chordae run from each papillary muscle (postero-medial and anterolateral) to both leaflets (anterior and posterior). The subvalular apparatus thickens and retracts with advancing disease. Because of the diffuse inflammation of the mitral apparatus, it is possible to have effective mitral stenosis below the level of the leaflets. The SVD is best evaluated in the parasternal long-axis view where tilting and gently adjusting the probe anteriorly or posteriorly will bring into focus the anterolateral or the posteromedial papillary muscle, respectively (Figure 8.3, Video 8.3a and 8.3b). Both of the papillary muscles may be seen together in a tilted two-chamber apical view (Figure 8.3d, Video 8.3e). It is important to note heterogeneity in thickening and retraction of the two papillary muscles as well as that of commissures (for example, unilateral or bilateral calcification) as it has implications for treatment. Scanning further apically from parasternal short-axis view, one can appreciate the thickening and retraction of subvalvular tissue, including both papillary muscles (Figure 8.3e, Video 8.3c). Given that mitral apparatus is a complex three-dimensional structure, it pays to inspect the valve and subvalvular structures in modified views (as explained above for SVD) to bring various structures into prominence.

The short-axis view is used for estimation of MV cross-sectional area (MVA). The foundation for a good short-axis view is an optimal parasternal long-axis view. It should lead to maximum excursion of the mitral leaflets and the valve should be in the center of the screen. From this point it is rotated to a short-axis view and the typical "fish-mouth" appearance of the mitral valve is seen. As mentioned earlier, the mitral apparatus is grossly distorted in MS and it may be difficult to appreciate an uneven three-dimensional structure by 2D echocardiography. Hence, a short-axis view should be flexible, both in terms of degrees of rotation as well as anterior and posterior tilt. For the estimation of cross-sectional area, a few salient points need to be borne in mind. First, the cross-section should be uninterrupted with no echo dropouts. Second, it should be the most apical section obtained with the above specification (Figure 8.4, Video 8.4). It is to be noted that this may indeed be at a level more apical than that of the valve itself, as in cases of significant subvalvular disease. Third, it should be in mid-diastole, easily surmised in the presence of ECG monitoring but also deducible

as the maximal outward excursion of the leaflets. Usually multiple estimations (at least three) should be done and averaged. This is especially important in atrial fibrillation (AF) and cases of incomplete commissural fusion, where flow characteristics may actually change the effective valve area.[2] Finally, the area seen within the commissures is also a part of the cross-sectional area and hence should be included in the measurement.

An accurate estimation of mitral valve area (MVA) may be difficult by 2D echocardiography due to constraints mentioned above. This is an inherent fallacy of assessing a three-dimensional structure by a 2D method. Three-dimensional echocardiography is more accurate for MVA estimation[4] as compared to 2D echocardiography. However, this difference may not be much in the hands of operators experienced in assessing rheumatic valves. If the estimated MVA does not fit with the overall echocardiographic picture, multiple measurements of MVA should be taken. For example, when the calculated MVA is moderate only and yet there is severe pulmonary hypertension (PAH) in presence of controlled heart rate and no other apparent cause for PAH. A useful semi-quantitative method for estimating MS severity is the mitral leaflet separation (MLS) index. This measures the distance between the tips of the mitral leaflets in diastole in parasternal long-axis and apical four-chamber view.[5] While there is significant overlap, averaged values of less than 0.8 cm and more than 1.2 cm can diagnose severe and non-severe MS reliably[6] (Figure 8.5).

It is equally important to look beyond the mitral valve when assessing individuals for MS. For one, the presence of co-existent valvular diseases as well as comorbid conditions are important in overall management of MS. As mentioned earlier, the presence of severe PAH should make one look carefully again if the calculated MVA is found at best moderate. The presence of a large atrium also implies significant MV pathology, but a severely enlarged LA should be a trigger to look for eccentric mitral regurgitation (MR), although pure MS can give rise to giant LA.

A note is also made of the comparative sizes of the right atrium and ventricle (RA and RV). In the absence of primary tricuspid valve disease, these chambers dilate in response to significant PAH as a consequence of MS. If dilated, it is essential to measure tricuspid annular diameter as this can have implications for patients undergoing MV

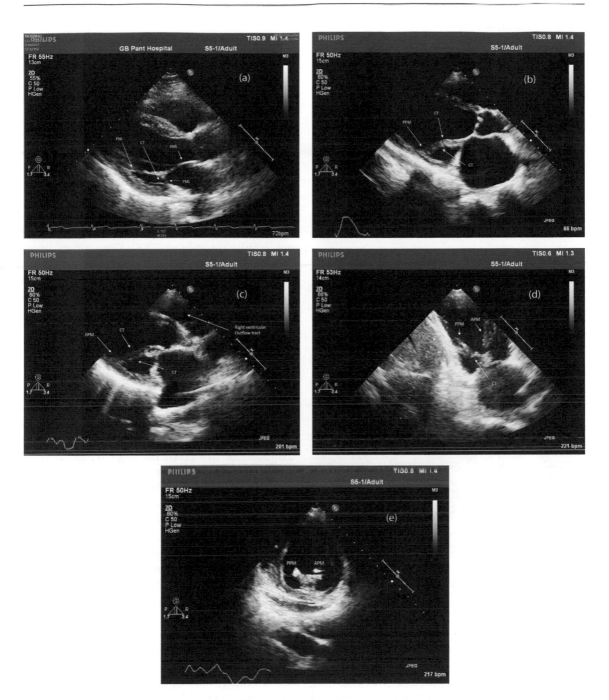

Figure 8.3 Involvement of subvalvular apparatus in rheumatic mitral stenosis. As compared to normal **(a)**, thickening and retraction of chordae and papillary muscles are seen in mitral stenosis. Tilting the probe posteriorly from PLAX **(b)** shows the posteromedial papillary muscle (PPM), while tilting anteriorly **(c)** brings anterolateral papillary muscle (APM) into focus. **(d)** a modified two-chamber apical view showing both the papillary muscles (PPM and APM together); **(e)** parasternal short-axis (PSAX) view at papillary level showing thickened subvalvular apparatus. CT, chordae tendinae.

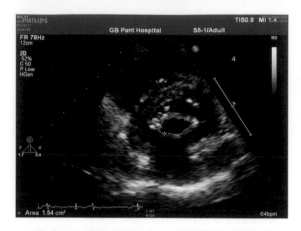

Figure 8.4 Estimation of mitral valve cross-sectional area (MVA) in parasternal short-axis view. The estimation is done in mid-diastole and the outline of the valve should be uninterrupted. The areas within the commissures should be included.

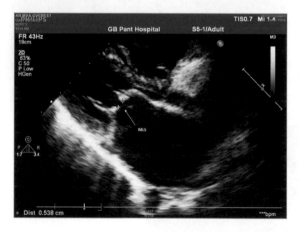

Figure 8.5 Mitral leaflet separation index (MLS) is the maximum distance between the leaflet tips in mid-diastole; a value of <0.8 cm is likely to denote severe MS.

surgery. Similarly, the morphology of interatrial septum, ventricular function, and the thickening of other valves, all features having management and prognostic implications, should be noted on 2D examination.

All patients should be carefully screened for the presence of spontaneous echo contrast (SEC) (Figure 8.6, Video 8.5a and 8.5b) or a thrombus in LA or left atrium appendage (LAA). SEC increases the risk of LA thrombus formation even among patients in sinus rhythm. While the LAA is best

visualized by transesophageal echocardiography (TEE), with practice one can get good views with transthoracic echocardiography (TTE) as well.[7] The LAA is best seen in the parasternal short-axis view with anterior tilt (Figure 8.7a). The body of LAA is seen even better sometimes if this view is made one intercostal space higher than usual short-axis position (Figure 8.7b, Video 8.6a). The orthogonal appearance of the LAA mouth is also seen very well by leftward tilt during apical two-chamber view (Figure 8.7c, Video 8.6b). TEE may be reserved for individuals who have poor transthoracic echogenicity or who have suspicious but not definite thrombi on TTE. A prominent linear bandlike structure, the warfarin ridge, with thickened tip, is often seen adjacent to the wall of the LAA and left superior pulmonary vein. While it may be confused with a thrombus, its typical location and similar echogenicity to other LA structures differentiates it from a thrombus.[8]

M-MODE ECHOCARDIOGRAPHY

M-mode was the first echocardiographic modality with which MS was evaluated. While no longer done routinely, it is very sensitive for the diagnosis of MS given the high temporal resolution it has for leaflet excursions, which are typically restricted in MS. The motion of mitral annulus and leaflet is complex and has various components during the cardiac cycle (Figure 8.8a). The anterior mitral leaflet inscribes an M shape on M-mode during diastole due to an early brisk diastolic anterior motion (E-wave) signifying rapid early filling of ventricle followed by near closure during mid-diastole when diastolic filling of ventricle eases (F-point). This is followed by an anterior motion again as the LA contracts causing A-wave followed by valve closure during isovolumic contraction (C-point). The posterior leaflet has a similar but opposite (posterior) motion with less amplitude, causing a W-formation. Rheumatic MS has a characteristic signature on the M-mode. Increased leaflet thickening can easily be appreciated on the M-mode (Figure 8.8b). The restricted movement of the leaflet causes decreased amplitudes of the E- and the A-waves. It also causes delayed opening of the valve and this along with the increased LA pressure causes the slope of E-wave to decrease. Raised transmitral

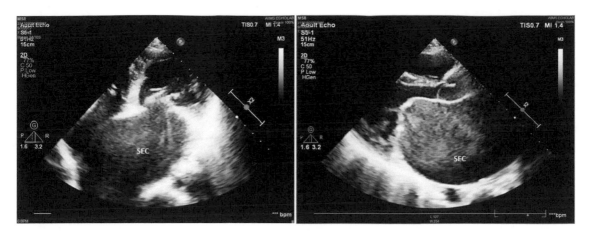

Figure 8.6 Spontaneous echo contrast (SEC) in the left atrium appearing like a dense smoke in apical 4 chamber view (left panel) and parasternal long axis view (right panel); the presence of SEC increases the risk of left-atrial thrombus formation.

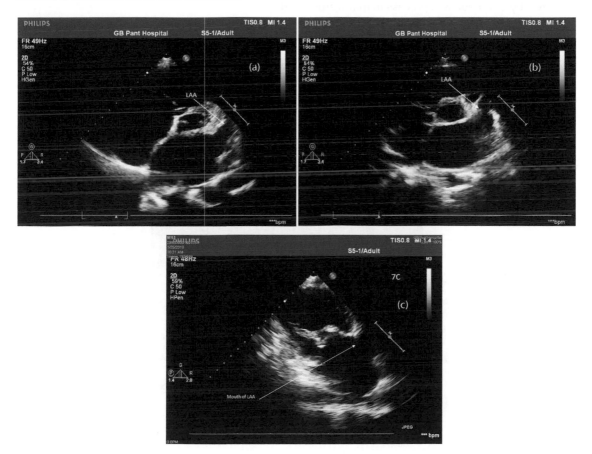

Figure 8.7 Imaging of the left atrial appendage (LAA) by transthoracic echocardiography. Usually the LAA is visualized in parasternal short-axis (PSAX) view with an anterior tilt, next to the aorta (a). Sometimes it is seen better when the same view is made one intercostal space higher (b). The mouth of the LAA can be also visualized by an anterior tilt in the apical four-chamber view and even better in the modified apical four-chamber view (c).

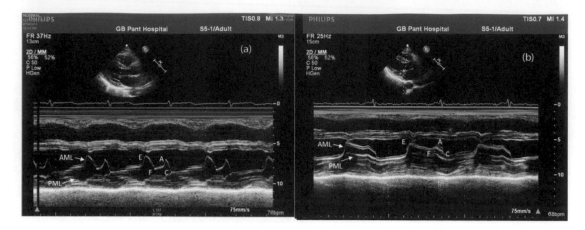

Figure 8.8 M-mode echocardiography of the mitral valve. The motion of the anterior mitral leaflet (AML) during a cardiac cycle is complex. With a normal valve **(a)**, the AML and posterior mitral leaflet (PML) inscribe different waveforms on the M-mode (see text). The movement of the AML and PML are affected by the rheumatic process in mitral stenosis **(b)**.

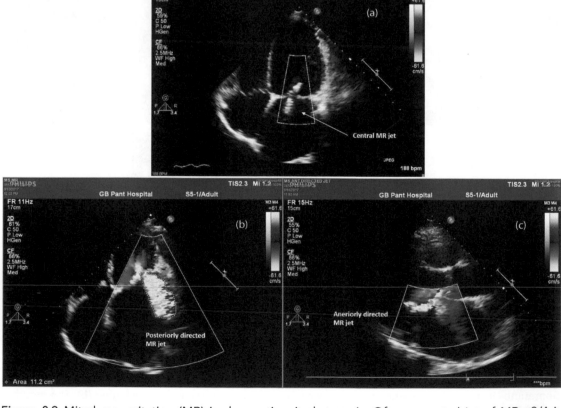

Figure 8.9 Mitral regurgitation (MR) in rheumatic mitral stenosis. Often a central jet of MR ≤2/4 in severity is due to fixed orifice and regresses after PTMC **(a)**. However, an eccentric jet is usually due to AML prolapse or subvalvular disease and can be directed posteriorly **(b)** or anteriorly **(c)**.

gradient even in mid-diastole causes the EF slope to decrease. The amplitude of the A-wave also decreases. Due to leaflet rigidity and thickening, the posterior mitral leaflet does not move posteriorly during diastole; rather, it parallels the motion of AML. This, along with decreased EF slope and thickened leaflets, are the hallmark of MS with good sensitivity for diagnosis. However, M-mode is semi-quantitative at best and the magnitude of changes described above does not track the mitral valve area closely, especially with mixed lesions and after mitral valvotomy.[9]

COLOR DOPPLER

Color doppler provides useful information about the presence of coexistent MR as well as clues to the severity of MS. MR may be central or eccentric. Patients with central MR with a grade of ≤2/4 can undergo PTMC (Figure 8.9a, Video 8.7a). This MR is usually due to a fixed mitral orifice and regresses after successful PTMC. More severe MR needs surgical intervention (Video 8.7b). Eccentric MR is often due to AML prolapse or severe SVD, which increase the risk of severe MR during PTMC (Figure 8.9b, Video 8.7c). Thus, even mild eccentric MR should lead to a consideration of surgical intervention if the patient is not high risk for surgery. A clue to significant MR is that the LA is inappropriately enlarged. Because of the enlarged LA, it is important to visualize the MR jet in several different orientations to get an idea about its eccentricity as well as magnitude. The assessment of MR should be done in at least apical four- and two-chamber views, parasternal long-axis view, and sometimes also in short-axis (commissural level) view (Figure 8.10a–c). The quantification of MR is done as in other causes of MR.[10] MR developing after PTMC can be severe and is usually diagnosed as a combination of clinical, hemodynamic, and echocardiographic features.

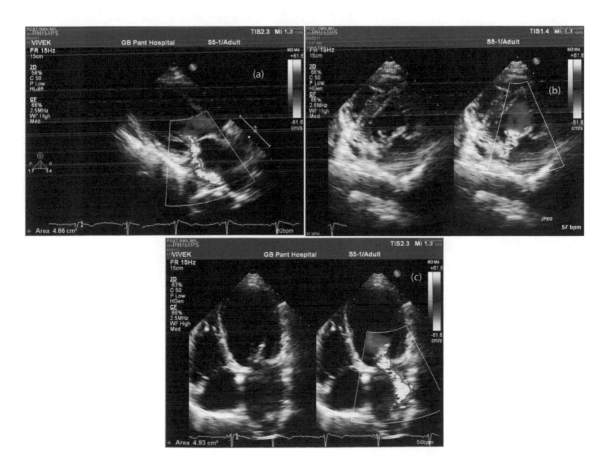

Figure 8.10 The jet of mitral regurgitation visualized in different transthoracic views; parasternal long-axis **(a)**, parasternal short-axis **(b)**, and apical four-chamber **(c)** view.

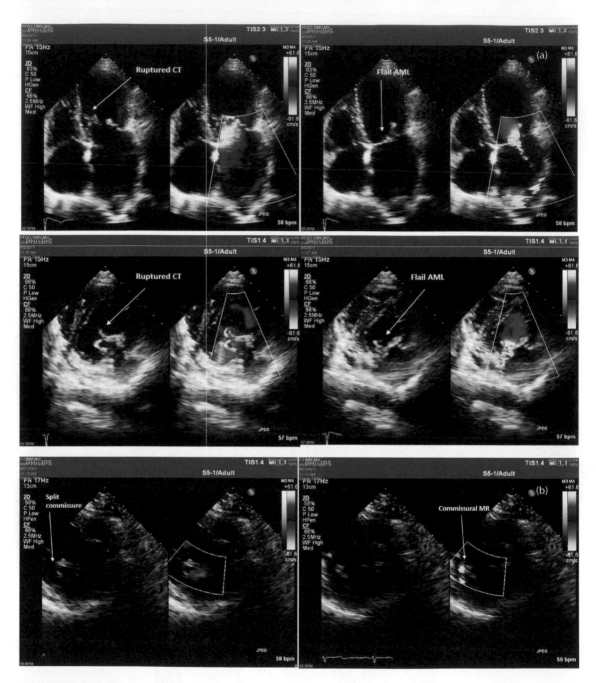

Figure 8.11 Development of mitral regurgitation (MR) after percutaneous transvenous mitral commissurotomy (PTMC). Severe MR due to chordal rupture after PTMC **(a)**. Development of commissural MR after PTMC **(b)**, seen on PSAX view, which regressed on follow-up. *(Continued)*

Post-PTMC MR requiring urgent attention is usually due to leaflet tear (Figure 8.11c, Video 8.8e) or chordal rupture (Figure 8.11a, Video 8.8c and 8.8d). However, as PTMC opens the valve by splitting commissures, a commissural MR (sometimes even severe) can often be seen (Figure 8.11b, Video 8.8a and 8.8b). However, this decreases with time due to the remodeling and fibrosis in the mitral valve. Commissural MR is best appreciated in a parasternal short-axis view.

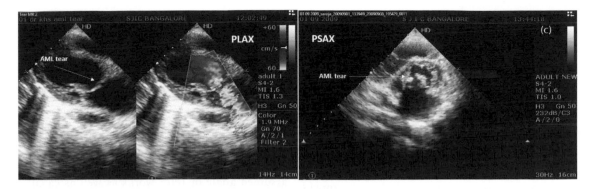

Figure 8.11 (Continued) Development of mitral regurgitation (MR) after percutaneous transvenous mitral commissurotomy (PTMC). Leaflet tear after PTMC **(c)** is the usual cause for MR requiring urgent surgery after PTMC.

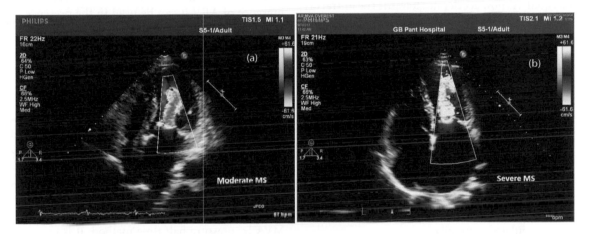

Figure 8.12 Different color Doppler pattern in case of moderate mitral stenosis **(a)** and severe mitral stenosis **(b)**; severe mitral regurgitation antegrade flow is more turbulent and has a mosaic pattern.

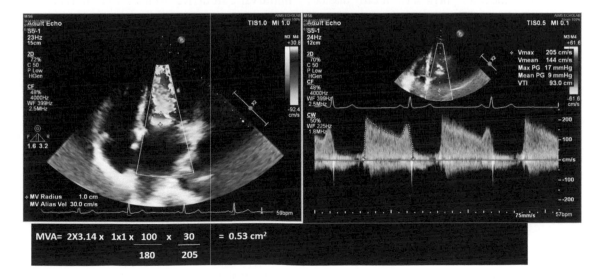

Figure 8.13 Estimation of mitral valve area by proximal isovelocity surface area (PISA) method.

Color doppler can also be used to estimate the severity of MS. A turbulent jet with a mosaic pattern suggests significant MS (Figure 8.12). However, this may not be so in cases with poor antegrade flow (decreased cardiac output, severe tricuspid valve disease) or increased LV stiffness. The pattern of this mosaic jet also gives an idea about subvalvular disease (SVD). Multiple antegrade jets suggest the presence of extensive SVD (Video 8.3d). A laminar flow after PTMC suggests a successful result.

The mitral valve area can also be calculated using the proximal isovelocity surface area (PISA) method.[11,12] The method is based on the continuity principle of conservation of mass, i.e., the stroke volume proximal and distal to the stenotic orifice must be equal. As flow accelerates towards the mitral orifice in MS, it causes multiple hemispheric shells of increasing velocity and decreasing radius to form. All blood cells in a particular shell of defined radius have the same velocity. Thus, the flow rate at a given hemispheric shell must be equal to the flow rate across the mitral valve. For calculating the velocity at the shell, the color scale is shifted towards the LV until a clear aliasing is seen and the aliasing velocity is noted at the red-blue interface of the hemispheric shell (Figure 8.13). Subsequently, the radius of the shell from the mitral valve is calculated. As the leaflets are doming in diastole and subtend an angle to the mitral annulus in MS, a correction angle needs to be calculated manually.

Diastolic flow rate at the isovelocity shell (mL/s) = $2\Pi r^2 \times$ (angle $\alpha/180°$) × "V" alias (cm/s), where r is the radius of the hemispheric shell in early diastole,

"V" alias is the aliasing velocity, and $\alpha/180°$ is the correction factor accounting for the angle α between the mitral leaflets.

$$MVA = 2\pi r^2 \times \left(\frac{Angle}{\alpha 180}\right) \times \frac{"V"alias\left(\frac{cm}{s}\right)}{Vmax}$$

[peak continuous doppler velocity across the MV (cm/s)]

However, it has been shown that an empirically assumed angle of 100° works as well as calculating the angle manually.[13] The value should be calculated over three to four beats and averaged. The PISA method correlates fairly well with planimetry and pressure half-time but is less accurate in the presence of AF.[14] It can be used in the presence of MR but is technically demanding and prone to error due to multiple measurements. It has been improvised with color M-mode, which allows simultaneous measurement of flow and velocity.[15]

CONTINUOUS WAVE DOPPLER

Continuous wave doppler interrogation of the mitral valve, despite its shortcomings, is one of the cornerstones in diagnosis and management of mitral stenosis. It is fast and easily reproducible. It provides the pressure gradients across the mitral valve in diastole and can also be used for estimation of the MVA by pressure-half-time method. It is preferred over pulsed wave doppler to ensure the recording of maximal velocities. The pressure gradients across the mitral valve are derived from the transmitral velocity

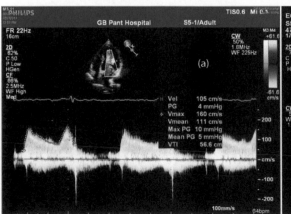
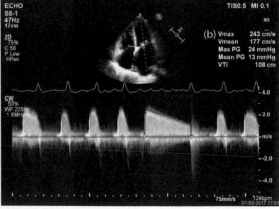

Figure 8.14 Estimation of atrioventricular pressure gradient by continuous-wave Doppler interrogation of flow across mitral valve. Pre-loaded software calculates both peak gradient (peak PG) and the mean diastolic gradient (mean PG). While the pattern is uniform in sinus rhythm **(a)**, it changes in atrial fibrillation **(b)**.

flow curve using the simplified Bernoulli equation $\Delta P = 4v^2$ (Figure 8.14).[16,17] Both instantaneous gradient as well as mean gradient (MDG) throughout diastole can be calculated and have been found to correlate well with gradients derived by transseptal catheterization.[18] The doppler interrogation is usually done in apical four-chamber view. To ensure accurate gradient, the ultrasound beam needs to pick up the maximally turbulent flow zone across MV. Hence, the continuous wave doppler interrogation is performed after seeing the color doppler flow across the mitral valve and aligned to zones with highest flow velocity to avoid underestimation of gradients. Sometimes the jet across the MV is eccentric, and better alignment is obtained in a two-chamber or any other modified apical view. If there are multiple jets, due to extensive SVD, the gradients of the maximal one should be taken. A good acoustic window, optimal gain settings, and higher sweep speed are also essential for an optimal doppler trace.

The gradients usually reported from the doppler trace are the peak diastolic gradient (PG) and the mean diastolic gradient (MDG) (Figure 8.14). These are usually calculated by pre-loaded software. PG is not a good indicator of severity as it is affected by heart rate, LA compliance and LV systolic and diastolic function.[19] MDG should be reported as it is the best indicator of hemodynamic severity. Heart rate should always be reported while recording gradients and in the case of AF an average taken from at least five beats. The MDG is affected by heart rate, cardiac output, and coexistent MR (which overestimates the gradient by increasing flow) and hence is not the best indicator of MS severity. It remains a useful complementary tool where accurate estimation of severity by cross-sectional area or pressure half-time (PHT) is not possible, and for routine follow-up of patients. An MDG of ≥5 mmHg is considered significant with MDG ≥10 mmHg indicating severe MS (for stable heart rates of 60–80 bpm).[2]

Pressure half-time (PHT) is obtained on the mitral inflow doppler trace and is defined as the time in milliseconds for the transmitral gradient to decrease by half of its original value in early diastole (Figure 8.15a). The concept was originally developed during cardiac catheterization studies[20] and subsequently adopted for doppler echocardiography by Hatle and colleagues,[21] who described it as doppler time for the peak velocity to

decrease by a factor of the square root of two. They then found an inverse relationship of this pressure half-time with MVA by the Gorlin equation and subsequently provided the equation for empirical calculation of MVA from PHT.[22] MVA (cm²) = $220/T_{1/2}$ (ms), where $T_{1/2}$ is the PHT on the deceleration slope of the E wave.

The MVA is calculated from pre-loaded software on the echo machine. The gain and filter settings should be optimized to get a clear trace that allows easy placement of the callipers and the sweep speed increased to 75–100 mm/s for accuracy. This is straightforward in many cases but may be difficult especially if an aortic regurgitation jet is interfering with the inflow stream. In such cases, careful positioning of the interrogation beam may still yield a uniform trace (Figure 8.15b). Further, many times the deceleration slope is not linear; rather, it is uneven with higher deceleration in the initial part (Figure 8.16). In such cases the deceleration slope in the mid-diastole (instead of early diastole) should be employed.[23] It may be impossible to calculate PHT in concave tracings and should be stated as such in the report. Similarly, very short cycles should be avoided for estimation in AF, where an average should be taken for multiple cycles. Initial studies demonstrated a good correlation of MVA obtained with this equation with that obtained by 2D planimetry and cardiac catheterization. However, it soon became clear that besides MVA, other hemodynamic factors also play a role in the determination of PHT.[24] These include LA compliance and initial LA diastolic pressure, as well as LV diastolic function. In uncomplicated MS, the effects of peak transmitral gradient on PHT are countered by those from atrioventricular compliance; thus, there is not much change in PHT. However, these factors assume significance with abrupt or significant hemodynamic changes, for example, immediately after PTMC (where there is sudden change in LA compliance and pressure), and with decreased LV compliance, for example, aortic regurgitation (Figure 8.17, Video 8.15), LV systolic dysfunction, LV hypertrophy, elderly population, etc.[2]

The use of the continuity equation for estimation of MVA. As for PISA, the continuity equation is based on conservation of mass, implying in this case that diastolic flow across LV inflow (i.e., MV) is equal to systolic flow across LV outflow or

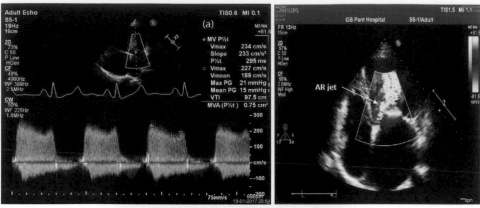

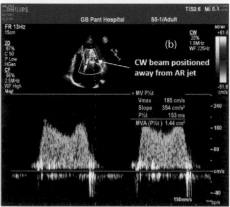

Figure 8.15 Estimation of mitral valve area (MVA) by the pressure half-time method (PHT) **(a)**. The ultrasound beam needs to be carefully positioned in case of co-existent AR **(b)** to get a smooth deceleration trace. P1/2t: pressure half-time.

stroke volume, provided there is no other egress of blood from LV (e.g., ventricular septal defect, AR, MR).

MVA $= \pi \, (D^2/4) \, (VTI_{Aortic}/VTI_{Mitral})$, where D is the diameter of the LV outflow in cm and VTI is velocity times integral of flow by pulsed doppler in cm[25] (Figure 8.18). It is not much used in clinical practice as it is time-consuming and prone to errors due to multiple measurements.

Mitral valve resistance. This is the ratio of the mean mitral gradient divided by the transmittal diastolic flow rate. Diastolic flow rate is calculated by dividing stroke volume by the diastolic filling period. It has been shown to correlate strongly with resting and stress pulmonary artery pressures[26] and outcomes of PTMC.[27] However, it is not used routinely in clinical practice as it does not provide incremental information to MVA, which is already a robust marker of the severity of MS.

ANCILLARY INFORMATION OBTAINED FROM ECHOCARDIOGRAPHY

Patients with MS should be evaluated for co-existing valvular lesions as well as other determinants of prognosis and management. The assessment of pulmonary artery pressures and its effects on the right-sided cardiac chambers is an integral part of echocardiographic examination in MS. While there is no strict correlation between MVA and PAH, generally pulmonary artery pressures increase with increasing severity of MS and can be used to prognosticate as well as decide management in borderline cases. The most common method to estimate PA systolic pressure is by calculating the maximum velocity (and thus gradient) of a regurgitant jet across the tricuspid valve and to add this gradient to presumed RA pressure (this is done by visualizing

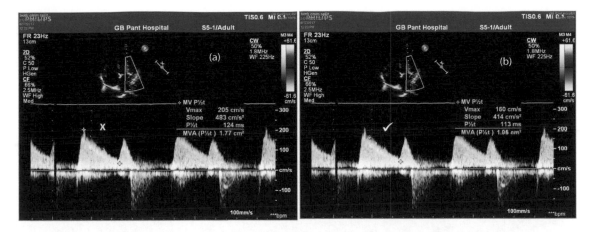

Figure 8.16 Estimation of mitral valve area (MVA) by pressure half-time method (PHT); the incorrect **(a)** and the correct **(b)** way in presence of non-linear deceleration slope.

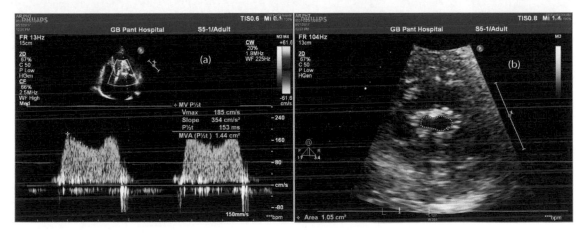

Figure 8.17 Overestimation of mitral valve area (MVA) by PHT in presence of AR **(a)** as compared to 2D echocardiography **(b)**. PHT, pressure half-time.

the inferior vena cava). Most cases of MS have tricuspid regurgitation (TR), allowing estimation of PA pressures. It is best to look for the TR gradient in multiple views besides the standard four-chamber apical view to get best alignment with an eccentric jet, for example, modified two-chamber apical view, tilted parasternal long-axis view, epigastric view, etc. Only the dense part of the spectral envelope should be used to calculate TR gradient (Figure 8.19).

The development of PAH (PASP >30 mmHg), at baseline or after exercise stress, implies significant MS that needs to be corrected while severe PAH (PASP >50 mmHg) due to MS should be addressed on a priority basis because of its impact on survival.[28] Severe PAH also leads to progressive

dilatation of the RA and RV, and the characteristic flattening of the interventricular septum causing a D-shaped LV (Figure 8.20, Video 8.9a and 8.9b). While PAH is a direct consequence of elevated pulmonary venous pressures in MS, severe PAH may have a "fixed" or persistent component, i.e., which does not reverse even after correction of MS. Also, organic tricuspid valve disease (stenosis, regurgitation, or both [Video 8.10b]) can be present in association with MS and should be carefully looked for. Severe tricuspid valve disease and RV dysfunction can lead to decreased forward cardiac output, which can have an impact on the estimation of severity of MS by affecting transmitral diastolic flow. With severe RV dilatation, it is important to measure the TV annulus diameter in

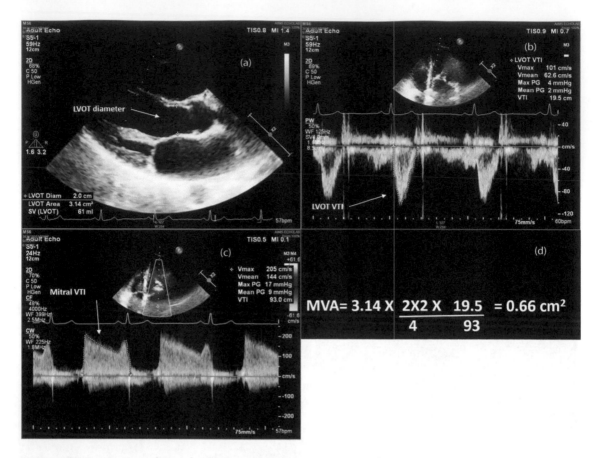

Figure 8.18 Estimation of MVA by the continuity equation. LVOT diameter is measured **(a)** in PLAX view, and LVOT VTI is estimated by pulsed Doppler in apical five-chamber view **(b)**. Mitral VTI is estimated in apical four-chamber view by continuous-wave Doppler across the mitral valve **(c)**. A continuity equation is used **(d)** to calculate MVA. MVA, mitral valve area; LVOT, left-ventricular outflow tract; VTI, velocity time integral.

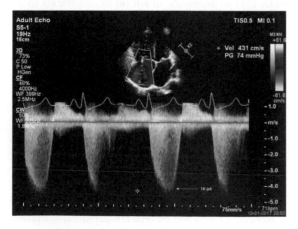

Figure 8.19 Estimation of pulmonary artery systolic pressure (PASP) by tricuspid regurgitation (TR) jet method; PASP is the systolic gradient across the tricuspid valve added to the estimated right-atrial pressure.

four-chamber apical view during diastole, in case the patient is destined for open heart surgery. A diameter of more than 40 mm is a strong marker for development or persistence of late TR after surgery and use of tricuspid annuloplasty.[29]

The presence of aortic valve disease is important to detect as significant disease has an impact on diagnosis as well as recommended management of MS (Figure 8.21, Video 8.10a). Significant aortic valve disease can lead to overestimation of MVA by PHT (Figure 8.17) as well as falsely low transmitral gradients.

Up to 10% of patients with MS can have significant LV systolic dysfunction that can be a direct consequence of MS (covered elsewhere) or due to other causes. It can again confound estimation of the severity of MS as well as have implications for management.

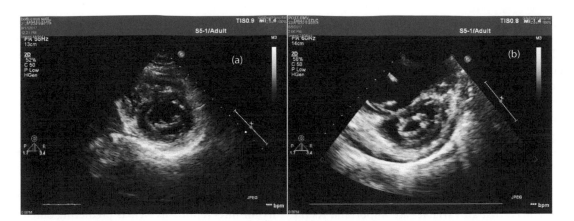

Figure 8.20 Flattening of the interventricular septum due to severe pulmonary artery hypertension with MS; as compared to its usual spherical shape **(a)**, the LV cavity assumes D-shape **(b)**.

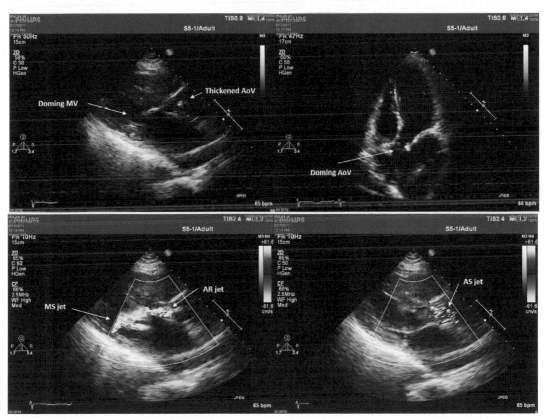

Figure 8.21 Top panel: 2-D echo showing thickened mitral and aortic valve. Bottom panel: Color doppler in same patient showing jets of mitral stenosis, aortic regurgitation, and aortic stenosis.

EVALUATION OF THE MITRAL VALVE APPARATUS FOR SUITABILITY OF PTMC

As PTMC is the preferred modality of treatment for MS, it is important to assess the suitability of the mitral valve apparatus for PTMC. There are only three absolute contraindications for a percutaneous PTMC; namely presence of LA thrombus, extensive bicommissural calcification, and severe MR (Grade 3–4). However, the outcomes of the procedure are dependent on the morphology of the mitral apparatus. These outcomes include acute success in achieving the desired increase in MVA, the development of iatrogenic severe MR, or both, as well as long-term events including attrition in MVA, event-free survival, etc. Accordingly, several echocardiographic scoring systems have been developed to screen patients for suitability of the procedure and predict acute and/or long-term event rates. Several points merit further explanation here. Most scoring systems use a combination of variables for predicting success as well as complications following PTMC, but not everyone is convinced that all variables are important. As the focus of PTMC is on commissural splitting, some investigators believe that commissural morphology alone (thickening, calcification, extent, symmetry) determines outcomes. Others believe that only the extent of subvalvular disease (SVD) determines outcomes. All scores are successful to some extent but there have been issues with their reproducibility in different populations and studies. Of note, we have seldom noticed individuals with MS in the current era presenting with valves with very suitable scores; in general, there is always highly uneven thickening as well as significant subvalvular disease of either or both papillary muscles.

Finally, several institutions and physicians now offer percutaneous mitral valvuloplasty to all eligible patients with MS, with standby mitral valve replacement (MVR) if required, in the absence of absolute contraindications. While the results are not optimal, they are usually acceptable[30] and delay the otherwise inevitable MVR for a few more years. This can be important in a comparatively younger population.

The Massachusetts General Hospital (MGH) score, or the Wilkins Score, is the oldest and the most commonly used score for assessing suitability for intervention as well as predicting outcomes (Table 8.1).[31] It scores the four variables on a scale of 1–4 with the range of the score being 4–16. No specific score is a complete contraindication for PTMC. The valve morphology becomes more adverse with an increasing score and a score ≥8 is generally considered suboptimal for percutaneous intervention. However, as it does not take into account commissural morphology and asymmetry of scarring, several studies have shown its poor ability to predict acute leaflet tear (and subsequent severe MR) and success following PTMC.

A simpler score was devised by Lung and Cormier,[32] which required measuring the length

Table 8.1 Components and scoring of the Wilkins or the MGH score

Grade	Mobility	Thickening	Calcification	Subvalvular disease
1	Highly mobile with only leaflet tip restricted	Near-normal thickness of 4–5 mm	Single area of increased echo brightness	Minimal thickening just below the leaflets
2	Leaflet mid and base have normal mobility	Midleaflet normal; considerable thickening of margins of 5–8 mm	Scattered area of echo brightness confined to leaflet margins	Thickening of the chordal structures extending to one-third of the chordal length
3	Valve moves forward in diastole, mainly from base	Thickening throughout the leaflet of 5–8 mm	Brightness extending to midportion of the leaflet	Thickening of the chordal structures extending to distal one-third of the chordal length
4	No or minimal forward movement of leaflet in diastole	Considerable thickening of the entire leaflet tissue of >8–10 mm	Extensive brightness throughout the leaflet tissue	Extensive thickening and shortening of all chordae extending down to the papillary muscles

Source: Adapted from Wilkins GT et al., *Br Heart J* 1988; 60:299–308.

of the chordae of anterior mitral leaflet (AML) in the parasternal long-axis view on echocardiography as well as performing a fluoroscopy for the presence of calcification (Table 8.2). Fluoroscopy was advised because of the difficulty

Table 8.2 Lung and Cormier risk score for commissurotomy

Grade	Description
1	Pliable non-calcific AML and mild subvalvular disease (thin chordae ≥10 mm long)
2	Pliable non-calcific AML and severe subvalvular disease (thickened chordae <10 mm long)
3	Calcification of mitral valve of any extent on fluoroscopy irrespective of SVD extent

Source: Lung B et al., Circulation 1996; 94:2124–30.

of differentiating calcification with nodular fibrosis on echocardiography.

A simple method to predict a candidate with poor outcomes post-PTMC (inadequate opening, restenosis, acute MR) is to examine calcium in each of the anterolateral and posteromedial commissures[33] (Figure 8.22, Video 8.11a–c). Commissural calcium was defined by bright echocardiographic density with acoustic shadowing. Calcium was said to be present if the brightness was more than compared to that of adjacent the aortic root. A score has been devised by giving a calcium score of 0 or 1 to each half commissure, with a total score thus ranging from 0 to 4 (Figure 8.22). Increasing commissural calcium with this score identifies a poor outcome after PTMC, especially among those with a Wilkins score of ≤8.[34] Padial and colleagues[35] devised a score consisting of extent and unevenness of individual leaflet thickness and calcification, commissural calcium, and subvalvular

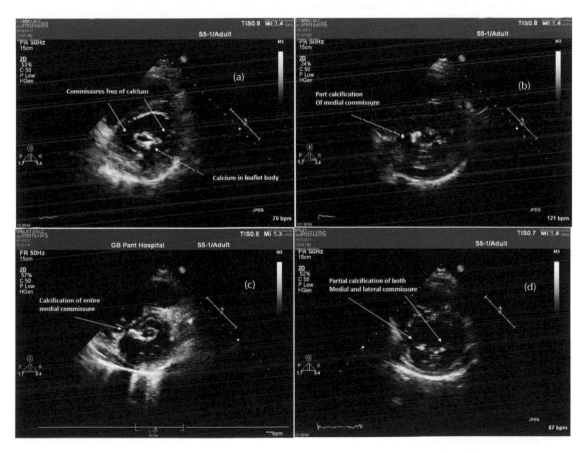

Figure 8.22 Spectrum of commissural calcification. (a) Calcification in leaflet body but not in commissures; (b) partial calcification of only medial commissure; (c) calcification of entire medial commissure; (d) bilateral spotty calcification of medial parts of both commissures.

disease to better predict the development of acute MR after PTMC (total score 0–16). The score was compared among those who developed MR versus those who did not, and a score of ≥10 had a good discriminatory value for this outcome. A real-time transthoracic three-dimensional echocardiography-based score has also been developed looking at the same determinants for individual leaflet,[36] but is not widely available and, with a poorer resolution, it's not clear whether it offers any advantage over a thoroughly conducted 2D echocardiogram. Nunes and colleagues[37] from the Harvard-MGH group developed a new score addressing the shortcomings of the Wilkins score and validated it in a separate patient population with good results. They tested the predictive ability of the Wilkins score as well as many other variables for prediction of acute success (an increase in MVA without an increase in MR) as well as long-term outcomes. Baseline MVA ≤1 cm^2, maximum leaflet displacement, commissural area ratio, and subvalvular thickening were the only factors found significant. Maximal leaflet displacement is the excursion distance of the domed restricted leaflets in systole from mitral annulus in a conventional four-chamber apical view. It typically sums up the effect of leaflet thickening, rigidity, calcification, and commissural fusion into one variable. Commissural area ratio incorporates the degree and symmetry of commissural fusion into one variable. The score was validated in an independent population by authors with similar predictive ability as in the original population. However, the overall calculation of score is lengthy and cumbersome. Bhalgat and colleagues[38] found that only subvalvular pathology, seen independently for each papillary muscle and summed into an easy score, was predictive of outcomes. In their study, none of the patients with extensive SVD had an acute favorable outcome (an increase in valve area and no significant MR). However, the score was not independently validated and is too simplistic for the prediction of all outcomes.

To summarize, detailed echocardiographic assessment of the mitral apparatus in severe MS is important for two objectives in the context of percutaneous intervention. First, candidates who are likely to have failed the procedure (no increase in valve area and/or severe MR requiring surgery) need to be identified so that they do not undergo a potentially harmful or unsuccessful procedure (see Box 8.1). The catastrophic event of acute MR is usually

due to leaflet perforation as the commissural MR is generally tolerated well and tends to decrease in the long-term due to progressive fibrosis. Leaflet perforation is due to unevenness of fibrosis/calcification in the valvular apparatus that will predispose certain points (interfaces of the mitral valve complex) for tearing. As the thicker portions refuse to give way, the brunt of asymmetric and large forces generated during balloon dilatation is borne by these weaker areas, especially with an inappropriately large balloon or a balloon in a high-pressure zone.[39] This asymmetry can exist within the leaflets and commissures, as well as on the interface between two components, for example, excessive thickening in commissures and/or subvalvular tissue in relation to leaflets, with the latter being less thick. It is the AML that mostly tears at a "hinge" point. This is why the Wilkins score may not predict procedural severe MR, while the Padial score (which takes into account leaflet heterogeneity) or the score proposed by Bhalgat and colleagues could.

Second, the acute success of the procedure is also determined by rigidity of the different components of the mitral apparatus while the principal determinant of long-term success is the acute gain in valve area. The Wilkins score may be good at predicting this (except in scenarios where a suitable score is co-existent with bad SVD or commissural calcification), and so would other scores. We are of the view that each component of the mitral apparatus should be examined and described in detail. Then one may choose, if at all, to summarize the findings with any one score. If that is a Wilkins score, then additionally one must describe commissural morphology and give a description of individual papillary muscles. The box suggests a practical way of assessing the mitral valve such that some patients are not offered PTMC at all, while others are prognosticated properly.

TRANSESOPHAGEAL ECHOCARDIOGRAPHY

Transesophageal echocardiography (TEE) is a useful imaging modality when the transthoracic windows are suboptimal for mitral valve assessment. While it has excellent and superior resolution for imaging posterior structures, it is not routinely recommended due to its invasive nature. Transesophageal echocardiography is superior to

BOX 8.1: Suggested assessment of mitral apparatus in mitral stenosis before percutaneous valvotomy

Ineligible for Percutaneous Dilatation

| Left-atrial clot | ≥2/4 MR | Extensive bicommissural calcification |

High risk of failure (valve not opened OR severe MR OR thromboembolism)

| Clot at mouth of LAA | Moderate MR | Commissural calcification | Severe SVD in both papillary muscles |

Likely to yield suboptimal results

| Severe leaflet asymmetry, thickening | Calcification anywhere | Asymmetric commissural involvement | Significant SVD |

Abbreviations: LAA, left-atrial appendage; MR, mitral regurgitation; SVD, subvalvular deformuty.

TTE for the imaging and assessment of the LAA (for its function and the presence of thrombus) and evaluating mitral regurgitation and is performed routinely in all patients with AF planned for PTMC to rule out an LAA clot (Figure 8.23, Video 8.12). In patients with sinus rhythm, a TEE is not routinely performed except in the presence of a prior embolic event, dense spontaneous echo contrast (SEC) in the LA, and suboptimal transthoracic imaging of the LAA. It can also be used for assessing commissures and subvalvular disease when these are not seen clearly by TTE. It is also used during PTMC for guiding transseptal puncture, balloon placement, and assessing MR and pericardial effusion.

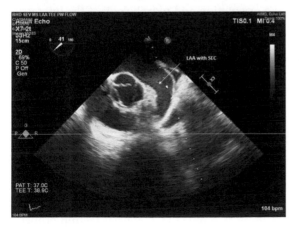

Figure 8.23 Transesophageal echocardiogram in a case with MS and indistinct visualization of LAA on 2D echocardiography; SEC can be seen in the LAA and left atrium. SEC, spontaneous echo contrast.

STRESS ECHOCARDIOGRAPHY

There are several patients who are diagnosed to have significant MS on screening and yet do not have any symptoms. Furthermore, in many patients the symptoms and the assessed severity do not correlate. Stress echocardiography (by exercise or dobutamine infusion) is very useful in the evaluation of such patients because of the pronounced influence of heart rate and exercise on the mitral diastolic gradients. The rise in left-atrial pressure (and pulmonary capillary wedge pressure) during exercise also depends on net atrioventricular compliance, besides absolute MVA.[40] Typically, mean mitral diastolic gradients (MDG) and pulmonary artery systolic pressure (PASP) are estimated during stress. Stress echocardiography can also be used to assess the impact of pregnancy, β-blockade, or simulate stress of non-cardiac surgery in indicated patients.[41] Semi-supine echocardiography is preferable to post-exercise echocardiography protocols as it allows estimation of hemodynamics throughout the examination. Objective limitation of exercise tolerance with a rise in MDG greater than 15 mmHg and a rise in PASP greater than 60 mmHg may be an indication for percutaneous valvotomy if the MV morphology is suitable.[42]

THREE-DIMENSIONAL ECHOCARDIOGRAPHY

Real-time three-dimensional echocardiography (3D echo) is a relatively new technology for visualizing intracardiac structures in various planes with reasonable accuracy. It uses a phased, matrix

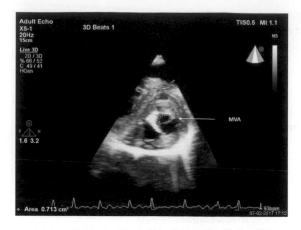

Figure 8.24 Calculation of mitral valve area (MVA) by real-time three-dimensional echocardiography.

array transducer probe and can be done by transthoracic and transesophageal route. Full-volume images of the mitral valve, usually in apical four-chamber view or parasternal long-axis view, are obtained for real-time or offline analysis. The volume acquisition can be rotated, steered, and sliced along all the three axes at any desired level, and the smallest mitral valve orifice visualized and measured using either atrial or ventricular view (Figure 8.24, Video 8.17). Three-dimensional echocardiography has been shown to more accurately measure mitral valve area (MVA) in comparison to 2D echo, at least in the hands of inexperienced operators. This has important implications for centers or regions where MS is seen infrequently. It has also been shown to better visualize the commissural opening, thus helping guide appropriate treatment, especially for a re-stenosed valve that could be narrowed due to valve rigidity per se rather than commissural fusion.[43] Finally, it is often feasible to obtain good 3D echo images when the 2D transthoracic images are suboptimal, even more so if 3D echo is transesophageal[44] On the flip side, 3D echo is not widely available in developing countries (where the actual burden of MS lies), the acquisition may be suboptimal with uncontrolled ventricular rates, and the spatial resolution still leaves a lot to be desired.

ECHOCARDIOGRAPHY DURING PREGNANCY

It is still not uncommon to encounter pregnant women with significant MS in developing countries. With increased preload and heart rate, the hemodynamic consequences of MS worsen during pregnancy. Thus, for the same mitral valve area, the transmitral gradient, tricuspid regurgitation, and chamber volumes may increase significantly during pregnancy, especially in the second and third trimester. Thus, the decision of performing PTMC/surgery or wait-and-watch with medical management is often more complex. This topic is covered in detail elsewhere in this book.

ECHOCARDIOGRAPHY DURING AND AFTER PERCUTANEOUS TRANSVENOUS MITRAL COMMISSUROTOMY

Echocardiography is indispensable before, during, and after PTMC. Pre-procedure echocardiography is required for: 1) the assessment of valve suitability for PTMC; 2) the assessment of MV hemodynamics (MVA, mean and end diastolic gradients); 3) the assessment of MR (presence, severity, mechanism); 4) the presence of LA/LAA appendage thrombus (Figure 8.25, Video 8.13a and 8.13b); and 5) pre-procedural PASP and RV function. In addition, two aspects need to be specifically noted. One is the presence of pericardial effusion (Figure 8.26, Video 8.16) at baseline (this may be due to congestive heart failure, carditis, or an unrelated cause). If this effusion is missed, the appearance of a pericardial effusion later in the procedure may be wrongly attributed to cardiac perforation, leading to the procedure being abandoned. The other is the orientation and morphology of the interatrial septum as it would help in transseptal puncture (TSP). The interatrial septum may bulge towards the RA (with high LA pressures) or sometimes also the other way (in the presence of severe PAH and/or tricuspid valve disease causing RA volume overload). TSP is usually done under fluoroscopic guidance. In challenging cases, echocardiographic guidance (TTE or TEE), may be needed for TSP, as in instances of thoracic deformities, severe bulging of the interatrial septum, or an aneursymal septum (Figure 8.27, Video 8.18). A transthoracic echocardiogram for this purpose needs more skill and training to profile the interatrial septum properly. Usually epigastric combined with apical and short-axis views (to visualize the aorta) are adequate.

Following TSP, a TTE may be performed to assess the site of septal puncture (appropriate, high, or low)

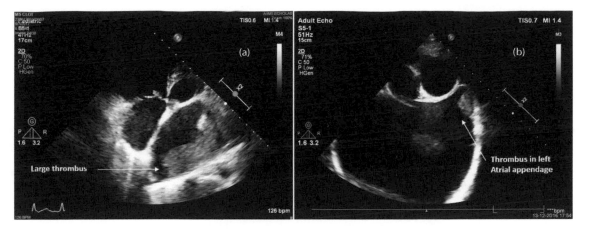

Figure 8.25 Presence of thrombus in LA **(a)** and LAA **(b)**.

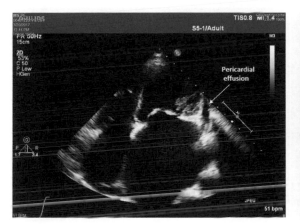

Figure 8.26 Presence of pericardial effusion in a case of severe MS.

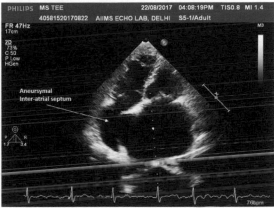

Figure 8.27 Aneurysmal interatrial septum in a case with severe MS.

and for the appearance of new PE. After each balloon inflation, TTE is usually performed to assess the success of PTMC (commissural splitting) and for the appearance of MR. MVA and mean gradients are assessed after each inflation. Grade 2/4 MR or an increase in MR by one grade is an indication for the termination of PTMC. Unexpected hemodynamic collapse or hypotension should lead to immediate performance of echo to rule out tamponade.

There can be large and unpredictable changes in atrial and ventricular compliance for up to 72 hours after PTMC. As mentioned earlier, this makes the PHT method for MVA estimation unreliable. Usually PHT underestimates the MVA during this period and proper measurement of cross-sectional MVA and visualization of split commissure(s) is the ideal method to decide about success of the procedure

(Figures 8.28 and 8.29, Video 8.19b). However, a PHT of less than 130 ms (Figure 8.16) has been shown to correlate with a good valve opening.[45]

After PTMC, 2D echo is used for following up patients for restenosis, progression or regression of MR, atrial septal defect, biventricular function, and PA pressure. Over the long term, a large number of individuals develop significant restenosis after having undergone an initial PTMC. Echocardiography in these individuals should focus on the predominant mechanism of restenosis as this will determine the treatment approach. While fusion of commissures (Video 8.20) can be addressed with a re-do PTMC, cases with severe subvalvular disease forming the effective stenotic orifice or severe valvular rigidity with split commissures should be offered mitral valve surgery.

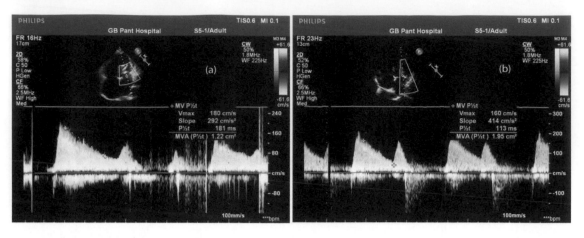

Figure 8.28 Pressure half-time (PHT) in a case of partially successful **(a)** and successful **(b)** BMV.

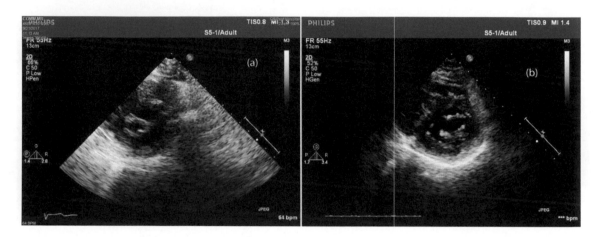

Figure 8.29 Commissural splitting after BMV; **(a)** shows only medial commissure being split while **(b)** shows both commissures split.

ASSESSMENT OF CO-EXISTENT VALVULAR LESIONS

Mitral regurgitation is often present along with MS and its careful assessment is required for appropriate management, as mentioned before. A mild central MR jet or a less-than-holosystolic jet, often due to fixed stenotic orifice, is acceptable for a percutaneous procedure. Usually this assessment should be carried out by an operator experienced in assessing rheumatic mitral valve disease. One clue to the presence of significant MR is a LA that is inappropriately large; such cases should be screened aggressively for eccentric MR jets in various standard and modified views.

Aortic valve disease is frequently seen in patients with MS, with aortic regurgitation (AR) being commoner than aortic stenosis (AS) (Figure 8.21). The severity of AS may be underestimated in the presence of severe MS due to decreased stroke volume. On the other hand, severe AR causes overestimation of MVA by PHT method, by changing LV compliance. While presence of severe AS is an indication for surgical treatment of the severe MS, we offer PTMC to patients with co-existent moderate AR (and sometimes even severe AR in the presence of high-surgical-risk or young patients) because the progression of AR in RHD may take several years. Hence, again, careful assessment of AR severity is very important for planning the management of severe MS.

The tricuspid valve is frequently secondarily involved in severe MS due to the presence of significant PAH. Primary involvement with tricuspid

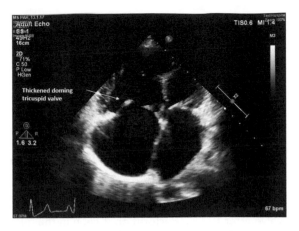

Figure 8.30 Presence of tricuspid stenosis (TS) along with severe MS.

stenosis (TS) (Figure 8.30), tricuspid regurgitation (TR), or a mixed lesion are also seen. In the presence of severe TS, the transmitral gradients may be low despite severe MS due to low forward output. Severe TS can usually be addressed in the same procedure as PTMC. Severe TV disease often causes RA volume overload and changes in orientation of intratrial septum—relevant details to notice while planning a PTMC procedure. A TV annulus of >40 mm or >21 mm/m² BSA is an indication for TV annuloplasty, even if the TR is mild.

VIDEOS

Video 8.1a: Parasternal long axis view of a typical case of rheumatic mitral stenosis. Both the leaflets are thickened. The posterior mitral leaflet is relatively fixed. The anterior mitral leaflet is unevenly thickened with restricted movement of the leaflet tip leading to doming of the valve. The anterior leaflet also has a mild prolapse. The chordae tendinae are thickened and fused. Left atrium is enlarged (corresponds to Figure 8.1a). https://youtu.be/n5AEy667V1Y

Video 8.1b: Parasternal short axis view of moderate mitral stenosis. Both the leaflets are thickened. Both the commissures, lateral more than medial, are also thickened (corresponds to Figure 8.1b). https://youtu.be/fN3fyV622VY

Video 8.2: Parasternal short axis view of a typical case of mitral stenosis. The "fish-mouth"

appearance is evident and both, posteromedial and anterolateral, commissures are thickened and fused. (corresponds to Figure 8.2b). https://youtu.be/AthfmMVrCJw

Video 8.3a: Modified parasternal long axis view tilted posteriorly to show subvalvular apparatus of posteromedial papillary muscle. The chordae tendinae are thickened, retracted and fused into two chords and papillary muscle appears pulled. Aortic valve is also thickened (corresponds to Figure 8.3b). https://youtu.be/wsiDnDGm3Tc

Video 8.3b: Modified parasternal long axis view tilted anteriorly to show subvalvular apparatus of the anterolateral papillary muscle. Pulmonary valve can be seen anteriorly. The chordae tendinae are thickened, retracted and fused into two chords and papillary muscle appears pulled (corresponds to Figure 8.3c). https://youtu.be/BQCzjleUZFl

Video 8.3c: Parasternal short axis view just below the mitral leaflet level showing significant subvalvular disease. Both the papillary muscles can be seen in crosssection (corresponds to Figure 8.3e). https://youtu.be/TvV_A_q9lrg

Video 8.3d: Modified apical 4-chamber view with colour doppler across mitral valve. There is severe mitral stenosis with significant subvalvular disease causing two jets of turbulent blood flow. https://youtu.be/jIJEWaRbT-o

Video 8.3e: Modified apical 2-chamber view showing significant mitral stenosis. The valve has bright echogenic areas suggesting spotty calcification. Both the papillary muscles are seen with subvalvular disease, fusion, and thickening of chordae in inferomedial papillary muscle and retraction in anterolateral papillary muscle (corresponds to Figure 8.3d). https://youtu.be/Bcg8Puu1MM4

Video 8.4: Parasternal short axis view at the mitral valve level in a case of very severe mitral stenosis. Mitral valve area should be calculated at the caudal most section of the valve where an uninterrupted valve outline can be traced. Thickened and fused lateral commissure can be also seen (corresponds to Figure 8.4). https://youtu.be/KON2V4ZR2jA

Video 8.5a: Spontaneous echo contrast (SEC) seen in apical 4-chamber view as echogenic "smoke" diffusing from left atrium to the left ventricle, in a case of mitral stenosis (corresponds to Figure 8.6). https://youtu.be/CEvzVw5leTA

Video 8.5b: Parasternal long axis view showing spontaneous echo contrast (SEC) in a case of severe mitral stenosis. The aortic valve is also thickened and doming (corresponds to Figure 8.6). https://youtu.be/qNS0HLg-kwY

Video 8.6a: Left atrial appendage seen in a modified parasternal short axis view (see text) (corresponds to Figure 8.7b). https://youtu.be /w9TVzx1ey7o

Video 8.6b: Apical 2-chamber view demonstrating the mouth of left atrial appendage in an orthogonal projection compared to parasternal short axis view. The left upper pulmonary vein (posterior to the appendage) and the ridge separating the two can also be seen (corresponds to Figure 8.7c). https://youtu.be/uSRksK5eFXA

Video 8.7a: Parasternal long axis view in a case of mitral stenosis showing a central jet of mild mitral regurgitation (corresponds to Figure 8.9a). https://youtu.be/JBBwN9TP15E

Video 8.7b: Apical 4-chamber view of severe mitral stenosis associated with severe eccentric jet of mitral regurgitation. The jet can be seen entering the pulmonary vein. https://youtu.be/IFQFd5SV73o

Video 8.7c: Parasternal long axis view in a case of severe mitral stenosis along with significant eccentric mitral regurgitation and severe enlargement of left atrium. Such jets can be highly eccentric and should be suspected in any case with severely enlarged left atrium (corresponds to Figure 8.9b). https://youtu.be/IeNSJkLFDjw

Video 8.8a: Parasternal short axis view of a mitral valve after PTMC. Two jets of mitral regurgitation can be seen: One central jet and the other due to splitting of lateral commissure (corresponds to Figure 8.11b) https://youtu.be/YcqeRdBKWQc

Video 8.8b: Apical 4-chamber view of a mitral valve after PTMC. Two jets of mitral regurgitation can be seen; one central jet and the other due to splitting of lateral commissure (corresponds to Figure 8.11b). https://youtu.be/zmgcH7ssrmE

Video 8.8c: Apical 4-chamber view of a mitral valve after PTMC. A torn chordae can be seen resulting in anterior mitral leaflet tip prolapse and severe mitral regurgitation (corresponds to Figure 8.11a). https://youtu.be/9dMZ-0VtYtQ

Video 8.8d: Parasternal short axis view of a mitral valve after PTMC. A torn chordae and possible damage to anterior mitral leaflet leads to severe mitral regurgitation (corresponds to Figure 8.11a). https://youtu.be/WRbhkpo9gSY

Video 8.8e: Parasternal long axis view of a mitral valve after PTMC. Perforation is seen in the mid-portion of anterior mitral leaflet leading to severe mitral regurgitation. The mitral valve has not opened (corresponds to Figure 8.11c). https://youtu.be/bonlDrweCzY

Video 8.9a: Parasternal long axis view of a case of severe mitral stenosis with severe pulmonary arterial hypertension. The right ventricle is enlarged and the interventricular septum is bowing towards the left ventricle (corresponds to Figure 8.20). https://youtu.be/E3XdfuzWF1E

Video 8.9b: Apical 4-chamber view of a case of severe mitral stenosis with severe pulmonary arterial hypertension. The right ventricle is larger than the left ventricle, and the tricuspid valve appears thickened (corresponds to Figure 8.20). https://youtu.be/Kyo9WWVGlZI

Video 8.10a: Parasternal long axis view with colour Doppler across mitral and aortic valve, showing mitral stenosis along with aortic valve disease. Turbulent jets can be seen for mitral stenosis and aortic regurgitation in diastole, and aortic stenosis in systole (corresponds to Figure 8.21). https://youtu.be/_TefHy-2d0c

Video 8.10b: Apical 4-chamber view of a case of mitral stenosis along with organic tricuspid valve disease. Right atrium and ventricle are dilated and there is severe low-pressure tricuspid regurgitation. https://youtu.be/XlX8NaEEy58

Video 8.11a: Parasternal short axis view at mitral valve level in a case of mitral stenosis. Calcification can be seen in the body of the posterior leaflet but not in the commissures (corresponds to Figure 8.22). https://youtu.be/AVBXFC16Ilc

Video 8.11b: The calcification of mitral leaflet tips can be appreciated in this parasternal long axis view with the gain settings turned down (corresponds to Figure 8.22). https://youtu.be /jVkqoZexftM

Video 8.11c: Parasternal short axis view at mitral valve level in a case of mitral stenosis. Calcification can be seen in the inner half of the medial commissure (corresponds to Figure 8.22). https:// youtu.be/oSKIo_vkl3k

Video 8.12: A typical transesophageal view of the left atrial appendage. Spontaneous echo contrast in the appendage and left atrium can also be seen (corresponds to Figure 8.23). https://youtu .be/aq4msWYPfQI

Video 8.13a: Parasternal short axis view tilted anteriorly to show the left atrial appendage. A discrete ball-shaped thrombus can be seen protruding from the mouth of the appendage (corresponds to Figure 8.25). https://youtu.be /KIHmaRArptM

Video 8.13b: Parasternal long axis view in a case of severe mitral stenosis with atrial fibrillation. A large thrombus can be seen occupying significant proportion of the left atrium (corresponds to Figure 8.25). https://youtu.be/ITMJgt7s7_w

Video 8.14: Parasternal short axis view at the level of mitral valve. Bright echogenic nodules can be seen on both the leaflet (three on the posterior and one on anterior). These nodules do not necessarily imply presence of active rheumatic inflammation. https://youtu.be/6bxXIKgYEUQ

Video 8.15: Parasternal long axis view in a case of mitral stenosis, essential systemic hypertension, and no significant aortic valve disease. Left ventricle has concentric hypertrophy, which can cause overestimation of mitral valve area by pressure half-time method. https://youtu.be /Yi9nE-ms_Wk

Video 8.16: Apical 4-chamber view showing severe mitral stenosis with buckling of anterior mitral leaflet and the typical hockey-stick appearance. There is pericardial effusion, which should be noted prior to PTMC procedure (corresponds to Figure 8.26). https://youtu.be/VgiW7gMrHeE

Video 8.17: Real-time 3D echocardiography of rheumatic mitral stenosis reveals typical fish mouth appearance (corresponds to Figure 8.24). https://youtu.be/ilNlFiUsY7E

Video 8.18: Parasternal short axis view at the aortic valve level in a case of mitral stenosis. The interatrial septum is bulging toward the right atrium. This needs to be noted prior to PTMC for planning trans-septal puncture (corresponds to Figure 8.27). https://youtu.be/CnThm6HrTsc

Video 8.19a: Parasternal short axis view at the mitral level in a case of mitral stenosis after a PTMC procedure. Lateral commissure is clearly split. Splitting of commissure is the predominant mechanism for increase in the mitral valve area after PTMC (corresponds to Figure 8.29). https:// youtu.be/eMVEV2xZyM4

Video 8.19b: Parasternal short axis view at the mitral level in a case of mitral stenosis after a PTMC procedure. Both medial and lateral commissures are clearly split. Splitting of commissure is the predominant mechanism for increase in mitral valve area after PTMC (corresponds to Figure 8.29). https://youtu.be/jx5TpMKB1JU

Video 8.20: Parasternal short axis view at the mitral level in a case of mitral stenosis after a PTMC procedure. Both the commissures are fused, implying possibility of success with a repeat PTMC procedure. https://youtu.be /tJChiTxDLvg

REFERENCES

1. Lang RM, Badano LP, Mor-Avi V et al. Recommendations for cardiac chamber quantification by echocardiography in adults: An update from the American Society of Echocardiography and the European Association of Cardiovascular Imaging. *J Am Soc Echocardiogr* 2015;28:1–39.
2. Baumgartner H, Hung J, Bermejo J et al. Echocardiographic assessment of valve stenosis: EAE/ASE recommendations for clinical practice. *J Am Soc Echocardiogr* 2009;22:1–23.
3. Nichol PM, Gilbert BW, Kisslo JA. Two-dimensional echocardiographic assessment of mitral stenosis. *Circulation* 1977;55:120–8.

4. Messika-Zeitoun D, Brochet E, Holmin C et al. Three-dimensional evaluation of the mitral valve area and commissural opening before and after percutaneous mitral commissurotomy in patients with mitral stenosis. *Eur Heart J* 2007;28:72–9.

5. Seow SC, Koh LP, Yeo TC. Hemodynamic significance of mitral stenosis: Use of a simple, novel index by 2-dimensional echocardiography. *J Am SocEchocardiogr* 2006;19:102–6.

6. Holmin C, Messika-Zeitoun D, Mezalek AT et al. Mitral leaflet separation index: A new method for the evaluation of the severity of mitral stenosis? Usefulness before and after percutaneous mitral commissurotomy. *J Am Soc Echocardiogr* 2007;20:1119–24.

7. Goswami KC, Narang R, Bahl VK, Talwar KK, Manchanda SC. Comparative evaluation of transthoracic and transesophageal echocardiography in detection of left atrial thrombus before percutaneous transvenous mitral commissurotomy. Do all patients need transesophageal examination? *Int J Cardiol* 1997(19);62:237–49.

8. McKay T, Thomas L. 'Coumadin ridge' in the left atrium demonstrated on three dimensional transthoracic echocardiography. *Eur J Echocardiogr* 2008;9:298–300.

9. Cope GD, Kisslo JA, Johnson ML, Behar VS. A reassessment of the echocardiogram in mitral stenosis. *Circulation* 1975;52:664–70.

10. Zoghbi WA, Adams D, Bonow RO et al. Recommendations for noninvasive evaluation of native valvular regurgitation: A report from the American Society of Echocardiography developed in collaboration with the Society for Cardiovascular Magnetic Resonance. *J Am Soc Echocardiogr* 2017;30:303–71.

11. Utsunomiya T, Ogawa T, Tang HA et al. Doppler color flow mapping of the proximal isovelocity surface area: A new method for measuring volume flow rate across a narrowed orifice. *J Am Soc Echocardiogr* 1991;4:338–48.

12. Rodriguez L, Thomas J, Monterroso V et al. Validation of the proximal flow convergence method: Calculation of orifice area in patients with mitral stenosis. *Circulation* 1993;88:1157–65.

13. Messika-Zeitoun D, Cachier A, Brochet E, Cormier B, Iung B, Vahanian A. Evaluation of mitral valve area by the proximal isovelocity surface area method in mitral stenosis: Could it be simplified? *Eur J Echocardiogr* 2007;8:116–21.

14. Rifkin RD, Harper K, Tighe D. Comparison of proximal isovelocity surface area method with pressure half-time and planimetry in evaluation of mitral stenosis. *J Am Coll Cardiol* 1995;26:458–65.

15. Messika-Zeitoun D, Fung Yiu S, Cormier B et al. Sequential assessment of mitral valve area during diastole using colour M-mode flow convergence analysis: New insights into mitral stenosis physiology. *Eur Heart J* 2003;24:1244–53.

16. Hatle L, Brubakk A, Tromsdal A, Angelsen B. Noninvasive assessment of pressure drop in mitral stenosis by Doppler ultrasound. *Br Heart J* 1978;40:131.

17. Holen J, Alasid R, Landmark K, Simonsen S. Determinant of pressure gradient in mitral stenosis with a noninvasive ultrasound Doppler technique. *Acta Med Scan* 1976;199:455.

18. Nishimura RA, Rihal CS, Tajik AJ, Holmes DR Jr. Accurate measurement of the transmitral gradient in patients with mitral stenosis: Asimultaneous catheterization and Doppler echocardiographic study. *J Am Coll Cardiol* 1994;24:152–8.

19. Thomas JD, Newell JB, Choong CY, Weyman AE. Physical and physiological determinants of transmitral velocity: Numerical analysis. *Am J Physiol* 1991;260:H1718–31.

20. Libanoff AJ, Rodbard S. Atrioventricular pressure half-time: Measure of mitral valve area. *Circulation* 1968;38:144–50.

21. Hatle L, Angelsen B, Tromsdal A. Noninvasive assessment of atrioventricular pressure half-time by Doppler ultrasound. *Circulation* 1979;60:1096–1104.

22. Hatle L, Angelsen B. *Doppler Ultrasound in Cardiology: Physical Principles and Clinical Applications*. Philadelphia: Lea & Febiger; 1982:83.

23. Gonzalez MA, Child JS, Krivokapich J. Comparison of two-dimensional and Doppler echocardiography and intracardiac hemodynamics for quantification of mitral stenosis. *Am J Cardiol* 1987;60:327–32.

24. Thomas JD, Weyman AE. Doppler mitral pressure half-time: A clinical tool in search of theoretical justification. *J Am Coll Cardiol* 1987;10:923–9.

25. Nakatani S, Masuyama T, Kodama K, Kitabatake A, Fujii K, Kamada T. Value and limitations of Doppler echocardiography in the quantification of stenotic mitral valve area: Comparison of the pressure half-time and the continuity equation methods. *Circulation* 1988;77:78–85.

26. Izgi C, Ozdemir N, Cevik C et al. Mitral valve resistance as a determinant of resting and stress pulmonary artery pressure in patients with mitral stenosis: A dobutamine stress study. *J Am Soc Echocardiogr* 2007;20:1160–6.

27. Sanati H, Zolfaghari R, Samiei N et al. Mitral valve resistance determines hemodynamic consequences of severe rheumatic mitral stenosis and immediate outcomes of percutaneous valvuloplasty. *Echocardiography* 2017;34:162–8.

28. Ward C, Hancock BW. Extreme pulmonary hypertension caused by mitral valve disease: Natural history and results of surgery. *Br Heart J* 1975;37:74–8.

29. Dreyfus GD, Corbi PJ, Chan KM, Bahrami T. Secondary tricuspid regurgitation or dilatation: Which should be the criteria for surgical repair? *Ann Thorac Surg* 2005;79:127–32.

30. Dreyfus J, Cimadevilla C, Nguyen V et al. Feasibility of percutaneous mitral commissurotomy in patients with commissural mitral valve calcification. *Eur Heart J* 2014;35:1617–23.

31. Wilkins GT, Weyman AE, Abascal VM, Block PC, Palacios IF. Percutaneous balloon dilatation of the mitral valve: An analysis of echocardiographic variables related to outcome and the mechanism of dilatation. *Br Heart J* 1988;60:299–308.

32. Lung B, Cormier B, Ducimetiere P et al. Immediate results of percutaneous mitral commissurotomy. A predictive model on a series of 1514 patients. *Circulation* 1996;94:2124–30.

33. Cannan CR, Nishimura RA, Reeder GS et al. Echocardiographic assessment of commissural calcium: A simple predictor of outcome after percutaneous mitral balloon valvotomy. *J Am Coll Cardiol* 1997;29:175–80.

34. Sutaria N, Northridge DB, Shaw TRD. Significance of commissural calcification on outcome of mitral balloon valvotomy. *Heart* 2000;84:398–402.

35. Padial LR, Freitas N, Sagie A et al. Echocardiography can predict which patients will develop severe mitral regurgitation after percutaneous mitral valvotomy. *J Am Coll Cardiol* 1996;27:1225–31.

36. Anwar AM, Attia WM, Nosir YF et al. Validation of a new score for the assessment of mitral stenosis using real-time three-dimensional echocardiography. *J Am Soc Echocardiogr* 2010;23:13–22.

37. Nunes MC, Tan TC, Elmariah S et al. The echo score revisited: Impact of incorporating commissural morphology and leaflet displacement to the prediction of outcome for patients undergoing percutaneous mitral valvuloplasty. *Circulation* 2014;129;886–95.

38. Bhalgat P, Karlekar S, Modani S et al. Subvalvular apparatus and adverse outcome of balloon valvotomy in rheumatic mitral stenosis. *Indian Heart J* 2015;67:428–33.

39. Chaturvedi V, Gupta MD, MPG. Subvalvular disease in patients undergoing balloon mitral valvotomy: A strong base is not always good. *Indian Heart J* 2015;67:416–8.

40. Schwammenthal E, Vered Z, Agranat O, Kaplinsky E, Rabinowitz B, Feinberg MS. Impact of atrioventricular compliance on pulmonary artery pressure in mitral stenosis: An exercise echocardiographic study. *Circulation* 2000;102:2378–84.

41. Picano E, Pibarot P, Lancelotti P et al. The emerging role of exercise testing and stress echocardiography in valvular heart disease. *J Am Coll Cardiol* 2009;54:2251–60.

42. Bonow RA, Carabello BA, Chatterjee K et al. ACC/AHA 2006 guidelines for the management of patients with valvular heart disease: A report of the American College of Cardiology/American Heart Association Task Force on Practice Guidelines. *J Am Coll Cardiol* 2006;48:e1–148.

43. Messika-Zeitoun D, Brochet E, Holmin C et al. Three-dimensional evaluation of the mitral valve area and commissural opening before and after percutaneous mitral

commissurotomy in patients with mitral stenosis. *Eur Heart J* 2007;28:72–9.

44. Dreyfus J, Brochet E, Lepage L et al. Real-time 3D transoesophageal measurement of the mitral valve area in patients with mitral stenosis. *Eur J Echocardiogr* 2011;12:750–5.

45. Messika-Zeitoun D, Meizels A, Cachier A et al. Echo-cardiographic evaluation of the mitral valve area before and after percutaneous mitral commissurotomy: The pressure half-time method revisited. *J Am Soc Echocardiogr* 2005;18:1409–14.

9

Cardiac catheterization

RAGHAV BANSAL AND GANESAN KARTHIKEYAN

INTRODUCTION

With the advance of two-dimensional and Doppler echocardiography in the 1990s the requirement of cardiac catheterization for the assessment of the severity of valvular lesions has greatly decreased. In today's era, hemodynamic evaluation for mitral stenosis (MS) with cardiac catheterization is reserved for selected patients, such as those with pulmonary arterial hypertension (PAH) out of proportion to the severity of stenosis, or patients in whom there is discrepancy between valve areas and gradients on echocardiography, or uncertainty in lesion severity in multivalve disease. Hemodynamic assessment is, however, recommended in patients undergoing percutaneous interventions, including percutaneous transvenous mitral commissurotomy (PTMC).

Apart from recording chamber pressures, analysis of pressure waveforms in the catheterization laboratory remains important for assessment of lesion severity and for a complete understanding of the associated hemodynamic derangements. Immediate changes in the left atrial (LA) and left ventricular (LV) pressure tracings following PTMC provide clues to assessing the success of the procedure and to detect the occurrence of mitral regurgitation (MR), which is an important complication of the procedure. This chapter will discuss the hemodynamic consequences of MS and the immediate changes following PTMC.

PATHOPHYSIOLOGY OF MITRAL STENOSIS

The normal mitral orifice area is approximately 4–6 cm^2. MS, most commonly occurring in the setting of rheumatic heart disease (RHD), causes constriction of the mitral orifice. The natural history entails a slow progression with a long asymptomatic period, with symptoms appearing only after the fall in mitral valve orifice area below 2.0 cm^2. A decrease below 1.0 cm^2 leads to critical MS and severe consequences. The central pathophysiologic mechanism involves the development of a diastolic gradient between the left atrium and left ventricle and a consequent increase in LA pressure. Left atrial pressure is then transmitted to the pulmonary circulation and leads sequentially to increases in pulmonary venous and right-sided pressures (Figure 9.1). Left-ventricular diastolic pressure remains normal or may be decreased, perhaps due to underfilling of the LV. Patients

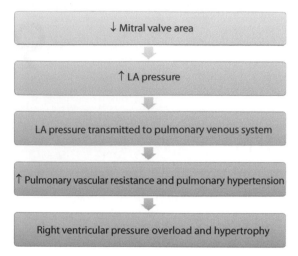

Figure 9.1 Pathophysiology of hemodynamic changes in mitral stenosis.

with MS typically pass through four hemodynamic stages:

1. Normal LA pressure
2. Normal LA pressure at rest with increase only during exercise but with preserved cardiac output on exercise
3. Increased LA pressure at rest with inability to increase cardiac output on exercise
4. Markedly increased LA pressure at rest with impaired cardiac output at rest

In the early stages of disease, with only small decreases in valve area, there may be no significant increase in transvalvular gradient at rest. However, with exercise the stenotic valve causes a significant rise in transvalvular gradient and a consequent rise in pulmonary venous pressure and symptoms. The exercise-induced rise in transvalvular gradient increases exponentially with decreasing mitral area. With significant MS, the transvalvular gradient remains elevated at rest.

MEASUREMENTS IN THE CATHETERIZATION LABORATORY

Importance of meticulous technique cannot be overemphasized so as to reduce hemodynamic artefacts and erroneous measurements. All pressure lines should be carefully flushed to clear any air bubbles and the circuit should be checked for kinks in the catheter or pressure tubing. The height of the pressure transducer should be adjusted to be level with the heart of the patient lying on the catheterization table (this corresponds roughly to the mid-axillary line).

Both venous (for right-heart hemodynamics) and arterial (for LV/systemic pressure recording) access should be obtained. All pressures should be measured with end-hole catheters. A balloon floatation end-hole catheter (Swan-Ganz catheter) is most commonly used for right-heart catheterization and remains the catheter of choice due to ease of use and accuracy in estimating pulmonary capillary wedge pressure (PCWP). Other catheters that can be used are the stiffer Lehman and Cournand catheters. Many patients with MS have associated severe tricuspid regurgitation and an enlarged right atrium, making it difficult to access the right ventricle and pulmonary arteries using balloon flotation catheters. In such instances, using stiffer catheters (including the Judkins right coronary catheter) over a wire may save time. For left-heart catheterization, LV pressures are obtained with a pigtail catheter placed through a retrograde approach. For obtaining an LA pressure waveform, transseptal puncture is required, which is usually done with a Brockenbrough needle within a long sheath (e.g., Mullin's sheath). LA pressures can be obtained by connecting the pressure line to the proximal end of the long sheath. During PTMC the central lumen of the balloon may also be used to record the LA pressure trace.

Ideally, for the calculation of valve gradient and area, simultaneous LA and LV pressures should be measured. However, this requires transseptal access, which is obtained only during PTMC. Alternatively, PCWP may be used as a surrogate measure of LA pressure. PCWP is obtained by inflating the balloon of a balloon-tipped end-hole catheter placed in a distal branch of the right or left pulmonary artery with the balloon completely occluding the lumen. It is important to correctly position the catheter in zone 3 of the lung. Errors in estimating PCWP arise both from overinflating the balloon, leading to a damped tracing, and underinflation, leading to incomplete wedging. The latter is common in the presence of severe PAH and dilated branch pulmonary arteries where incomplete occlusion results in a summation of the pulmonary arterial waveform and PCWP waveform, and overestimation of PCWP and transmitral gradients. A good PCWP waveform is characterized by:

1. Well-defined *a*- and *v*-waves
2. Mean PCWP being generally less than the PA diastolic pressure (but possibly equal to or within 5 mmHg of the diastolic PA pressure)
3. *v*-waves of PCWP peak after the T-wave of the simultaneously recorded ECG
4. Oximetric sampling from the catheter showing an O_2 saturation ≥95%

It is important to recognize some important differences between the PCWP and LA waveforms while using PCWP as a substitute for LA pressure. There is a phase delay in transmission of pressure from LA to the pulmonary venous circulation. The PCWP tracing is therefore delayed by 50–150 ms compared to the LA tracing. This may lead to overestimation of valve gradient (Figure 9.2). Second, PCWP is more damped with less-prominent waveforms and a less steep and deep *y*-descent. In a mechanically ventilated patient, PCWP may overestimate LA pressure due to the positive pressure transmitted to the pulmonary circulation.

Even with these limitations, PCWP remains a commonly used surrogate for LA pressure estimation due to its ease and decreased time of catheter manipulation in the LA. In routine practice, at lower wedge pressures (<25 mmHg) there is good correlation between LA pressure and PCWP, but considerable error may occur at higher pressures.[1] To correct for the phase variation, the PCWP waveform may be shifted manually to the left until the peak of the *v*-wave coincides or just precedes the LV downstroke (Figure 9.2). In a study of ten patients by Lange et al., the use of phase-adjusted PCWP in place of LA pressure resulted in similar calculations of transvalvular gradients and mitral valve area.[2] However, according to some authors, adjustment for phase variation might overestimate the gradient and remains controversial.[3] Transseptal catheterization should be considered for obtaining true LA-LV gradients in the presence of severe PAH, poor-quality wedge waveform, discrepant non-invasive gradients, or prior prosthetic valve implantation.

Left-atrial pressure waveform analysis

Increased LA pressure with a prominent *a*-wave is one of the earliest findings in MS. However, with longstanding MS, atrial compliance is decreased due to fibrosis and stiffening associated with exposure to longstanding high LA pressures. Therefore, *v*-waves may also become prominent even in the absence of MR (Figure 9.3). Large *v*-waves in the absence of MR strongly correlate with diminished exercise tolerance and are a predictor of PAH.[4,5] Left-ventricular filling is impaired due to the obstruction at the mitral valve level, which leads to a decreased slope of the *y*-descent. This is important to differentiate from the prominent *v*-wave of MR where the *y*-descent is steep and there is equalization of LA pressure and LV pressure in mid-diastole (diastasis). Diastasis is not achieved in severe MS and there remains a LA-to-LV gradient even at the end diastole. In normal individuals, the contribution of atrial contraction to ventricular filling is less than 25% as most of the filling is completed in early diastole.[6] Intuitively, the contribution of atrial contraction should increase in MS as ventricular filling is not completed in early diastole. However, in patients with severe MS, despite the increased LA pressure and slowed rate of deceleration of transmitral flow, the contribution of atrial contraction is paradoxically decreased.[7,8] Atrial contribution to LV filling decreased from 29% in mild MS to 9% in severe MS. This is perhaps because the mitral valve offers increased resistance throughout the diastole, including during the period of atrial contraction. However, the exact reason for this phenomenon remains unclear.

With the onset of atrial fibrillation (AF) there is acceleration of atrial dilatation and impairment of left-atrial contractile function. This leads to absence of *a*-wave and a prominent *v*-wave (Figure 9.4). Hemodynamically, the atrium has two functions: a reservoir and conduit function; and a contractile function. The contribution of contractile function, even though small in patients with severe MS, is completely lost in AF. However, the hemodynamic decompensation associated with the onset of AF may be more likely a result of the rapid ventricular rate rather than the loss of atrial contraction.[7] Heart rate is an important determinant of transvalvular gradient. Even in sinus rhythm, tachycardia

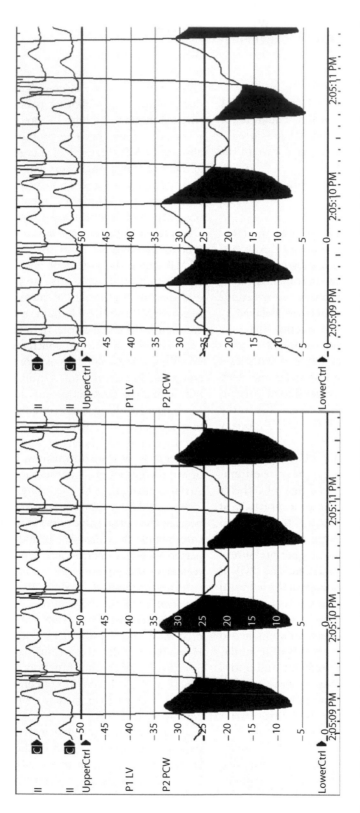

Figure 9.2 Overestimation of transmitral gradient with use of PCWP due to the presence of phase delay. The left side of the figure shows gradient (calculated to be 15 mmHg) between PCWP and LV trace. In the right side of the figure PCWP trace was adjusted for the phase delay by shifting the PCWP trace to the left so that the peak of the v-wave coincides with the downstroke of the LV trace. The calculated gradient subsequently decreased to 13 mmHg.

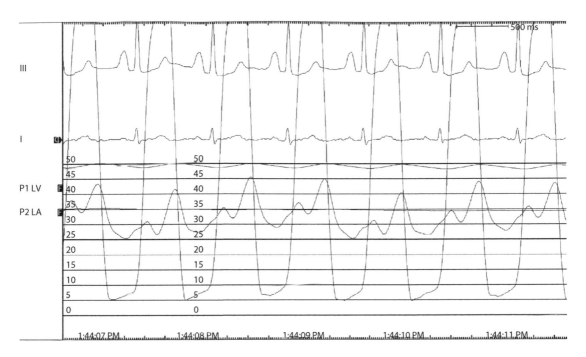

Figure 9.3 Simultaneous LA and LV pressure recording in a patient with severe MS with normal sinus rhythm. The patient is in normal sinus rhythm. Left-atrial pressure waveform shows prominent *a*-wave. There is significant transvalvular diastolic gradient, which remains even at the end of diastole. There is slow *y*-descent and slow rise in LV diastolic pressure.

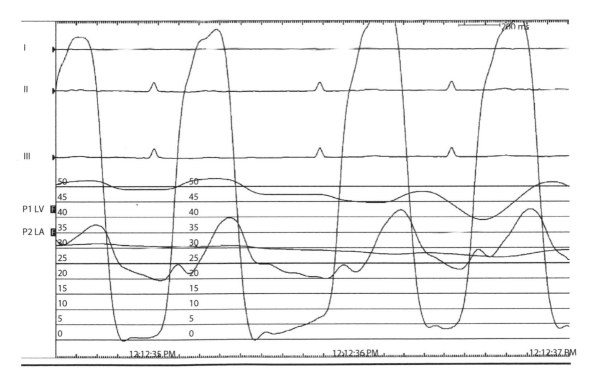

Figure 9.4 Simultaneous LA and LV pressure recording in a patient with severe MS with AF. Note the absence of *a*-wave and prominent *v*-wave on the LA pressure waveform.

can convert an anatomically mild MS into a physiologically severe MS by decreasing the diastolic filling period and increasing the LA-LV gradient.

Pulmonary artery pressure

Pulmonary artery (PA) pressure is elevated only during exercise in mild to moderate MS. However, in severe MS, PA pressure may be increased at rest. Pulmonary hypertension is determined by increased pulmonary venous pressure in concordance with the raised LA pressure and due to the increased pulmonary vascular resistance (PVR). Elevated PVR in MS is mainly "reactive," due to pulmonary arteriolar constriction, but secondary obliterative changes in the pulmonary vascular bed may contribute to a lesser extent in longstanding MS. Varying degrees of PA and RV systolic pressure elevation are noted during cardiac catheterization. Pressures may reach supra-systemic levels in some patients with critical MS (Figure 9.5). The RA pressure waveform is marked by prominent *a*-wave due to a decrease in right-ventricular compliance, which can be seen even in moderate pulmonary hypertension. The presence of tricuspid regurgitation may lead to prominent *cv*-waves in the RA trace.

Left-ventricular pressure and cardiac output

Left-ventricular diastolic filling is impaired in patients with MS in proportion to the severity of stenosis. This can be seen as a delayed rise in the diastolic pressure waveform of the LV. The LV end-diastolic pressure (LVEDP), however, remains normal in most patients, but may be elevated in some cases. In a recent study of 107 patients undergoing PTMC, 32.7% of the patients had raised LVEDP (≥15 mmHg).[9] Raised LVEDP in MS is a marker of MR or impairment of LV diastolic or systolic function. There is an early diastolic movement of the interventricular septum towards the LV (left and posterior) secondary to the rapid unrestricted RV filling as compared to the obstructed mitral inflow. This phenomenon is exaggerated in patients with severe PAH, which may sometimes lead to impairment in LV diastolic function.

Left-ventricular systolic dysfunction is an unexpected but known occurrence in MS. The prevalence of LV systolic dysfunction in MS is still unsettled,

but has been reported in up to 33% of cases in some studies.[10] The causes of LV systolic dysfunction in MS remain unclear. Chronic inflammation secondary to rheumatic fever was one of the earliest factors implicated by Fleming and Wood.[11] Others attributed it to the mitral valve thickening and subvalvular scarring leading to tethering of the LV wall. Other mechanisms proposed for LV systolic dysfunction include LV remodelling because of neurohormonal activation secondary to decreased cardiac output in severe MS, and due to concomitant diseases, such as aortic stenosis, hypertension, and coronary artery disease.

Cardiac output is dependent on stroke volume and heart rate. There is restriction of the rise in stroke volume with exercise in patients with severe MS. With an increase in heart rate, due to a decrease in diastolic filling, there is further impairment of stroke volume. It is important to note that a similar increase in cardiac output is produced at the cost of a much greater increase in LA pressure and pulmonary venous pressure in a patient with a smaller mitral valve area as compared to one with a larger valve area. Patients with critical MS may have reduced stroke volume even at rest.

The important hemodynamic changes in mitral stenosis have been summarized in Table 9.1.

QUANTIFICATION OF MITRAL STENOSIS AND CALCULATION OF VALVE AREA

The severity of MS can be reliably assessed in the cardiac catheterization laboratory. The transvalvular gradient is obtained by simultaneous recording of LA and LV pressures at a fast speed (100 mm/sec) and at a scale of 0–50 mmHg. In the modern-day laboratory, measurement of the gradient and the diastolic filling period is automated by computer software (Figure 9.6). The gradient should be measured as an average of five cardiac cycles in normal sinus rhythm and as an average of ten cardiac cycles in AF. By convention, a gradient of more than 10 mmHg is considered as severe, 5–10 mmHg as moderate, and less than 5 mmHg as mild MS. It is important to remember that conditions like anemia, thyrotoxicosis, anxiety, and pregnancy, which increase cardiac output, will also lead to increased gradients. Thus, the gradient is dependent on the hemodynamic status of the patient and may give a false assessment of severity.

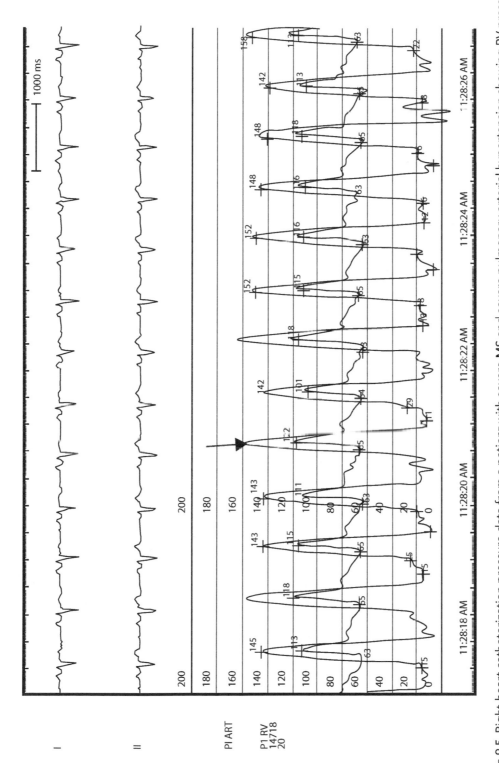

Figure 9.5 Right-heart catheterization pressure data from a patient with severe MS and severe pulmonary arterial hypertension showing RV pressure (arrow) exceeding femoral artery pressure.

Table 9.1 Summary of hemodynamic changes in mitral stenosis

- Increased LA pressure with prominent a-wave and sometimes prominent v-wave
- Decreased slope of y-descent
- Persistent gradient between LA and LV during diastole
- Increased PA pressure at exercise/rest according to severity
- Prominent a-wave with decreased slope of y-descent on RA tracing

Mitral valve area is calculated by Gorlin's formula. This formula was derived by Dr. Richard Gorlin and his father on autopsy-based specimens based on Toricelli's law, developed for hemodynamic systems with fixed rounded orifices.[12] According to Toricelli's law:

$$F = A \times V \times Cc$$

where F is the flow rate, A is the orifice area, V is the velocity of flow, and Cc is the coefficient of orifice contraction. The coefficient was added to compensate for the fact that the cross-sectional area of the stream is less than the true area of the orifice. Rearranging the equation gives:

$$A = F/V \times Cc$$

According to hemodynamic principles,

$$V = Cv \sqrt{2g} \times h$$

where V is the velocity of flow, Cv is the coefficient of velocity correcting for the energy loss as pressure energy is converted to kinetic energy, h is the pressure gradient in cm H_2O, and g is the gravitational constant (980 cm/sec^2).

Combining these two equations:

$$A = F/Cv \times \sqrt{2gh} \times Cc = F/C \times 44.3 \times \sqrt{h}$$

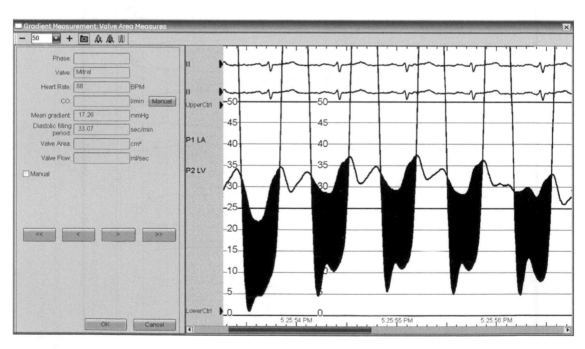

Figure 9.6 Calculation of the mean diastolic gradient and diastolic filling period from the simultaneous LA-LV pressure trace from the same patient in Figure 9.3. Mean diastolic gradient is the area enclosed between the LA and LV pressure trace (shaded area). The diastolic filling period is the duration (in seconds) between the early and late diastolic cross-points of LV and LA pressure tracings. Mean diastolic gradient was automatically calculated by the computer software to be 17.3 mmHg and diastolic filling period to be 33.07 sec/min.

where C accounts for Cv and Cc, and h is the mean transvalvular gradient in mmHg. In this equation, F represents the flow through the orifice. Antegrade flow through the valve occurs only during the diastole. Therefore, dividing the cardiac output (in mL/min) by the product of diastolic filling period (in sec/min) and heart rate (in beats/min) gives us the value of flow F. The empiric constant C was given a value of 0.7 by Gorlin but was later adjusted to 0.85 after comparing the calculated and actual valve areas. Gorlin's formula is as follows:

$$MVA = \left(\frac{CO/DFP \times HR}{44.3 \times 0.85 \times \sqrt{\text{mean gradient}}} \right)$$

where
MVA = Mitral valve area (cm₂)
CO = Cardiac output (cm₃/min)
HR = Heart rate (bpm)
mean gradient = average diastolic gradient across mitral valve (mmHg)
DFP = Diastolic filling period (seconds per beat, measured between initiation of diastole [PCWP/LV crossover] and end of diastole [peak of R wave on ECG])
44.3 × 0.85 = 37.7 is an empiric constant

A mitral valve area of <1.5cm^2 is considered as severe MS according to the 2014 ACC/AHA valvular heart disease guidelines.[13]

A simplified version of the Gorlin formula for quick calculations in the catheterization laboratory has also been proposed and is known as Hakki's formula.[14] This formula ignores the empiric constant, the heart rate, and the diastolic filling period:

Valve area = Cardiac output/ √ Pressure gradient

This formula is easy to remember and apply. However, it leads to significant discrepancies when compared to Gorlin's formula, especially in the presence of tachycardia (>100/min).

Limitations of Gorlin's formula

1. Gorlin's formula was derived from idealized flow dynamics through a narrow orifice and is an oversimplification of the actual hemodynamics. Also, it makes assumptions to create a mathematical formula applicable in clinical practice.

Therefore, it gives, at best, an estimate of the valve area even with accurate measurements.
2. An important clinically relevant assumption during derivation of Gorlin's formula is that the area of a stenotic valve remains constant in changing hemodynamic conditions, which may not be true. Low flow state is a condition where Gorlin's formula remains inaccurate.
3. Cardiac output measurement is done with Fick's principle in most laboratories and is based on the arteriovenous difference of oxygen content and assumed oxygen consumption. There is large variation in oxygen consumption from individual to individual and also from time to time. The use of assumed oxygen consumption can introduce large unexpected errors. Measurement of oxygen saturations with faulty sample collection technique and inaccurate calibration of the blood gas machine is also a source of error. Even in the most stringent conditions, the cardiac output calculated by assumed oxygen consumption can vary by 10%–15%.
4. Atrial fibrillation: Gorlin's formula was developed for normal sinus rhythm. Mean diastolic gradient varies from beat to beat in AF and it becomes important to take an average of at least ten beats.
5. Mitral regurgitation: the presence of MR leads to increased transvalvular flow as compared to the actual cardiac output. This would lead to an underestimation of the valve area and overestimation of the severity of MS. Coexistent MR presents a significant limitation of Gorlin's formula.

Mitral valve resistance has been proposed as an alternative hemodynamic indicator to valve area. The inherent advantage of this parameter is that it takes care of the assumption that the area remains constant during changing hemodynamic states. Its variability has been shown to be less than Gorlin's area, in changing hemodynamic conditions induced by a change in heart rate with isoproterenol infusion.[15] Resistance is calculated with the formula:

$$R = \Delta P/Q$$

where ΔP is the pressure gradient across the resistance and Q is the flow through the resistance.

ΔP is the mean transvalvular gradient and Q is the antegrade flow through the valve calculated similarly to Gorlin's equation.

$$\text{Mitral valve resistance}\left(\text{dynes} \times \frac{\text{sec}}{\text{cm}^5}\right)$$
$$= \left(\frac{1.333 \times \text{Mean gradient [mmHg]}}{\text{CO} \times \text{DFP} \times \text{HR}}\right)$$

where CO = cardiac output (cm³/min); HR = heart rate (bpm); mean gradient = average diastolic gradient across mitral valve (mmHg); DFP = diastolic filling period (sec/beat) (measured between initiation of diastole [PCWP/LV crossover] and end of diastole [peak of R wave on ECG]); 1.333 is a constant to convert from mmHg to dynes/cm².

Mitral valve resistance remains underutilized as a tool due to its lower acceptance. This may be due to the fact that the unit of mitral valve resistance is difficult to conceptualize as compared to the valve area.

Hemodynamics after PTMC

Successful PTMC leads to an immediate increase in mitral valve area and a consequent drop in the transmitral pressure gradient. This leads to an immediate decrease in LA volume so that the stiff LA wall is no more maximally stretched and there is a significant fall in mean LA pressure. In a study analyzing 85 patients for changes in LA compliance immediately after PTMC, Kapoor et al. demonstrated significant rapid increase in calculated LA compliance.[16] However, it should be noted that there is no immediate change in LA wall characteristics after PTMC and the change in calculated LA compliance is a mere consequence of decrease in the LA wall stretch secondary to a fall in LA pressure. These rapidly changing LA pressure-volume parameters may make echocardiographic assessment of valve area by pressure half-time method less reliable as the slope of the LA pressure decay may take time to stabilize.[17] However, the assessment of gradients and valve area by planimetry at the end of the procedure remains fairly accurate. Immediate success is defined by an increase in mitral valve area to more than 1.5 cm². Mitral valve area doubles after PTMC in most successful cases and there is reduction in transvalvular gradient by >50%, ideally to less than 5 mmHg.

Immediately after a successful PTMC there is a significant reduction in transmitral gradient and equalization of LV end diastolic pressure with

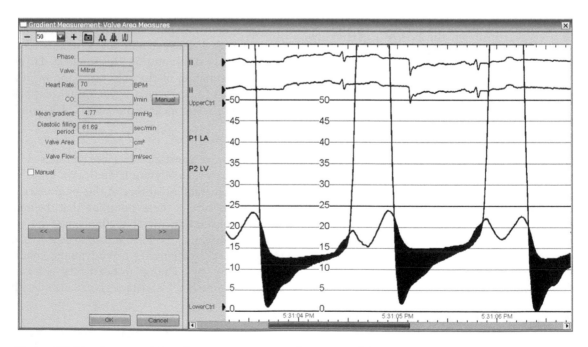

Figure 9.7 Simultaneous LA and LV pressure traces after successful PTMC in the same patient as in Figure 9.3. Note the absence of any increase in v-wave suggestive of absence of significant MR. Mean diastolic gradient decreased from 17.3 mmHg to 4.8 mmHg.

LA pressure (Figure 9.7). There is a rapid change in atrial stretch due to a fall in mean LA pressure reflected as a sudden decrease in the height of earlier prominent v-waves (in the absence of MR). The v-wave is the most dynamic component of the LA pressure trace during PTMC and needs to be carefully monitored to judge procedural success and also to recognize the most important complication of PTMC: MR. The occurrence of significant MR is marked by an increase in LA pressure and increase in v-wave height. There is either de novo prominence of v-wave if it was previously absent or its peak is increased to more than the baseline value if it was already prominent. However, the height of the v-wave is not an accurate marker of the severity of MR. It is helpful to remember that v-waves of MR have a rapid downslope resulting in a steep y-descent (Figure 9.8).

Cardiac output is improved after PTMC due to improved LV filling and an increase in stroke volume. There is usually an increase in LVEDP immediately after successful PTMC. This is often transient and reverts back to normal but LVEDP may remain persistently elevated in those with persistent LV systolic dysfunction.[18] However, significant MR is marked by a drop in forward cardiac output. The cardiac output should be calculated before and after the procedure separately for the calculation of valve area. A left-to-right shunt may occur at the atrial level at the transseptal puncture site. The incidence is reported to be in the range of 10%–25%.[19] In a case series of 68 patients undergoing successful PTMC, left-to-right shunts were detected immediately after the procedure in 25% by oximetric analysis. Using the indicator dilution method, which is more sensitive, a shunt was detected in 62% of the patients. The mean of ratio of pulmonary blood flow to systemic blood flow (Qp/Qs) was 1.3 and it was greater than 1.5 in only 9% of the patients.[20] On follow-up at six months, this shunting persisted in 84% of the patients, although with decreased severity.[20] The left-to-right shunt may interfere with accurate calculation of cardiac output by the thermodilution method and the more time-consuming Fick's method has to be used.[21] To minimize this error due to shunting, all measurements should ideally be taken before the catheter is removed from across the interatrial septum. But in practice, both SVC and mixed venous saturations (PA saturation) are taken separately and the magnitude of shunt

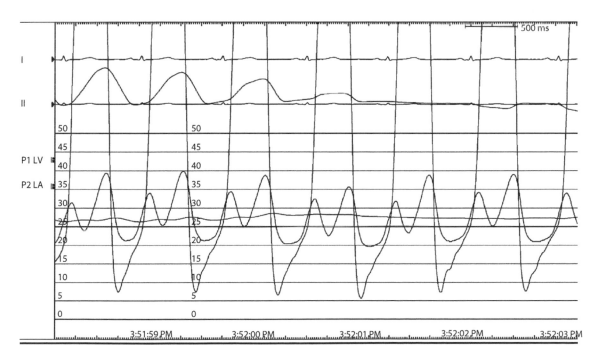

Figure 9.8 Simultaneous LA and LV pressure recording in a patient with severe MS just after PTMC showing prominent v-waves with steep y-descent suggestive of MR. Also note the raised LV end diastolic pressure.

is calculated. The systemic blood flow (Qs) is used to calculate the mitral valve area, thus minimizing the error due to the shunt.

There is an immediate reduction in PA pressure consequent to the fall in LA pressure after a successful PTMC. It has been demonstrated that this fall in mean PA pressure is around 50% with a successful procedure.[22] Though the PA pressure does not normalize immediately, it continues to decrease over a period of time due to the gradual drop in PVR. Dev et al. studied the time course of changes in PA pressure in 53 patients with severe MS undergoing PTMC and showed that most of the changes were complete by the end of the first week followed by a negligible fall afterwards.[23] In a case series of 559 patients of severe MS undergoing successful PTMC, there was complete normalization of the PA pressure immediately post-valvuloplasty in patients who had mild PAH at baseline ($n = 345$ [62%]) in contrast to patients with moderate to severe PAH. However, patients with moderate and severe PAH at baseline ($n = 188$ [33%] and $n = 31$ [5%], respectively) had a substantial regression of PAH at a mean follow-up of 12 months. This occurred secondary to a gradual decrease in PVR even when the PCWP and transmitral gradient remained constant in the follow-up period.[24] Pulmonary arterial pressures regress even when they are supra-systemic prior to PTMC. Among 45 patients with severe MS and systemic or supra-systemic PA pressure who had a successful PTMC, there was a significant immediate decline in PA pressure.[25] In summary, there is an immediate rapid fall in PA pressures after successful PTMC, which continues to regress over time and may reach normal levels in many patients.

CONCLUSION

The central pathophysiologic mechanism in MS is obstruction at the mitral valve level during diastolic LV filling leading to increased LA pressure and secondary changes in the pulmonary circulation. The hemodynamic hallmark of severe MS is the presence of a diastolic gradient between the LA and LV, which persists at end diastole. The LA pressure trace is marked by a prominent *a*-wave in the presence of sinus rhythm. A prominent *v*-wave may be present in longstanding MS due to decrease in atrial compliance. Left-ventricular end diastolic

pressure is usually normal in MS but, when elevated, points to the presence of LV systolic or diastolic dysfunction. Gorlin's formula can be used to calculate the valve area with fair accuracy but is unreliable in the presence of significant MR. Acute MR is an important complication of PTMC and can be easily diagnosed in the catheterization laboratory from a careful inspection of the LA pressure trace. Elevated PA pressures are expected to fall immediately after a successful PTMC, although normalization may take more time in patients with greater severity of MS and severe PAH to begin with.

REFERENCES

1. Walston A, Kendall ME. Comparison of pulmonary wedge and left atrial pressure in man. *Am Heart J* 1973;86:159–64.
2. Lange RA, Moore DM, Jr, Cigarroa RG, Hillis LD. Use of pulmonary capillary wedge pressure to assess severity of MS: Is true left atrial pressure needed in this condition? *J Am Coll Cardiol* 1989;13:825–31.
3. Nishimura RA, Rihal CS, Tajik AJ, Holmes DR Jr. Accurate measurement of transmitral gradient in patients with MS: A simultaneous catheterization and Doppler echocardiography. *J Am Coll Cardiol* 1994;24:152.
4. Park S, Ha JQ, Ko YG et al. Magnitude of left atrial v wave is the determinant of exercise capacity in patients with MS. *Am J Cardiol* 2004;94:243–5.
5. Ha JW, Chung N, Jang Y et al. Is the left atrial v wave the determinant of peak pulmonary artery pressure in patients with pure MS? *Am J Cardiol* 2000;85:986–91.
6. Prioli A, Marino P, Lanzoni L et al. Increasing degrees of left ventricular filling impairment modulate left atrial function in humans. *Am J Cardiol* 1998;82:756–61.
7. Meisner JS, Keren G, Pajaro OE et al. Atrial contribution to ventricular filling in MS. *Circulation* 1991;84:1469–80.
8. Karthikeyan G. The value of rhythm control in MS. *Heart* 2006;92:1013–16.
9. Eleid M, Nishimura R, Lennon R, Sorajja P. Left ventricular diastolic dysfunction in patients with MS undergoing percutaneous mitral balloon valvotomy. *Mayo Clin Proc* 2013;88(4):337–44.

10. Gash AK, Carabello BA, Cepini D et al. Left ventricular ejection performance and systolic muscle function in patients with MS. *Circulation.* 1983;67(1):148–54.

11. Fleming HA, Wood P. The myocardial factor in mitral valve disease. *Br Heart J* 1959;21:117–22.

12. Gorlin R, Gorlin SG. Hydraulic formula for calculation of the area of the stenotic mitral valve, other cardiac valves, and central circulatory shunts. *Am Heart J* 1951;41:1–29.

13. Nishimura RA, Otto CM, Bonow RO, Carabello BA, Erwin JP, Guyton RA et al. 2014 AHA/ACC guideline for the management of patients with valvular heart disease. *J Am Coll Cardiol* 2014;63(22):e57–e185.

14. Hakki AH, Iskandrian AS, Bemis CE et al. A simplified formula for the calculation of stenotic cardiac valve areas. *Circulation* 1981;63:1050–5.

15. Beyer RW, Olmos A, Bermudez RF, Noll HE. Mitral valve resistance as a hemodynamic indicator in MS. *Am J Cardiol* 1992;69:775–9.

16. Kapoor A, Kumar S, Shukla A, Tewari S, Garg N, Goel P, Sinha N. Determinants of left atrial pressure in rheumatic MS: Role of left atrial compliance and "atrial stiffness." *Indian Heart J* 2004;56:27–31.

17. Thomas JD, Wilkins GT, Choong CY, Abascal VM et al. Inaccuracy of mitral pressure half-time immediately after percutaneous mitral valvotomy. Dependence on transmitral gradient and left atrial and ventricular compliance. *Circulation* 1988;78:980–93.

18. Yasuda S, Nagata S, Tamai J et al. Left ventricular diastolic pressure-volume response immediately after successful percutaneous transvenous mitral commissurotomy. *Am J Cardiol* 1993;71:932–7.

19. Palacios JF, Block PC. Atrial septal defect during percutaneous mitral valvotomy (PMV): Immediate results and follow-up (abstract). *Circulation* 1988;78(suppl II):II–529.

20. Cequier A, Bonan R, Serra A, Dyrda I, Crepeau J, Dethy M, Waters D. Left-to-right atrial shunting after percutaneous mitral valvuloplasty. Incidence and long-term hemodynamic follow-up. *Circulation* 1990;81:1190–7.

21. Wilkinson JL. Haemodynamic calculations in the catheter laboratory. *Heart* 2001;85:113–20.

22. Shrivastava S, Mathur A, Dev V, Saxena A, Venugopal P, Sampathkumar A. Comparison of immediate hemodynamic response to closed mitral commissurotomy, single-balloon, and double-balloon mitral valvuloplasty in rheumatic MS. *J Thorac Cardiovasc Surg* 1992;104:1264–7.

23. Dev V, Shrivastava S. Time course of changes in pulmonary vascular resistance and the mechanism of regression of pulmonary arterial hypertension after balloon mitral valvuloplasty. *Am J Cardiol* 1991;67:439–42.

24. Fawzy ME, Hassan W, Stefadouros M, Moursi M, El Shaer F, Chaudhary MA. Prevalence and fate of severe pulmonary hypertension in 559 patients with severe MS undergoing mitral balloon valvotomy. *J Heart Valve Dis* 2004;13:942–8.

25. Bahl VK, Chandra S, Talwar KK, Kaul U, Sharma S, Wasir HS. Balloon mitral valvotomy in patients with systemic and supra-systemic pulmonary artery pressures. *Cath Cardiovasc Diagn* 1995;36:211–5.

PART 3

Management

10

Assessment of severity and treatment strategy

RAVI S. MATH

ASSESSMENT OF SEVERITY

The assessment of severity of any valvular pathology is based on the development of symptoms or complications as well as the severity at which intervention improves symptoms.[1] Cardiac surgery has favorably altered the course of the natural history of mitral stenosis (MS). However, the natural history studies of MS that predated the arrival of cardiac surgery have been primarily based on symptomatology rather than on an assessment of severity of MS based on mitral valve area (MVA).[2] It could not be assessed whether the the symptoms developed due to progression of disease or due to other secondary sequelae. Some of the complications of MS

such as atrial fibrillation (AF) and stroke have been shown not to be consistently related to the severity of MS. Similarly, the exact level of left atrial (LA) pressure at which pulmonary edema may develop in an individual varies and is further modified by lymphatic drainage. Paul Wood had noted in his seminal paper on MS: "Certainly pulmonary edema was just as likely to occur in a patient with an average or relatively large orifice (provided it was within the critical range) as with extreme stenosis; auricular fibrillation, hemoptysis, and systemic embolism were also indifferent to the size of the orifice."[3] As such, the grading of MS, although intuitive, is to some extent arbitrary. The classification of MS as mild, moderate, and severe is based on theoretical thresholds of pulmonary edema at a certain cardiac output, heart rate, and MVA. It should be emphasized that the mitral valve gradient is directly proportional to the square of mitral flow in diastole (cardiac output) and inversely proportional to the time in diastole (heart rate). Thus, even patients with mild MS may develop pulmonary edema. With this background, it is essential to remind ourselves that the management of MS should not be based solely on arbitrary cut-off values of MVA but rather on the hemodynamic and symptomatic status of the individual patient. MS should be viewed as a disease spectrum.

Clinical stages and mitral valve area

The normal MVA is 4–6 cm^2.[4] A mitral valve (MV) gradient is rare in patients with a MVA >2 cm^2. In the past, MS was classified as mild, moderate, and severe using MVA cut-offs of >1.5 cm^2, and 1–1.5 cm^2, and <1 cm^2, respectively (Table 10.1).[5] A MVA of >2 cm^2 was considered very mild MS.[6] Some authorities denoted moderate and severe MS as significant MS (MVA <1.5 cm^2).[7] It was noted that symptomatic patients with MS could have a valve area of >1 cm^2.[8] Their mean pulmonary artery pressure (PAP) and pulmonary capillary wedge pressure (PCWP) were high, both at rest and exercise (albeit lower than those with MVA <1 cm^2).[8] These patients (i.e., those with MVA >1 cm^2) derived the same benefit from percutaneous transvenous mitral commissurotomy (PTMC)

as those with a MVA of <1 cm^2. There was a similar improvement in hemodynamics, exercise time, functional class, and event-free survival in both groups. This has led to a reclassification of MS (Table 10.2).[1] A new staging system has been proposed similar to the heart failure staging system. Patients are classified as being in Stage A to D, ranging from at-risk patients (Stage A) to progressive obstruction (Stage B), to severe asymptomatic (Stage C), and symptomatic MS (Stage D). The definition of "severe" MS has now been based on the severity at which symptoms occur and at a level when interventional treatment improves symptoms. Severe MS has now been defined as ≤1.5 cm^2, unlike previous guidelines, where it was ≤1.0 cm^2. Patients with a MVA of ≤1.0 cm^2 are considered to have very severe MS. This makes comparisons with historical cohorts problematic.

The calculation of MVA is performed by transthoracic echocardiography (TTE). Traditionally, this has relied upon planimetry by two-dimensional TTE.[9] Planimetry is performed at the tips of the MV leaflets. This requires an expert echocardiographer as changes in the depth or angle of the ultrasound beam can significantly overestimate the MVA. Further, planimetry may not be feasible in patients with a poor echocardiographic window or heavy calcifications. Some of these limitations may be overcome using three-dimensional echocardiography (3D echo). This underscores the need for due diligence while performing the echo with appropriate attention paid to the MV gradients, the pulmonary artery pressure, and the left- and right-ventricular functions while assessing the severity of MS. In some patients with non-diagnostic echocardiographic studies or where there is a discordance between clinical and echocardiographic findings, cardiac catheterization is needed.

Clinical evaluation

The evaluation of a patient with MS begins with a thorough history and physical examination. Clinical evaluation can diagnose moderate to severe MS with an accuracy of 92%.[6] The electrocardiogram and chest X-ray are extremely useful in supporting the clinical diagnosis as well as in assessing any complications. Patients with severe MS may be asymptomatic whereas patients with mild MS may become symptomatic in the setting of anemia, infection, pregnancy, or AF with

---

Table 10.1 Mitral stenosis severity as per ACC/AHA 2006 guidelines[a]

Mild MS	MVA >1.5 cm^2, mean gradient <5 mmHg,[a] PASP <30 mmHg
Moderate MS	MVA 1–1.5 cm^2, mean gradient 5–10 mmHg,[a] PASP 30–50 mmHg
Severe MS	MVA <1.0 cm^2, mean gradient >10 mmHg,[a] PASP >50 mmHg

Source: Data from Bonow RO et al., Circulation 2006; 114:e84–231.

[a] Valve gradients are dependent upon transvalvular flow. The gradients suggested in this table assume a normal cardiac output and may not pertain to patients with abnormally high or low transvalvular flows. Criteria are applicable when HR is between 60–90 bpm. MVA: mitral valve area.

Table 10.2 Stages and severity of mitral stenosis

Stage	Definition	Valve anatomy	Valve hemodynamics	Hemodynamic consequences	Symptoms
A	At risk of MS	Mild diastolic valve doming	Normal transmitral flow velocity	None	None
B	Progressive MS	1. Rheumatic valve changes with commissural fusion and diastolic doming of the mitral valve leaflets 2. Planimetered MVA >1.5 cm²	1. Increased transmitral flow velocities 2. MVA >1.5 cm² 3. Diastolic pressure half-time <150 ms	1. Mild-to-moderate LA enlargement 2. Normal pulmonary pressure at rest	None
C	Asymptomatic severe MS	1. Rheumatic valve changes with commissural fusion and diastolic doming of the mitral valve leaflets 2. Planimetered MVA ≤1.5 cm² with very severe MS (MVA ≤1.0 cm² with very severe MS)	1. MVA ≤1.5 cm² (MVA ≤1.0 cm² with very severe MS) 2. Diastolic pressure half-time ≥150 ms (diastolic pressure half-time ≥220 ms with very severe MS)	1. Severe LA enlargement 2. Elevated PASP >30 mmHg	None
D	Symptomatic severe MS	1. Rheumatic valve changes with commissural fusion and diastolic doming of the mitral valve leaflets 2. Planimetered MVA ≤1.5 cm²	1. MVA ≤1.5 cm² (MVA ≤1.0 cm² with very severe MS) 2. Diastolic pressure half-time ≥150 ms (diastolic pressure half-time ≥220 ms with very severe MS)	1. Severe LA enlargement 2. Elevated PASP >30 mmHg	1. Reduced exercise tolerance 2. Exertional dyspnea

Source: Nishimura RA et al., J Am Coll Cardiol 2014;63:e57–185.

fast ventricular rates. More often, a symptomatic patient will have significant MS.

Physical findings suggestive of severe MS are a short A2-opening snap (OS) interval (<0.08 secs) and a long diastolic murmur (especially with pre-systolic accentuation) and evidence of pulmonary hypertension (loud P2 and parasternal heave) in absence of other causes.[4,6] The ECG may show LA enlargement, right axis deviation, right-ventricular hypertrophy with or without AF.[4,6] The chest X-ray may show evidence of LA enlargement (as a double atrial, shadow, straightening of left-heart border, or widening of carinal angle), pulmonary venous hypertension (as equalization/cephalization of blood flow, interstitial or alveolar edema) and pulmonary arterial hypertension (as dilated pulmonary artery or right-ventricular enlargement).[4,6] In a scenario where the physical or radiologic findings are suggestive of severe MS and the echocardiographic findings are discordant, it is essential to reconsider the echocardiographic findings or to look for precipitating factors.

MANAGEMENT STRATEGY

The management strategy of MS depends on the symptomatic status of the patient and the MVA (Figures 10.1 and 10.2).

Asymptomatic patient with mitral valve area of >1.5 cm²

Asymptomatic or minimally symptomatic patients with MS have a ten-year survival rate of 80%, with 60% showing no progression.[2,10,11] Thus, in an asymptomatic patient with documented mild MS (MVA >1.5 cm², mean gradient <5 mm), no further work-up is needed.[1] A history, physical examination, chest X-ray, and ECG should be obtained at yearly intervals. An echocardiogram may be obtained at three-to-five-year intervals or whenever there is a change in symptom status or clinical evaluation. Ambulatory ECG recording (24-hour Holter or event recorder) is indicated in patients with palpitations to detect paroxysmal AF.

Asymptomatic patient with mitral valve area of 1.0–1.5 cm²

As mentioned previously, patients with a MVA of <1.5 cm² are now considered to have severe MS.

While some patients are genuinely symptomatic, other patients may be asymptomatic. Some patients may readjust their lifestyle to a more sedentary level or an elevated pulmonary vascular resistance and/or low cardiac output may prevent symptoms from occurring. In such patients, an exercise test with Doppler echocardiography is useful. This may be accomplished by supine bicycle or treadmill exercise.[1,5] Although most of the data are available with the latter, the former allows hemodynamic data to be obtained at various stages of exercise. Bicycle or arm ergometry exercise testing can also be done during cardiac catheterization. Objective limitation of exercise with a rise in pulmonary artery systolic pressure (PASP) of >60 mmHg, a transmitral gradient of >15 mmHg, or a PCWP of >25 mmHg with symptoms is an indication for percutaneous valvotomy.[5]

Patients with clinical evidence of pulmonary artery hypertension (PAH) have worse survival. Symptomatic patients with severe PAH have a mean survival of less than 3 years.[12] Given these poor outcomes, asymptomatic patients with PASP of >50 mmHg at rest may also be considered for PTMC if the anatomy is suitable.[5,7] Successful PTMC has been shown to reduce and normalize the elevated PA pressure in the majority of patients over long-term follow-up. The higher the PA pressure, the greater the reduction.

Should genuinely asymptomatic patients with MVA of 1–1.5 cm² be considered for PTMC? Theoretically, the argument is that intervention early in the course of the disease may alter the course of the disease by decreasing the likelihood of new-onset AF or an embolic event, which may often be the first manifestation of MS. Early in the course of the disease, the valve score is lower, the valves are more pliable, and there is less LA enlargement, enabling a more successful procedural outcome with PTMC.[4,13] One retrospective study evaluated the risk of deferring valvotomy (surgical) in patients with moderate MS without symptoms; 105 patients were followed up for a mean period of 4.5 years and approximately 21% (one-fifth) had an embolic event.[14] This study was in an era of surgical valvotomy and before the advent of routine anticoagulation for AF. Two studies have evaluated the role of PTMC (a less morbid procedure) in asymptomatic patients. In the first study, 237 patients in New York Heart Association (NYHA) class I–II with a mean age of 46 ± 12 years underwent

PTMC.[15] The mean valve area was 1.1 ± 0.2 cm^2 (≤ 1.5 cm^2 in all cases). PTMC was successful in 94% of cases with a mean post-procedure MVA of 1.9 ± 0.3 cm^2. The 20-year actuarial survival without re-intervention and in NYHA class I–II was $41 \pm 4\%$ and for patients older than 50 years it was $50 \pm 6\%$. On multivariate analysis, young age and a large MVA post procedure were predictors of good late functional outcomes. The second study consisted of 244 consecutive asymptomatic patients (mean age 51 ± 11 years) with moderate rheumatic MS (MVA 1–1.5 cm^2).[16] PTMC was performed in 108 patients and the rest were followed conservatively. PTMC was successful in 97% of patients. Over a median follow-up of 8.8 years, estimated actuarial 11-year event-free survival rate was $89 \pm 4\%$ and $69 \pm 5\%$ ($p < 0.001$) in the PTMC and conservative groups, respectively. This difference was not evident in those without AF or without previous embolism (discussed later). There was, however, a worsening of the echo score in the conservative group.

It is important to note that the operators in both these studies were highly skilled, with high success and low complication rates. There is an inherent bias in such observational studies. If at all, these results apply to high-volume centers with skilled operators in young patients with favorable valve morphology. However, currently, there are no randomized trials evaluating a strategy of early intervention vs. medical therapy in such asymptomatic patients. One needs to take into consideration the indolent natural history in asymptomatic patients, the rarity of sudden death and the small but definite possibility of iatrogenic complications including death or need for mitral valve replacement (MVR). Current guidelines do not recommend any intervention for patients who are genuinely asymptomatic except for those at high thromboembolic risk (discussed later).[1,7] A history, physical examination, chest X-ray, and ECG should be obtained at yearly intervals. An echocardiogram may be obtained at one-to-two-year intervals.

Asymptomatic patient with new-onset atrial fibrillation/embolic event (MVA 1.0–1.5 cm^2)

Approximately 40% of patients with MS develop AF.[1] The ten-year survival with AF is 25% as against 46% for those in sinus rhythm.[11] AF may develop as an isolated event in an otherwise-asymptomatic patient, but often heralds the onset of a symptomatic phase in MS. An embolic event may be the first manifestation of MS. Systemic embolism occurs in 10%–20% of patients, which again is related to the presence of AF.[1,10] Thus, it appears intuitive to intervene in patients with new-onset AF or those presenting with an embolic event.

Successful PTMC has not been shown to revert AF[17] but it has enabled patients to persist in sinus rhythm.[18] Further, in a subgroup of patients with AF (LA size <45 mm, duration of AF < one year), successful PTMC was associated with increased probability of cardioversion.[19] On the other hand, successful PTMC has been shown to have a favorable impact on certain risk factors that predispose to embolic events. There is a reduction in spontaneous echo contrast and LA size along with a reduction in coagulation activation in LA. In a prospective study, among the 402 patients in AF, PTMC was shown to be an independent negative predictor for systemic embolism.[20] In another prospective study of 244 asymptomatic patients[16] with moderate MS (MVA 1.0–1.5 cm^2), there were five embolic events among patients who underwent PTMC ($n = 106$) vs. 19 events in those who were followed conservatively ($n = 138$) over a median follow-up of 8.3 years. The estimated actuarial 11-year embolism rate was significantly lower in the PTMC group ($7 \pm 3\%$ vs. $23 \pm 4\%$, $p = 0.0013$) with a hazard ratio of 0.309 ($p = 0.02$). Thus, in asymptomatic MS patients with a MVA of <1.5 cm^2 who develop new-onset AF or have had an embolic event, PTMC may be performed in those with favorable valve anatomy (ACC 2014 Class 2b indication, ESC 2012 Class 2a indication). In such cases, PTMC should be preceded by four weeks of anticoagulant therapy and a transesophageal echocardiography (TEE) just before the procedure should rule out a thrombus in LA/LAA. The presence of dense spontaneous contrast has been shown to be the strongest predictor of thromboembolic events. Its presence is also an indicator for the need of PTMC. In patients with unfavorable anatomy for PTMC, MVR is not recommended in asymptomatic patients with new-onset AF/previous embolic event, given the morbidity and mortality associated with the procedure. One exception could be patients with repeated episodes of embolism.

Another indication for PTMC in this group are patients who are in need of a major non-cardiac surgery or those who wish to become pregnant. Both these situations are associated with increased heart rate, risk of blood loss, and fluid imbalance, which may precipitate pulmonary edema.

Asymptomatic patient with mitral valve area of <1.0 cm²

A MVA of <1.0 cm² has been termed as very severe MS.[1] As in the previous scenario (MVA 1–1.5 cm²), there are no studies comparing a strategy of early intervention vs. medical therapy and very few studies have evaluated the role of PTMC in such a scenario. However, it is generally accepted that there will be a true reduction in functional capacity at this valve area, even if not clinically obvious. Further, it is preferable to intervene before severe PAH occurs. Current guidelines recommend PTMC in asymptomatic patients with a MVA of <1.0 cm² with favorable valve anatomy.[1]

If the valve morphology is not suitable for PTMC, MVR is not recommended in asymptomatic patients given the morbidity and mortality associated with the procedure. Such patients should be followed up with a yearly echocardiogram. An exception here is an asymptomatic severe MS patient with severe PAH (PASP >60–80 mmHg), where MVR may be recommended to prevent right-heart failure.

Symptomatic patient with mild mitral stenosis (MVA >1.5 cm²)

Usually patients with mild MS are asymptomatic. There are some patients with mild MS who are symptomatic. This may occur due to various reasons. For a given valve area, the transmitral gradient may be higher in the obese or those with a large body surface area.[1,21] The relation of PCWP to MVA is also variable. Finally, there may be errors in the non-invasive assessment of MVA. When there is a discrepancy between the clinical symptoms and echocardiographic findings, exercise testing with Doppler or invasive hemodynamic assessment is recommended. Objective limitation of exercise with a rise in PASP of >60 mmHg, a transmitral gradient of >15 mmHg, or PCWP of >25 mmHg with symptoms is an indication for PTMC if the valve morphology is suitable. It is essential to rule out other causes for symptoms in such patients such as diastolic dysfunction, pulmonary embolism, etc.[21] Such patients should be managed medically.

There is currently no recommendation for PTMC for asymptomatic patients with mild MS and AF. These patients (mild MS with AF) may become symptomatic with rapid ventricular rates. With rapid ventricular rates, the MV gradients are higher and assessment of MVA by planimetry is difficult. In such patients, it is essential to control the ventricular rates and reassess the severity of MS. If the MVA is >1.5 cm² and the patient has become asymptomatic after rate control, such a patient should be managed medically. If such a patient remains symptomatic, an attempt to restore sinus rhythm should be made first.

Symptomatic patient with significant mitral stenosis (MVA <1.5 cm²)

Once symptoms develop, the prognosis of MS becomes poor if left untreated. The 10-year survival of NYHA class II, III, and IV was 69%, 33%, and 0%, respectively, among 271 symptomatic patients.[11] No medical therapy has been shown to relieve the mechanical obstruction in MS. The obstruction may be relieved by valvotomy or MVR. Valvotomy (surgical or percutaneous) relieves the stenosis by splitting the fused commissures, thereby reducing the transmitral gradient and increasing the MVA.

SELECTION OF TREATMENT STRATEGY

Valvotomy may be accomplished by surgical or percutaneous approach. Surgical valvotomy may be achieved by closed mitral valvotomy (CMV) or by open mitral valvotomy (OMV).

Closed mitral valvotomy

Closed mitral valvotomy is performed on a beating heart via a transatrial or transventricular route using a dilator across the mitral valve. Large series with long-term follow-ups have documented the role of CMV in favorably altering the natural history of MS. In 1964, Ellis et al. published a 12-year follow-up study of 1571 patients who underwent CMV.[22] The 10-year survival for Class III and IV patients was between 60% and 80%, a marked improvement compared to medical therapy. A study of 3724 consecutive patients from India found an actuarial survival rate of 93%, 89%, and 84% at 12, 18, and 24 years, respectively (99% of patients were in NYHA class III–IV at the time of surgery).[23] The indications for CMV are the same as for PTMC. A favorable valve anatomy is a prerequisite. However, the results of CMV are inferior to those of PTMC or OMV. This procedure continues to be performed in developing countries. It is indicated only if PTMC is not available or the technical expertise for PTMC is lacking. The presence of a LA/LAA thrombus and ≥ grade 3 mitral regurgitation (MR) is a contraindication.

Open mitral valvotomy

Open mitral valvotomy is performed under cardiopulmonary bypass. Its advantage over CMV is that it enables direct visual inspection of MV enabling direct splitting of commissures, splitting of fused chordae tendinae and papillary muscles, and debridement of calcific deposits. Thrombectomy with removal of LA thrombi and ligation/amputation of the LA appendage may be performed. Moderate to severe tricuspid regurgitation (TR) can be repaired, avoiding a prosthetic valve. Long-term successful outcomes have been reported with OMV with ten-year actuarial survival of 81%–90%.[24-26] MVR for restenosis was required in 7%–16% of patients over 10 years. Given the observational nature of these studies, their reporting is prone to bias. The procedure is dependent on the skills of the operating surgeon. Although MVR is a much simpler and more durable operation than OMV, MVR is associated with lower survival as compared with OMV (10-year survival of 98% vs. 93%) due to thromboembolism, anticoagulation-related complications, and other prosthetic valve-related complications that outweigh the durability of MVR.[27] OMV is indicated in patients who are in NYHA class III–IV when valve anatomy is unfavorable for PTMC (echo score >8, heavy calcification) or when PTMC cannot be performed (presence of LA/LAA clot). Given the morbidity and mortality associated with surgical commissurotomy, these procedures are not recommended for patients who are in NYHA class I or II except for those at high risk of thromboembolism or hemodynamic decompensation. Patients with an LA/LAA appendage clot in NYHA class I–II can be treated with anticoagulation for 2 to 6 months and reassessed for suitability for PTMC.[28] If a repeat TEE shows dissolution of the clot, PTMC may be performed. If the thrombus persists, surgery is performed. Recently, some centers have performed PTMC even in the presence of LA/LAA clot following a minimum six weeks of anticoagulation.

If MV cannot be repaired due to severe deformity or there is preexisting moderate to severe MR, MVR is indicated. In view of the morbidity and mortality associated with MVR and the potential long-term complications associated with a prosthetic valve such as prosthetic valve thrombosis, infective endocarditis, or hemorrhagic complications with anticoagulation, the threshold for MVR is higher than for PTMC. It is limited to NYHA class III and IV patients.[1] The operative mortality rate is between 4% and 7%,[29,30] but may reach as high as 11%.[29] The risk of surgery increases with NYHA class IV patients. Hence, it is important to avoid progression of these patients to NYHA class IV symptoms. Even if the patient does present in NYHA class IV, surgery should not be denied as the outlook without surgery is very poor. PTMC can be an alternative in such cases after careful discussion (see later discussion on PTMC). The type of valve inserted will depend on the patient's age and the risk of anticoagulation but is being progressively more dictated by patient choice. If the patient has longstanding AF and must be anticoagulated anyway, a mechanical valve may be inserted. On the other hand, a young patient in sinus rhythm may opt for a bioprosthetic valve to avoid the hazards of anticoagulation with an understanding of the need for future redo surgery for valve deterioration. A maze procedure may be performed at the time of MVR, although its success in a purely rheumatic population is less certain than in a non-rheumatic population. The indications for MVR are as follows: 1) severely symptomatic patients (NYHA class III/IV) with severe MS (MVA <1.5 cm^2) who are not high-risk for surgery and who are not candidates for, or have failed, previous PTMC (Class 1 indication); 2) patients with severe MS (MVA <1.5 cm^2) undergoing other cardiac surgery (e.g., aortic valve surgery, CABG, etc.) (Class 2 IIa indication); 3) mitral valve surgery and LAA excision may be considered for patients with severe MS (MVA ≤1.5 cm^2, stages C and D) with recurrent embolic events despite adequate anticoagulation (Class 2 IIb indication).

Percutaneous transvenous mitral commissurotomy

Percutaneous transvenous mitral commissurotomy (PTMC) was first performed by Inoue in 1984,[31] followed by Lock in 1985.[32] When compared to its surgical counterpart, PTMC is less traumatic; avoids the need for thoracotomy, general anesthesia, or blood transfusions; requires a shorter hospital stay[33,34]; and is less expensive (when hardware is reused).[33] Furthermore, PTMC can be repeated without additional risk, unlike repeat CMV or OMV, which are associated with higher morbidity and mortality. Today, PTMC is the procedure of choice for relieving MS with surgery being reserved for patients who are not candidates for PTMC or have failed PTMC.[1,7] Unlike surgical valvotomy, PTMC is indicated in NYHA class II patients as well, given the less morbid nature of the procedure. However, its effect on the natural history in NYHA class II patients is less clear. It may be performed antegrade via a transseptal route or retrograde using a steerable guidewire. It can be performed using an hourglass-shaped balloon (triple-lumen Inoue balloon or double-lumen Accura balloon), a single or double peripheral angioplasty balloon, or a reusable commissurotome/valvulotome. The three techniques produce a similar outcome, but the hourglass-shaped balloons are preferred.

PATIENT SELECTION

The selection of the optimal patient for PTMC is based on echocardiography. Various scores have been utilized to aid in the selection of the ideal patient. The Wilkins score has been most widely used. A score of <8 with no more than moderate MR is the best candidate for PTMC. However, this does not exclude patients with less favorable valve anatomy from PTMC.[1,7] Patients with higher scores can still achieve a good result but the success rates are lower. In such a scenario, it is essential to assess other clinical characteristics. Those patients who are at a high surgical risk may be offered PTMC despite unfavorable anatomic characteristics (e.g., elderly, kyphoscoliosis, renal failure, cardiac failure, chronic obstructive airway disease, etc.). As PTMC relieves MS by the splitting of commissures, bicommisural calcification is an absolute contraindication for PTMC. Other absolute contraindications are the presence of LA/LAA thrombus and presence of MR of grade 3–4 severity.[1,5] In patients with LA/LAA thrombus who are not in NYHA class III–IV or if the thrombus is not mobile or at an imminent risk of embolization, PTMC can be performed after anticoagulation for 2 to 6 months (discussed earlier).[28] PTMC is a relative contraindication if the obstruction is subvalvular without any commissural fusion.

INDICATIONS

The current indications for PTMC are as follows:[1]

1. Symptomatic patients (NYHA class II–IV) with severe MS (MVA ≤1.5 cm^2) (Class 1 indication) or asymptomatic patients with very severe MS (MVA ≤1.0 cm^2) (Class 2a indication) with a favorable valve morphology in the absence of LA thrombus and moderate-severe MR
2. Asymptomatic patients with severe MS (MVA ≤1.5 cm^2) with new-onset AF and suitable valve anatomy (Class 2b indication)
3. Symptomatic patients with MVA >1.5 cm^2 and hemodynamically significant MS during exercise (mean MV gradient >15, PCWP >25 mmHg) (Class 2b indication)
4. Severely symptomatic patients (NYHA class III–IV) with severe MS (MVA ≤1.5 cm^2) with suboptimal valve anatomy and high risk for surgery (Class 2b indication)

PTMC OUTCOMES

Successful PTMC has been defined as a post-procedure valve area of >1.5 cm^2 (without higher than grade 2 MR), in the absence of major complications that require emergency surgery.[1] Some studies have also utilized a 50% increase in the baseline area as a measure of success.[36] A number of studies enrolling a large number of patients have evaluated the success rates of PTMC[37-46] (Table 10.3). The results of these studies may not be entirely comparable on account of differences in age, clinical characteristics, and valve morphology. Studies from the United States and Europe had older patients, with greater co-morbidities and worse valve morphology as compared to studies from Asia or South America. While varying success rates have been reported, large cohorts have reported rates of greater than 90%. Successful PTMC results in a doubling of MVA[4,35,36] (from approximately 1 to 2 cm^2). There is a 50%–60% reduction in transmitral gradient and an immediate reduction in mean LA and PA pressure.[5] Even patients with systemic or suprasystemic PAP have an immediate significant drop in PAP after successful PTMC.[47] A reduction in PAP is associated with improvement in tricuspid regurgitation in some but not all patients. Mortality in experienced hands is rare (<1%). Cardiac tamponade rates are around 1% (Table 10.4). Severe MR remains the dreaded complication. Reported rates range from

Table 10.3 Acute outcomes after PTMC in large series

Author, Year	Country	Number	Age (years)	Success	Pre-PTMC MVA (cm^2)	Post-PTMC MVA (cm^2)
Palacios,[37] 1986–2000	Boston, USA	879	55 ± 15	71.7%	0.9 ± 0.3	1.9 ± 0.7
Lung,[38] 1986–1995	France	1514	45 ± 15	89	1.04 ± 0.23	1.92 ± 0.31
Tomai,[39] 1991–2010	Rome, Italy	527	55.3 ± 11.6	91.5	0.99 ± 0.2	1.9 ± 0.4
NHLBI,[40] 1987–1989	USA	738	54 ± 15	76	1.0 ± 0.3	2.0 ± 0.8
Ben Farhat,[41] 1987–1998	Tunisia	654	33.6 ± 13	98	1.0 ± 0.2	2.2 ± 0.4
Arora,[42] 1987–2000	Delhi, India	4850	27.2 ± 11.2	91	0.7 ± 0.2	1.9 ± 0.3
Fawzy,[43] 1989–2005	Saudi Arabia	562	31 ± 11	96.4	0.92 ± 0.17	1.95 ± 0.29
Manjunath,[44] 2005–2007	Bangalore, India	2622	26 ± 9	98	0.9 ± 0.2	1.9 ± 0.2
Sharma,[45] 1999–2005	Lucknow, India	2330	32 ± 11	93%	0.82 ± 0.15	1.69 ± 0.21
Chen,[46] 1985–1994	China	4832	36.8 ± 12.3	99.3	1.1 ± 0.3	2.1 ± 0.2

Table 10.4 Acute complications after PTMC

Author, Year	Country	Number	Death	Tamponade	Severe MR (MVR)	Thrombo-embolism
Palacios,[37] 1986–2000	Boston, USA	879	0.6	1	9.4 (3.3)	1.8
Lung,[38] 1986–1995	France	1514	0.4	0.3	3.4	0.3
Tomai,[39] 1991–2010	Rome, Italy	527	0.4	0.4	4.9 (4.9)	0.2
NHLBI,[40] 1987–1989	USA	738	1.6	4	3 (1.3)	4
Ben Farhat,[41] 1987–1998	Tunisia	654	0.4	Na (0.7)	5	1.5
Arora,[42] 1987–2000	Delhi, India	4850	0.2	0.2	1.4 (1.1)	0.1
Fawzy,[43] 1989–2005	Saudi Arabia	562	0	0.1	1.6	0.5
Manjunath,[44] 2005–2007	Bangalore, India	2622	0.19	1.52	1.22 (0.76)	0.6
Sharma,[45] 1999–2005	Lucknow, India	2330	0.5	0.6	5.4 (0.6)	0.2
Chen,[46] 1985–1994	China	4832	0.12	0.8	1.4	0.48

2%–10% with a need for urgent MVR in up to 5% of cases (<1% in experienced centers). It is mainly seen in those with unfavorable morphology and may be due to commissural, leaflet or chordal tears. It may be reduced by using a stepwise approach to balloon dilation and avoiding balloon entrapment in subvalvular structure. Atrial septal defect (ASD) following PTMC is common (66% by TEE) but most of these are small (mean diameter 4 mm).[48] Only 1%–2% have a significant ASD, and most ASDs close spontaneously by 6 months (residual ASD 8%).

The predictors of successful PTMC are multifactorial[36,38] with valve morphology being one of the most important. The parameters include echo score, extent and location of valve calcification, pre-procedure MVA, and pre-procedure degree of MR. Patient-related factors include gender (women have worse outcomes), age, NYHA class, previous commissurotomy, and AF. Procedural aspects include balloon size, type of balloon (hour-glass vs. double balloon), and operator experience.

In patients with unsuccessful PTMC, there is no or transient functional improvement. In patients with insufficient valve opening, cardiac surgery is required either immediately or on a deferred basis as per the patient's clinical status. Patients with severe MR in heart failure or cardiogenic shock need cardiac surgery on an emergent basis. Those who tolerate severe MR also have a poor outlook and cardiac surgery is often needed in a few weeks to months.

IMMEDIATE OUTCOMES IN PATIENTS WITH UNFAVORABLE MORPHOLOGY

Initial studies with PTMC in patients with unfavorable valve morphology indicated poor results, with success rate as low as 52%–64%.[49,50] These patients had higher rates of MVR or death on follow-up leading to a recommendation of MVR in such a group of patients. With accumulating experience and the use of the stepwise balloon dilatation technique, there has been an improvement in the results even among this group of patients. Bouleti et al.[51] noted a success rate of 80% in calcified valves (vs. 93% in noncalcified valves). Kumar et al.[52] noted a success rate of 93% in patients with severe subvalvular disease despite these patients having a lower valve area and higher PAP. However, patients with unfavorable anatomy have lower event-free

survival on long-term follow-up. Over a 12-year follow-up, survival with and without repeat intervention were lower in patients with an echo score >8 when compared with those with a score of <8 (82% vs. 57% and 38% vs. 22%, respectively).[37] In calcified valves, long-term survival at 20 years was 50% for calcified valves vs. 81% for non-calcified valves with good functional result noted in 12% and 38%, respectively.[51] Thus, while PTMC is associated with acceptable outcomes in patients with unfavorable anatomy, these patients need careful follow-up with greater need for MVR. On the other hand, if a patient with an unfavorable anatomy wishes to undergo MVR, the same may be offered to him/her.

LONG- AND VERY-LONG-TERM OUTCOMES OF OBSERVATIONAL STUDIES

Long-term results in patients with successful PTMC have been expressed in various parameters such as overall mortality, cardiovascular mortality, cardiovascular (CV) survival without cardiac surgery, CV survival without reintervention (i.e., without surgery or PTMC), and good functional class (CV survival without reintervention and in NYHA class I–II) (Tables 10.5 and 10.6).

Ten-year actuarial survival has ranged from 87% to 97%,[41,53] with survival without reintervention ranging from 67% to 80%.[41,53,54] Most of the patients remain in NYHA functional class I–II (approximately 60%).[53,55] At 20 years, overall and cardiovascular survival is 75%–86% and 85%–91%, respectively, for a mean age of 48–55 years at the time of intervention.[39,56,57] However, event rates start to increase. Cardiovascular survival without reintervention and cardiovascular survival without surgery was 38% and 46% at 20 years.[56,57] For patients younger than 50 years, these figures are 45% and 57%, respectively.[56,57] Thus, almost half of the patients remain free from surgery even at 20 years.

The most common reason for late functional deterioration is restenosis. Of patients with late functional deterioration, 97% have restenosis.[53] Restenosis is defined as a MVA of <1.5 cm² or a >50% loss of the initial gain in valve area. Studies have given varied results depending on patient characteristics. In older patients, it has been reported to occur in as high as 39% of patients at 7 years.[55] In younger patients, the ten-year actuarial probability

Table 10.5 Long-term results of large series with successful PTMC (10-year follow-up)[a]

Author, Year	Institution	Number[b]	Mean follow-up (years)	10-year overall actuarial survival	10-year survival without reintervention	Good functional class (NYHA I–II)	Restenosis (10-year actuarial)
Iung,[53] 1986–1995	France	912	4	87	67	61	12%
Ben Farhat,[41] 1987–1998	Tunisia	654	5 ± 3	97	72		16 (34)
Fawzy,[56] 1989–2003	Saudi Arabia	493	5		80		17 (32)
Hernandez,[57] 1989–1995[c]	Spain	561	3.2 1.9	95[c]	69	61	39

[a] Success definition: MVA of ≥1.5 cm^2 with MR of ≤2/4.
[b] Patients with successful PTMC.
[c] Seven-year outcomes.

Table 10.6 Very-long-term results of large series with successful PTMC (20-year follow-up)[a]

	Bouleti et al.[56,57]	Tomai et al.[39]	Fawzy et al.[43]
Number	912	482	547
Mean age	48	55.4	31
Follow-up (maximum years)	20	20	19
Follow-up (mean years)	12	11	9
Echo score	NA	7.9	8
Reintervention	38	33	31
Overall survival	75	86	
CV survival	85	91	
CV survival without reintervention	38	36	
CV survival without reintervention and in NYHA class I–II	33	21	28

[a] Success definition: MVA of ≥1.5 cm2 with MR of ≤2/4.

of restenosis is 22%–34%.[41,54] However, after 10 years, the rates tend to rise markedly. At 15 and 19 years, this rate is 48% and 74%, respectively, for younger patients.[58] Repeat PTMC has been performed after restenosis following surgical/percutaneous valvotomy.[59,60] Approximately one in four patients who need reintervention are suitable for repeat PTMC.[56] Success rates for reintervention vary from 82% to 93% in patients with suitable morphology.[59,60] Following a successful repeat PTMC, one out of three patients remain free from surgery for 20 years.[60]

The long-term predictors of poor outcome include older age, male sex, higher NYHA class at presentation, AF, a higher echo score (>8) and lower valve area (MVA <1.8 cm^2) after PTMC.[39,43,57] The degree of PAH and degree of TR before PTMC are inversely related to the immediate and long-term outcome of PTMC. A post-MVA of >1.8 cm^2 is associated with high event-free rates in the long term.[39,43,61]

Thus, similar to surgical series, PTMC has been associated with good very long-term outcomes. However, comparison with surgical series is difficult in view of differing clinical and morphological characteristics. Most surgical series enrolled younger patients with pliable valves and no calcification/subvalvular disease. There have been six randomized trials that have compared surgical and percutaneous mitral valvotomy.

RANDOMIZED CONTROLLED TRIALS OF PTMC VS. OMV/CMV

There have been six randomized trails that have compared PTMC with surgical valvotomy (Table 10.7).[62–67] Three trials compared PTMC with CMV,[62–64] two trials compared PTMC with OMV (Table 10.8),[65,66] and one trial compared PTMC, CMV, and OMV together.[67] The average age of patients enrolled in these trials was between 20 and 30 years, except for one trial that enrolled older patients (mean age 47–49 years).[66] All trials enrolled patients with pliable valves only.

Patel et al.[62] randomized 45 patients to PTMC vs. CMV. They noted that PTMC was associated with a greater increase in MVA (2.1 ± 0.7 cm^2 vs. 1.3 ± 0.3 cm^2) and greater increase in exercise time as compared with PTMC. The safety of PTMC and CMV were comparable.

Turi et al.[63] randomized 40 patients with severe MS to PTMC ($n = 20$) and CMV ($n = 20$). They noted a similar improvement in MVA with both procedures (1.6 ± 0.6 cm^2 vs. 1.6 ± 0.7 cm^2). This improvement was sustained and comparable at the eight-month follow-up. Once again, the safety of PTMC and CMV were comparable.

Arora et al.[64] randomly compared 100 patients undergoing PTMC to another 100 patients undergoing CMV (mean age 19 years). Both procedures led to similar improvement in post-procedure MVA (2.39 ± 0.9 cm^2 vs. 2.2 ± 0.9 cm^2 for PTMC and CMV, respectively). At a mean follow-up of 22 months, echocardiographic restenosis was low in both groups (5% vs. 4% in PTMC and CMV, respectively).

Reyes et al.[65] enrolled 60 patients in a randomized trial comparing PTMC ($n = 30$) with OMV ($n = 30$) with severe MS and favorable anatomy. Both PTMC and OMV resulted in similar improvement in MVA post-procedure (2.1 ± 0.6 cm^2 vs.

Table 10.7 Randomized trials of PTMC vs. CMV/OMV-immediate results

Author, Year	Procedure	Number	Age	Echo score	Post-procedure MVA (cm^2)	MR (%)	SE	Death
Patel et al.,[62] 1991	PTMC vs. CMV	23 vs. 22	30 vs. 26	6 vs. 6	2.1 ± 0.7 vs. 1.3 ± 0.3	4.3 vs. 4.5	0 vs. 0	0 vs. 0
Turi et al.,[63] 1991	PTMC vs. CMV	20 vs. 20	27 vs. 28	7.2 vs. 8.4	1.6 ± 0.6 vs. 1.6 ± 0.7	5 vs. 5	0 vs. 0	0 vs. 0
Arora et al.,[64] 1993	PTMC vs. CMV	100 vs. 100	19 vs. 20	NA	2.39 ± 0.94 vs. 2.2 ± 0.85	14 vs. 12		
Reyes et al.,[65] 1994	PTMC vs. OMV	30 vs. 30	30 vs. 31	6.7 vs. 7.0	2.1 ± 06 vs. 2.0 ± 0.6	6.6 vs. 0	0 vs. 0	0 vs. 0
Ben Farhat et al.,[67] 1998	PTMC vs. OMV vs. CMV	30 vs. 30 vs. 30	29 vs. 27 vs. 28	6.0 vs. 6.0 vs. 6.1	2.2 ± 0.4 vs. 2.2 ± 0.4 vs. 1.6 ± 0.4	3.3 vs. 0 vs. 0	0 vs. 0 vs. 0	0 vs. 0 vs. 0
Cotrufo et al.,[66] 1999	PTMC vs. OMV	111 vs. 82	46 vs. 49	7.6 vs. 8.1	1.84 ± 0.31 vs. 2.28 ± 0.33	2.7 vs. 0	0 vs. 0	0 vs. 0

Table 10.8 Randomized trials of PTMC vs. CMV/OMV-long-term results

Author, Year	Follow-up	Procedure	MVA	Restenosis	Reintervention	NYHA Class I
Reyes et al.,[65] 1994	3 years	PTMC vs. OMV	2.4 ± 0.4 vs. 1.8 ± 0.4	10 vs. 13	NA	72 vs. 57
Ben Farhat et al.,[67] 1998	7 years	PTMC vs. OMV vs. CMV	1.8 ± 0.4 vs. 1.8 ± 0.4 vs. 1.3 0.3	6.6% vs. 6.6% vs. 37%	10 vs. 7 vs. 50	87 vs. 90 vs. 33
Cotrufo et al.,[66] 1999	3 vs. 4 years	PTMC vs. OMV	2.05 ± 0.35 vs. 1.81 ± 0.33	28 vs. 18	12 vs. 4	67 vs. 84

2.0 ± 0.6 cm^2) with comparable safety. Over a follow-up of 3 years, the improvement in MVA area was more sustained in the PTMC group as compared to the OMV group (2.4 ± 0.4 cm^2 vs. 1.8 ± 0.4 cm^2). Restenosis rates were low and similar (three patients in PTMC and four in OMV group). Given the lower cost, avoidance of thoracotomy and the better MVA associated with PTMC, the authors concluded that PTMC should be preferred over OMV.

Ben Farhat et al.[67] conducted a prospective, randomized trial comparing PTMC vs. CMV vs. OMV with 30 patients in each group with severe pliable MS. There was a greater increase in MVA with PTMC and OMV (2.2 ± 0.4 cm^2 and 2.2 ± 0.4 cm^2) than (CMV 1.6 ± 0.4 cm^2). Residual MS (MVA <1.5 cm^2) occurred more commonly with CMV (0% with PTMC and OMV vs. 27% with CMV). There was no death and thromboembolism. There was no difference in MR. Patients were followed for 7 years, at which point echocardiographic MVA was similar after PTMC and OMV (1.8 ± 0.4 cm^2) and greater than after CMV (1.3 ± 0.3 cm^2; $p < 0.001$). Restenosis (MVA <1.5 cm^2) occurred in 6.6% after PTMC or OMV vs 37% after CMV. The authors concluded that PTMC and OMV give excellent and comparable results in the short and long term and are better than CMV. Given the lower cost and lack of thoracotomy and cardiopulmonary bypass, PTMC should be the treatment of choice.

Finally, Cotrufo et al.[66] randomized 193 patients to PTMC (111 cases) vs. OMV (82 cases). These patients were older than those enrolled in previous RCTs (mean age 46 and 49 years, study conducted in Italy). In contrast to all the previous studies, they noted a higher MVA with OMV as compared with PTMC (2.28 ± 0.33 cm^2 vs. $1.84 \pm$ 0.31 cm^2) immediately after the procedure. At a 3- to 4-year follow-up, the MVA continued to remain higher in the OMV group (2.05 ± 0.35 cm^2 vs. 1.81 ± 0.33 cm^2) and more patients in the OMV group had a lower NYHA functional class. Thus, the authors concluded that, while both procedures achieve good results with low complications, OMV should be preferred in view of the greater MVA in the long-term follow-up while PTMC should be reserved for high-risk surgical cases.

In summary, of the four trials that compared PTMC and CMV, two reported similar efficacy,[63,64] while two others noted greater post procedure MVA with PTMC.[62,67] This benefit of PTMC over CMV was sustained up to 7 years. Thus, clearly, when compared to CMV, PTMC is preferred. There could be some mechanistic reasons behind the unfavorable outcomes of CMV. The increase in MVA after CMV is by no means uniform or universal. The blades used in CMV open in one plane and apply pressure only at two diametrically opposite points on the mitral orifice.[67] On the other hand, the inflated balloon applies pressure uniformly on the overall mitral orifice. The balloon with its circumferential dilatation and radial stretching serves as a better dilator. In fact, Kaul et al.[68] compared the dilatation capabilities of the Inoue balloon and Tubbs' dilator by introducing them via the transventricular route on the operating table during CMV. The Inoue balloon achieved greater reduction in the transmitral gradient as compared to the Tubbs' dilator. Further, they noted that, on finger palpation, the Inoue balloon achieved more complete opening as compared to the Tubbs' dilator.

When PTMC was compared with OMV, of the three studies, one noted that PTMC achieved better results than OMV,[65] another noted similar results,[67] while the third noted better results

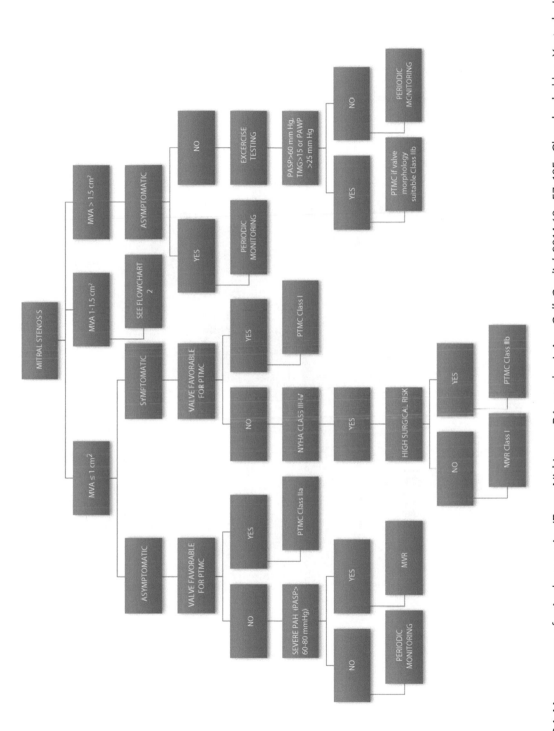

Figure 10.1 Management of mitral stenosis. (From Nishimura RA et al., *J Am Coll Cardiol* 2014;63:e57–185; Chandrashekhar Y et al., *Lancet* 2009;374:1271–83; Bonow RO et al., *Circulation* 2006;114:e84–231; Vahanian A et al., *Eur Heart J* 2012;33:2451–96.)

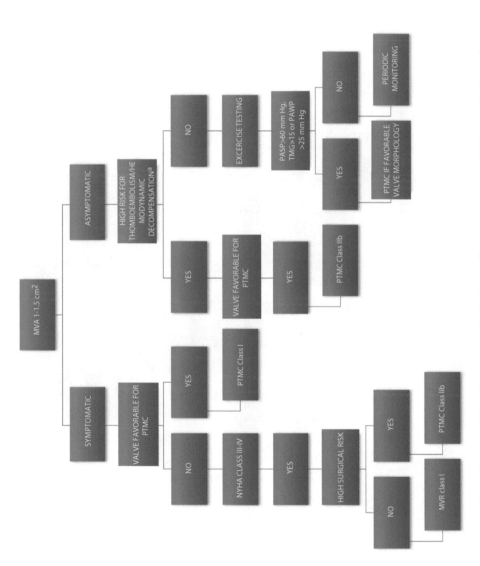

Figure 10.2 (continued from Figure 10.1). [a] Thromboembolic risk indicates new-onset AF, h/o embolism, dense spontaneous echo contrast in LA. Hemodynamic decompensation risk indicates PASP >50 mmHg at rest, need for major non-cardiac surgery, planned pregnancy. PTMC should be performed by experienced operators in such cases.

with OMV in terms of immediate post-procedure MVA.[66] The last study had older patients with a slightly higher MV echo score. While PTMC achieves commissural opening alone, OMV also ameliorates the aspect of leaflet thickening, rigidity, and subvalvular disease. It must be noted here that even in the third study,[66] long-term restenosis, reintervention, and survival were similar in the PTMC and OMV arms. Thus, given the avoidance of thoracotomy and cardiopulmonary bypass and similar efficacy, PTMC is preferred over OMV. However, in patients with very severe subvalvular disease, OMV is a good option. Figures 10.1 and 10.2 describe a flowchart for the approach to patients with mitral stenosis.

The PTMC technique and hardware has remained essentially unchanged over the past three decades. It has a steep learning curve. In high-volume centers with experienced operators, it has high success and low complication rates. While making recommendations for PTMC, this needs to be taken into consideration. Over the years, the indications of PTMC have expanded, encompassing patients with unfavorable anatomy and clinical characteristics. The systematic use of the stepwise Inoue technique, echo guidance, and cumulative experience with the procedure has ensured that, despite unfavorable anatomy, the results of PTMC have been maintained over the years.

CONCOMITANT VALVE DISEASE

Mitral regurgitation

As the rheumatic process may involve any of the four valves in any combination, mitral stenosis often co-exists with other valve involvement. Probably, the most common occurrence is the mixed mitral stenosis and regurgitation.[5] The two are never balanced and this may lead to a dilemma in choosing the optimum management strategy. The presence of LV volume overload indicates that MR is the dominant lesion, whereas if the LV volume is normal, MS tends to predominate. In the former, the high transvalvular flow leads to high transmitral gradient. This does not represent true severe MS. From an interventional standpoint, PTMC is the treatment of choice when significant MS co-exists with Grade 1–2 MR, while MR of Grade 3–4 is a contraindication for PTMC.

Successful PTMC has been performed in selected cases of Grade 3 MR when the MR jet is central. Finally, MVR/OMV remains a suitable option in the presence of severe MR with significant MS.

Tricuspid valve disease

Tricuspid regurgitation (TR) is an important concomitant lesion. It is often functional, resulting from dilatation of the right ventricle secondary to pulmonary hypertension. It tends to improve and often disappears after successful relief of MS.[69] At times, the TR does not regress and may lead to right-heart failure with increased long-term morbidity and mortality. There is some debate as to optimal management of patients with severe MS with severe functional TR. While MV surgery can address both issues simultaneously (MVR/repair with tricuspid valve [TV] annuloplasty), PTMC does not directly correct the TR. On the other hand, MV surgery is associated with increased morbidity and mortality. There are no randomized studies that have assessed this issue. One retrospective study evaluated 92 consecutive patients with severe MS and severe functional TR who underwent either PTMC ($n = 48$) or MVR with TV annuloplasty ($n = 44$).[70] Over a period of 57 months follow-up, there was no difference in mortality. However, there were seven cases of heart failure that needed surgical correction in the PTMC group (none in the surgical group). Mild/absent TR was noted in 98% of the surgical group vs. 46% in the PTMC group. There was also a greater reduction in RV size in the surgical arm. Multivariate analysis revealed that TV annuloplasty and sinus rhythm were predictors for improvement of TR. The authors concluded that the surgical option is preferred especially in the presence of AF or RV enlargement. A more practical approach would be to perform PTMC if the valve is pliable and to follow up the patient with regular TTE for regression of TR. If the TR persists, surgery (TV repair) should be performed. On the other hand, if the patient needs to undergo MV surgery, it is preferable to perform TV annuloplasty even if the TR is mild when the tricuspid annulus is dilated (>40 mm or >21 mm/m^2 BSA) or a prior recent history of right-heart failure.[1] In patients with severe organic TR with MS, surgery is the preferred option.

Coexisting rheumatic tricuspid stenosis (TS) can be addressed with balloon dilatation at the time of PTMC.[71] Coexisting tricuspid regurgitation (in addition to TS) secondary to severe PAH is not a contraindication to tricuspid valve dilation. However, coexisting severe TR due to organic tricuspid valve disease requires surgical correction.

Aortic valve disease

Combined mitral and aortic stenosis (AS) is relatively uncommon. MS protects the LV from increased wall stress imposed by AS. The low cardiac output in severe MS leads to a state of low-flow, low-gradient AS potentially leading to underestimation of the severity of AS. The history and symptoms in combined significant MS and AS are those of mitral stenosis.[72] Combined MS and AS is more common in females. Symptoms occur earlier and palpitations, dyspnea, and peripheral embolism are common. Angina and syncope are infrequent. The clinical signs of MS and AS may easily be discerned or one lesion may mask the other (often findings of AS mask MS).[72,73] Findings of MS such as loud S1, OS, and mid-diastolic murmur may be diminished or absent, being dominated by the harsh AS murmur. Likewise, the findings of AS such as late peaking pulse, heaving apex, systolic thrill, and systolic murmur may not be evident. At times, the murmur of AS may become evident only after control of heart failure. The recognition of severe AS in patients of severe MS is important while selecting patients for valvotomy. Sudden relief of MS may place a hemodynamic burden on the unprepared and previously protected LV, leading to heart failure. Urrichio et al. reported three patients who, following successful CMV, developed progressive heart failure and had a fatal outcome over 2 years from unrecognized or uncorrected AS.[74] Calculation of aortic valve area either by TTE (continuity equation) or cardiac catheterization is essential to assess the severity of AS in combined severe AS and MS. In combined severe AS and MS, it is essential that both the valves are addressed. Double valve replacement (DVR) appears to be one straightforward solution. While such a scenario is common, it needs to be emphasized that the operative mortality for DVR is substantial

(mortality double for DVR). Further, the long-term morbidity and mortality associated with DVR is significantly worse as compared to single valve replacement. Thus, if feasible, mitral valve repair (OMV/PTMC) associated with aortic valve replacement (AVR) appears to be an alternative to DVR. Percutaneous techniques have been used to address combined MS and AS. Simultaneous aortic and mitral balloon valvuloplasty has been performed if the anatomy of both valves is suitable.[75] Antegrade, retrograde, and combined antegrade-retrograde techniques have been described with good success rates. It needs to be stressed that the aortic valve in RHD is often calcified and regurgitant, making it unsuitable for balloon valvotomy. In such a case, percutaneous aortic valve replacement has been performed along with PTMC, if the surgical risk is prohibitive. Percutaneous replacement of both the aortic and mitral valves has also been reported when both the valves are severely calcified. When the AS is less than severe, PTMC alone is sufficient. The AS can be followed up until it becomes severe.

MS and aortic regurgitation (AR) often coexist. Some degree of AR is seen in 30% to 50% of patients of MS undergoing intervention, but severe AR is seen in only 10% of patients.[76] Combination of severe MS and severe AR have opposite loading effect on LV. As MS restricts LV filling, the increase in stroke volume associated with AR is blunted.[77] Wide pulse pressure and LV S3 are absent. The LV dimensions may be only mildly enlarged. All of these may lead to underestimation of AR severity. Further, AR leads to significant shortening of pressure half-time and overestimation of the MVA.[78] This overestimation increases with increasing grades of AR. Hence, planimetry rather than pressure half-time should be used to assess the MVA. The apical diastolic murmur may be mistaken for an Austin Flint murmur. For patients with mild-moderate AR with severe MS, PTMC is recommended.[79] Concomitant AR does not affect procedural success or patient outcome. On long-term follow up, only a minority of patients with moderate AR require AV surgery.[80] In patients with severe AR and severe MS, it is preferable to perform PTMC first rather than refer the patient for DVR, given the morbidity/mortality associated with the later. If symptomatic improvement occurs, AVR can be delayed. On the other hand, if LV dysfunction (LVEF <50%) or LV dilatation (LV end systolic diameter >50 mm) is present, both valves need to be addressed (DVR or AVR with OMV/PTMC).

REFERENCES

1. Nishimura RA, Otto CM, Bonow RO et al. American College of Cardiology/American Heart Association Task Force on Practice Guidelines. 2014 AHA/ACC guideline for the management of patients with valvular heart disease. *J Am Coll Cardiol* 2014;63:e57–185.

2. Selzer A, Cohn KE. Natural history of mitral stenosis: A review. *Circulation* 1972;45:878–90.

3. Wood P. An appreciation of mitral stenosis: II. Investigations and results. *Br Med J* 1954;1:1113–24.

4. Chandrashekhar Y, Westaby S, Narula J. Mitral stenosis. *Lancet* 2009;374:1271–83.

5. Bonow RO, Carabello BA, Kanu C et al. ACC/AHA 2006 guidelines for the management of patients with valvular heart disease. *Circulation* 2006;114:e84–231.

6. Rahimtoola SH, Durairaj A, Mehra A, Nuno I. Current evaluation and management of patients with mitral stenosis. *Circulation* 2002;106:1183–8.

7. Vahanian A, Alfieri O, Andreotti F et al. Guidelines on the management of valvular heart disease (version 2012). *Eur Heart J* 2012;33:2451–96.

8. Orrange S, Kawanishi D, Lopez B et al. Severe mitral stenosis with valve area >1.0 cm²? *Eur Heart J* 1998;19(suppl):15319Abst.

9. Baumgartner H, Hung J, Bermejo J et al. American Society of Echocardiography; European Association of Echocardiography. Echocardiographic assessment of valve stenosis: EAE/ASE recommendations for clinical practice. *J Am Soc Echocardiogr* 2009;22:1–23.

10. Rowe JC, Bland EF, Sprague HB, White PD. The course of mitral stenosis without surgery: Ten- and twenty-year perspectives. *Ann Intern Med* 1960;52:741–9.

11. Olesen KH. The natural history of 271 patients with mitral stenosis under medical treatment. *Br Heart J* 1962;24:349–57.

12. Ward C, Hancock BW. Extreme pulmonary hypertension caused by mitral valve disease. Natural history and results of surgery. *Br Heart J* 1975;37:74–8.

13. Iung B, Gohlke-Bärwolf C, Tornos P et al. Working Group on Valvular Heart Disease. Recommendations on the management of the asymptomatic patient with valvular heart disease. *Eur Heart J* 2002;23:1253–66.

14. Bannister RG. The risks of deferring valvotomy in patients with moderate mitral stenosis. *Lancet* 1960;2:329–33.

15. Bouleti C, Iung B, Brochet E et al. What are long-term results of percutaneous mitral commissurotomy in patients with few or no symptoms? *Arch Cardiovasc Dis. Supplements* 2013;5:52–3.

16. Kang DH, Lee CH, Kim DH et al. Early percutaneous mitral commissurotomy vs. conventional management in asymptomatic moderate mitral stenosis. *Eur Heart J* 2012;33:1511–7.

17. Langerveld J, van Hemel NM, Kelder JC et al. Long-term follow-up of cardiac rhythm after percutaneous mitral balloon valvotomy. Does atrial fibrillation persist? *Europace* 2003;5:47–53.

18. Fawzy ME, Shoukri M, Al Sergani H et al. Favorable effect of balloon mitral valvuloplasty on the incidence of atrial fibrillation in patients with severe mitral stenosis. *Catheter Cardiovasc Interv* 2006;68:536–41.

19. Hu CL, Jiang H, Tang QZ et al. Comparison of rate control and rhythm control in patients with atrial fibrillation after percutaneous mitral balloon valvotomy: A randomised controlled study. *Heart* 2006;92:1096–1101.

20. Chiang CW, Lo SK, Ko YS et al. Predictors of systemic embolism in patients with mitral stenosis. A prospective study. *Ann Intern Med* 1998;128:885–9.

21. Sorajja P, Borlaug BA. Severe heart failure in the setting of relatively mild mitral stenosis: The role of invasive hemodynamic assessment. *Catheter Cardiovasc Interv* 2008;72:739–48.

22. Ellis LB, Harken DE. Closed valvuloplasty for mitral stenosis: A twelve-year follow-up study of 1571 patients. *N Engl J Med* 1964;270:643–50.

23. John S, Bashi VV, Jairaj PS et al. Closed mitral valvotomy: Early results and long-term follow-up of 3724 consecutive patients. *Circulation* 1983;68:891–6.

24. Halseth WL, Elliott DP, Walker EL et al. Open mitral commissurotomy. A modern re-evaluation. *J Thorac Cardiovasc Surg* 1980; 80:842–8.

25. Kay PH, Belcher P, Dawkins K, Lennox SC. Open mitral valvotomy: Fourteen years' experience. *Br Heart J* 1983;50:4–7.

26. Choudhary SK, Dhareshwar J, Govil A et al. Open mitral commissurotomy in the current era: Indications, technique, and results. *Ann Thorac Surg* 2003;75:41–6.

27. Cotrufo M, Renzulli A, Vitale N et al. Long-term follow-up of open commissurotomy vs bileaflet valve replacement for rheumatic mitral stenosis. *Eur J Cardiothorac Surg* 1997;12:335–9.

28. Silaruks S, Thinkhamrop B, Kiatchoosakun S et al. Resolution of left atrial thrombus after 6 months of anticoagulation in candidates for percutaneous transvenous mitral commissurotomy. *Ann Intern Med* 2004;104:101–5.

29. Reames BN, Ghaferi AA, Birkmeyer JD et al. Hospital volume and operative mortality in the modern era. *Ann Surg* 2014;260:244–51.

30. D'Agostino RS, Jacobs JP, Badhwar V et al. The Society of Thoracic Surgeons Adult Cardiac Surgery Database: 2017 update on outcomes and quality. *Ann Thorac Surg* 2017;103:18–24.

31. Inoue K, Owaki T, Nakamura T et al. Clinical application of transvenous mitral commissurotomy by a new balloon catheter. *J Thorac Cardiovasc Surg* 1984;87:394–402.

32. Lock JE, Khalilullah M, Shrivastava S et al. Percutaneous catheter commissurotomy in rheumatic mitral stenosis. *N Engl J Med* 1985;313:1515–18.

33. Reyes VP, Raju BS, Wynne J et al. Percutaneous balloon valvuloplasty compared with open surgical commissurotomy for mitral stenosis. *N Engl J Med* 1994;331:961–7.

34. Ben FM, Ayari M, Maatouk F et al. Percutaneous balloon vs surgical closed and open mitral commissurotomy: Seven-year follow-up results of a randomized trial. *Circulation* 1998;97:245–50.

35. Carabello BA. Modern management of mitral stenosis. *Circulation* 2005;112:432–7.

36. Nunes MC, Nascimento BR, Lodi-Junqueira L et al. Update on percutaneous mitral commissurotomy. *Heart* 2016;102:500–7.

37. Palacios IF, Sanchez PL, Harrell LC et al. Which patients benefit from percutaneous mitral balloon valvuloplasty? Prevalvuloplasty and postvalvuloplasty variables that predict long-term outcome. *Circulation* 2002;105:1465–71.

38. Iung B, Cormier B, Ducimetiere P et al. Immediate results of percutaneous mitral commissurotomy. A predictive model on a series of 1514 patients. *Circulation* 1996;94:2124–30.

39. Tomai F, Gaspardone A, Versaci F et al. Twenty-year follow-up after successful percutaneous balloon mitral valvuloplasty in a large contemporary series of patients with mitral stenosis. *Int J Cardiol* 2014;177:881–5.

40. The National Heart, Lung, and Blood Institute Balloon Valvuloplasty Registry. Complications and mortality of percutaneous balloon mitral commissurotomy. *Circulation* 1992;85:2014–24.

41. Ben-Farhat M, Betbout F, Gamra H et al. Predictors of long-term event-free survival and of freedom from restenosis after percutaneous balloon mitral commissurotomy. *Am Heart J* 2001;142:1072–9.

42. Arora R, Kalra GS, Singh S et al. Percutaneous transvenous mitral commissurotomy: Immediate and long-term follow-up results. *Catheter Cardiovasc Interv* 2002;55:450–6.

43. Fawzy ME, Shoukri M, Fadel B et al. Long-term (up to 18 years) clinical and echocardiographic results of mitral balloon valvuloplasty in 531 consecutive patients and predictors of outcome. *Cardiology* 2009;113:213–21.

44. Manjunath CN, Srinivasa KH, Ravindranath KS et al. Balloon mitral valvotomy in patients with mitral stenosis and left atrial thrombus. *Catheter Cardiovasc Interv* 2009;74:653–6.

45. Sharma J, Goel PK, Pandey CM et al. Intermediate outcomes of rheumatic mitral stenosis post-balloon mitral valvotomy. *Asian Cardiovasc Thorac Ann* 2015;23:923–30.

46. Chen CR, Cheng TO. Percutaneous balloon mitral valvuloplasty by the Inoue technique: A multicenter study of 4832 patients in China. *Am Heart J* 1995;129:1197–1203.

47. Bahl VK, Chandra S, Talwar KK et al. Balloon mitral valvotomy in patients with systemic and suprasystemic pulmonary artery pressures. *Cathet Cardiovasc Diagn* 1995;36:211–5.

48. Manjunath CN, Panneerselvam A, Srinivasa KH et al. Incidence and predictors of atrial septal defect after percutaneous transvenous mitral commissurotomy – a transesophageal echocardiographic study of 209 cases. *Echocardiography* 2013;30:127–30.

49. Tuzcu EM, Block PC, Griffin B et al. Percutaneous mitral balloon valvotomy in patients with calcific mitral stenosis: Immediate and long-term outcome. *J Am Coll Cardiol* 1994;23:1604–9.

50. Post JR, Feldman T, Isner J, Herrmann HC. Inoue balloon mitral valvotomy in patients with severe valvular and subvalvular deformity. *J Am Coll Cardiol* 1995;25:1129–36.

51. Bouleti C, Iung B, Himbert D et al. Relationship between valve calcification and long-term results of percutaneous mitral commissurotomy for rheumatic mitral stenosis. *Circ Cardiovas* Interv 2014;7:381–9.

52. Sreenivas Kumar A, Kapoor A, Sinha N et al. Influence of sub valvular pathology on immediate results and follow up events of Inoue balloon mitral valvotomy. *Int J Cardiol* 1998;67:201–9.

53. Iung B, Garbarz E, Michaud P et al. Late results of percutaneous mitral commissurotomy in a series of 1024 patients. Analysis of late clinical deterioration: Frequency, anatomic findings, and predictive factors. *Circulation* 1999;99:3272–8.

54. Fawzy ME, Hegazy H, Shoukri M et al. Long-term clinical and echocardiographic results after successful mitral balloon valvotomy and predictors of long-term outcome. *Eur Heart J* 2005;26:1647–52.

55. Hernandez R, Banuelos C, Alfonso F et al. Long-term clinical and echocardiographic follow-up after percutaneous mitral valvuloplasty with the Inoue balloon. *Circulation* 1999;99:1580–6.

56. Bouleti C, Iung B, Himbert D et al. Reinterventions after percutaneous mitral commissurotomy during long-term follow-up, up to 20 years: The role of repeat percutaneous mitral commissurotomy. *Eur Heart J* 2013;34:1923–30.

57. Bouleti C, Iung B, Laouénan C et al. Late results of percutaneous mitral commissurotomy up to 20 years: Development and validation of a risk score predicting late functional results from a series of 912 patients. *Circulation* 2012;125:2119–27.

58. Fawzy ME. Long-term results up to 19 years of mitral balloon valvuloplasty. *Asian Cardiovasc Thorac Ann* 2009;17:627–33.

59. Iung B, Garbarz E, Michaud P et al. Percutaneous mitral commissurotomy for restenosis after surgical commissurotomy: Late efficacy and implications for patient selection. *J Am Coll Cardiol* 2000;35:1295–1302.

60. Bouleti C, Iung B, Himbert D et al. Long-term efficacy of percutaneous mitral commissurotomy for restenosis after previous mitral commissurotomy. *Heart* 2013;99:1336–41.

61. Song JK, Song JM, Kang DH et al. Restenosis and adverse clinical events after successful percutaneous mitral valvuloplasty: Immediate post-procedural mitral valve area as an important prognosticator. *Eur Heart J* 2009;30:1254–62.

62. Patel JJ, Shama D, Mitha AS et al. Balloon valvuloplasty vs closed commissurotomy for pliable mitral stenosis: A prospective hemodynamic study. *J Am Coll Cardiol* 1991;18:1318–22.

63. Turi ZG, Reyes VP, Raju BS et al. Percutaneous balloon vs surgical closed commissurotomy for mitral stenosis: A prospective, randomized trial. *Circulation* 1991;83:1179–85.

64. Arora R, Nair M, Kalra GS, Nigam M, Khalilullah M. Immediate and long-term results of balloon and surgical closed mitral valvotomy: A randomized comparative study. *Am Heart J* 1993;125:1091–4.

65. Reyes VP, Raju BS, Wynne J et al. Percutaneous balloon valvuloplasty compared with open surgical commissurotomy for mitral stenosis. *N Engl J Med* 1994;331:961–7.

66. Cotrufo M, Renzulli A, Ismeno G et al. Percutaneous mitral commissurotomy vs open mitral commissurotomy: A comparative study. *Eur J Cardiothorac Surg* 1999;15:646–51.

67. Ben Farhat M, Ayari M, Maatouk F et al. Percutaneous balloon vs surgical closed and open mitral commissurotomy: Seven-year follow-up results of a randomized trial. *Circulation* 1998;97:245–50.

68. Kaul A, Bhattacharya S, Borker S et al. Transventricular mitral valve dilator: An improved design concept. *J Thorac Cardiovasc Surg* 1995;110:856–9.

69. Skudicky D, Essop MR, Sareli P. Efficacy of mitral balloon valvotomy in reducing the severity of associated tricuspid valve regurgitation. *Am J Cardiol* 1994;73:209–11.

70. Song H, Kang DH, Kim JH, Park KM et al. Percutaneous mitral valvuloplasty vs surgical treatment in mitral stenosis with severe tricuspid regurgitation. *Circulation* 2007;116(11 Suppl):I246–50.

71. Bahl VK, Chandra S, Goel A et al. Versatility of Inoue balloon catheter. *Int J Cardiol* 1997;59:75–83.

72. Katznelson G, Jreissaty RM, Levinson GE et al. Combined aortic and mitral stenosis: A clinical and physiological study. *Am J Med* 1960;29:242–56.

73. Morrow AG, Awe WC, Braunwald E. Combined mitral and aortic stenosis. *Br Heart J* 1962;24:606–12.

74. Uricchio JF, Likoff W. Effect of mitral commissurotomy on coexisting aortic-valve lesions. *N Engl J Med* 1957;256:199–204.

75. Pillai AA, Ramasamy C, Saktheeshwaran M et al. Balloon valvuloplasty in rheumatic aortic valve stenosis: Immediate and long-term results. *Cardiovasc Interv Ther* 2015;30:45–50.

76. Unger P, Rosenhek R, Dedobbeleer C, Berrebi A, Lancellotti P. Management of multiple valve disease. *Heart* 2011;97:272–7.

77. Gash AK, Carabello BA, Kent RL et al. Left ventricular performance in patients with coexistent mitral stenosis and aortic insufficiency. *J Am Coll Cardiol* 1984;3:703e11.

78. Flachskampf FA, Weyman AE, Gillam L et al. Aortic regurgitation shortens Doppler pressure half-time in mitral stenosis: Clinical evidence, in vitro simulation and theoretic analysis. *J Am Coll Cardiol* 1990;2:396e404.

79. Chen CR, Cheng TO, Chen JY et al. Percutaneous balloon mitral valvuloplasty for mitral stenosis with and without associated aortic regurgitation. *Am Heart J* 1993;125:128e37.

80. Sanchez-Ledesma M, Cruz-Gonzalez I, Sanchez PL et al. Impact of concomitant aortic regurgitation on percutaneous mitral valvuloplasty: Immediate results, short-term, and long-term outcome. *Am Heart J* 2008;156:361–6.

11

Medical management

RAJNISH JUNEJA AND NEERAJ PARAKH

INTRODUCTION

Mitral stenosis (MS) is essentially a mechanical obstruction, which is unrelieved by any form of medical therapy. However, patients with milder and asymptomatic disease can be managed with some supportive therapy. In addition, reduction in symptoms like dyspnea and palpitations can be achieved by at least one grade in NYHA class II and III patients with severe MS awaiting mechanical relief. Similarly, patients with advanced pregnancy who for various reasons are not candidates for percutaneous transvenous mitral commissurotomy (PTMC) could receive palliative therapy with drugs. However, many experts believe in a fairly significant incidence of "flash" pulmonary edema during pregnancy and thus prefer intervention over medical management for pregnant MS patients. Prevention of progression of MS and preventing restenosis after surgical or percutaneous valvotomy by drug therapy is an approach that has not been systemically explored. There have been some attempts to modify the natural history of MS through the use of drugs to suppress fibrosis, inflammation, and calcification, but overall evidence is scarce.[1,2] Similarly, valve calcification is not a simple marker of "disease duration," as many patients even in their second or third decade of life present with significant valvular calcification, whereas others may never show calcification over the valve leaflets or commissures. The reasons for "juvenile MS" are also unexplored, as well as why such patients invariably have advanced subvalvular disease.

Currently, the aim of medical therapy for MS is to reduce recurrences of rheumatic fever, provide prophylaxis for infective endocarditis, reduce symptoms of pulmonary congestion (breathlessness, cough), control the ventricular rate and reduce thromboembolic complications (Table 11.1). In general, the guiding principles for the management of congestive heart failure, rheumatic heart disease (RHD), infective endocarditis, thromboembolism, etc., need to be followed and these are discussed in specific sections (see Chapters 6 and 18). Specific therapy for MS, especially the need for heart rate control to optimize diastolic filling time, is needed due to the characteristic hemodynamic implications of MS. Exercise testing may sometimes be of help in deciding about the need for intervention in a borderline patient who has no symptoms and a valve area bordering 1.5 cm^2.

Table 11.1 Medical therapy for mitral stenosis

Aim	Drug
Lifestyle modification	Salt restriction Limited exercise
Secondary prevention of rheumatic fever	Benzathine penicillin I/M; alternatives: penicillin V, sulfadiazine, erythromycin (only for proven severe allergic reactions with injectable penicillin or non-availability)
Infective endocarditis prophylaxis	Recommended only if prosthetic mitral valve or associated mitral regurgitation
Decongestion	Thiazides, frusemide, torsemide, spironolactone (only if symptoms dictate)
Heart rate control	β-blockers, preferably metoprolol succinate; alternatives: diltiazem, verapamil, digoxin, ivabradine
Disease modification	No definitive therapy. ? Statins

EXERCISE TESTING

Patients with MS exhibit a certain degree of dynamic valve reserve. This dynamic reserve is defined as the maximum exercise burden that the stenotic orifice is able to sustain before clinical symptoms or hemodynamic impairment becomes evident. Exercise testing provides additional information in asymptomatic patients or in patients in whom MS severity and symptoms do not seem to correlate. Decisions regarding intervention versus continuation of medical therapy needs exercise testing in these patients. The resting transmitral gradient and pulmonary arterial pressure may not necessarily reflect the actual severity of the disease. It is debatable whether the severity of MS should be expressed as mitral valve area or as pressure gradients across the valve. While expressing area as an anatomical measurement does not give any further information about its functional status, there are no clear cutoff values of gradients at which one can grade the severity of MS, especially because gradients are highly heart rate-dependent and, even in severe MS, heart rates of <50 bpm could actually decrease the end diastolic gradient to as low as 5 mmHg. However, it is generally agreed that obstructions are better expressed as resistance.[3]

Exercise testing may provide the necessary clues in determining the severity of MS, assessing its hemodynamic impact and explaining exercise-induced symptoms. Objective limitation of exercise with a rise in pulmonary artery systolic pressure (PASP) of >60 mmHg, a transmitral gradient of >15 mmHg, or a pulmonary capillary wedge pressure (PCWP) of >25 mmHg with symptoms are indications for intervention in otherwise-asymptomatic patients with MS.[4] Asymptomatic patients with a mitral valve area (MVA) between 1.0 and 1.5 cm^2 and symptomatic patients with mild MS (MVA >1.5 cm^2) require exercise testing for determining management strategy. It is essential to rule out other causes for symptoms in these patients, such as anemia, diastolic dysfunction, pulmonary embolism, and occasionally left-ventricular systolic dysfunction.[5] In addition, stress testing is useful in evaluating women with MS who are contemplating pregnancy.[6] As mentioned earlier, results of exercise testing should be interpreted with caution. Exercise leads to an increase in cardiac output, that in turn causes more blood to flow across the mitral valve every minute. The increase in blood flow itself can lead to an increase in the MVA. It is not very clear as to how much a diseased calcified stenotic mitral valve can actually open, especially with valvular and often severe tunnel-like subvalvular stenosis. However, a rise in gradients is often impressive even with minimal increase in heart rates and can provide invaluable information vis-à-vis management.

DIET AND ACTIVITY

The patient may be asked to decrease his/her salt intake if pulmonary vascular congestion is severe. In general, current diuretics have enough potency to take care of the excess sodium load incurred in normal diets and, hence, strict dietary restriction of salt is not required. In most patients with MS, recommendations for exercise are symptom-limited. Patients should be encouraged to pursue a low-level aerobic exercise program for maintenance of cardiovascular fitness.[4] Many patients with mild MS will remain symptom-free even with strenuous exercise. Those with very severe MS may have sudden, marked exercise-induced elevations in left-atrial pressure precipitating pulmonary edema. The long-term sequelae of repeated exercise-induced elevation in left-atrial pressure and pulmonary venous hypertension are well characterized in terms of pulmonary interstitial changes and, in extreme cases, alveolar edema and hemorrhage. Subsequent elevation of pulmonary arterial pressure (that is in general always reversible, unlike severe precapillary hypertension) often leads to right-ventricular hypertrophy and functional tricuspid regurgitation, which gradually resolve after a successful mitral valve dilatation.[7,8]

SECONDARY PREVENTION OF RHEUMATIC FEVER

Since rheumatic heart disease is the most common etiology for MS, secondary prevention for rheumatic fever is an essential part of treatment. It is unclear how much MS progression can be delayed by regular secondary prophylaxis. Regular secondary prophylaxis reduces the clinical severity and mortality of mitral regurgitation (MR), prevents involvement of other valves, and decreases the chance of developing MR over pre-existent MS. The progression of MS is a complex process related mostly to the turbulence generated at the valve and subvalvular level. Progressive subvalvular disease and calcification could be related to rheumatic fever recurrence, but there is a lack of clear documentation in prospective studies. Intramuscular benzathine penicillin reduces streptococcal pharyngitis by 71%–91% and reduces recurrent rheumatic fever by 87%–96%.[9] Table 11.2 describes various antibiotic regimens for secondary prevention of rheumatic fever. Patients with persistent valvular disease should receive prophylaxis for 10 years after the last episode of acute rheumatic fever or until 40 years of age, whichever is longer. Some high-risk patients may require longer

Table 11.2 Antibiotic regimens for secondary prevention of rheumatic fever

Antibiotic	Dose Child (≤27 kg)	Dose Adult (or >27 kg)	Route of administration
Benzathine penicillin	6 MU[a] Every two weeks	1.2 MU Every three weeks[b]	Single deep intramuscular injection
Penicillin V	–	250 mg BD	Oral
For penicillin allergy			
Sulfonamide: "sulfadiazine"	500 mg OD	1000 mg OD	Oral
For sulfonamide or penicillin allergy			
Erythromycin	–	250 mg BD	Oral
Azithromycin[c]	6 mg/kg OD (up to 250 mg)	250 mg OD	Oral

[a] For children, Indian recommendations are for administration every two weeks.[10]

[b] In a high-risk population, administration every three weeks is justified and recommended in populations in which the incidence of rheumatic fever is particularly high and those who have recurrent acute rheumatic fever despite adherence to an every-four-weeks regimen.

[c] Limited data; should exercise caution while using alternative antibiotics, as streptococci may develop resistance against penicillin, that has not happened in the last 70 years of its use.

(even lifelong) prophylaxis, depending upon the severity of valvular disease and the potential for exposure to group A streptococci.

DECONGESTION

Diuretics reduce left-atrial pressure and pulmonary congestion. They help in ameliorating symptoms of breathlessness, cough, and hemoptysis. Thiazide (hydrochlorthiazide) and loop (frusemide, torsemide) diuretics may be used depending upon the degree of congestive symptoms. Excessive use of diuretics will impair cardiac output by decreasing the preload of the already undefiled left ventricle. It is important to understand that diuretics offer only symptomatic benefit. Indiscriminate use of diuretics in all patients of severe MS as a strategy to prevent complications of fluid overload has never been shown to improve long-term survival. In fact, given the likelihood of potassium loss with overzealous diuresis, it may harm the patient. The addition of spironolactone not only potentiates the diuresis but also helps in potassium homeostasis. The disease-modifying role of spironolactone is not established in MS.

HEART RATE CONTROL

Even though there have been no large-scale prospective studies of appropriate heart rate (HR) control in MS with normal sinus rhythm (NSR) or atrial fibrillation (AF), it is generally appreciated that the control of ventricular response of AF is important in improving the patient's symptoms, especially fatigue and dyspnea. Even in patients with sinus rhythm, optimal control of ventricular rate (resting rates close to 60/min and exercise rates ≥100 bpm) with β-blockers is an important adjunct in the management of symptoms. Theoretically, the logic of slowing heart rates is obvious—a longer diastolic filling period decreases end diastolic and mean diastolic gradients, thus decreasing left-atrial pressure and pulmonary venous hypertension. Since left-ventricular systolic function in the majority of patients with MS is normal, the negative inotropic effect of β-blockers is of little consequence. Patients with mild MS rarely have any symptoms, while exercise may cause symptoms in moderate MS. Such patients could also be candidates

for ventricular rate control. In general, we prefer to use long-acting metoprolol succinate taken once or twice daily to achieve target heart rates; β-blockers obviate the need for diuretics in such patients. Even in patients with severe MS awaiting intervention, HR control is useful as a temporary measure for adequate relief in symptoms (improve by at least one grade). The symptoms of pulmonary venous congestion in MS are highly dependent on the diastolic filling period. Negative chronotropic agents prevent an increase in HR and thus improve the diastolic filling period.[11-13] Catheterization studies with β-blockers have demonstrated a reduction in left-atrial pressure and PCWP in patients with MS at rest and during exercise, but their effect on cardiac output and maximum O_2 consumption has been unpredictable.[14,15] Any possible improvement in the cardiac output, because of better ventricular filling, is countered by negative inotropic and negative chronotropic effect of β-blockers. A greater dependence on sympathetic drive for the maintenance of effective cardiac output in MS may be one of the mechanisms. Thus, complex interplay of various factors is responsible for the variable effect of HR control in patients with MS. The results from clinical studies with HR controlling agents have shown that despite a reduction in exercise HR in patients with MS and sinus rhythm, the effect on effort tolerance remains unpredictable (Table 11.3).[16-23] Patient selection in these studies has been quite heterogeneous, and explains the contradictory results of effect of HR control on effort tolerance in MS. Studies with patients having good baseline effort tolerance showed no further benefit with use of β-blockers,[18-20] whereas studies with patients having poor baseline effort tolerance showed beneficial effect with use of β-blockers.[21-23] Use of β-blockers in selected patients with MS and sinus rhythm, whose symptoms worsen markedly with exercise, is a Class 2b recommendation. Selective sinus node-blocking agents like ivabradine has also been compared with β-blockers. In two studies it was better than β-blockers in improving effort tolerance while in the other two studies its effect was neutral (Table 11.4).[24-27] Ivabradine is at least as good as β-blockers in HR control and improving effort tolerance in patients with mild to moderate MS and may be used if β-blockers are contraindicated/not tolerated. Therapeutic utility of digoxin and calcium channel blockers in

Table 11.3 Various studies in mitral stenosis and sinus rhythm with rate controlling drugs

Study	N	Study design	Drug	Exercise time[a]			Maximum HR (beats/min)		
				Baseline	Drug	p value	Baseline	Drug	p value
Klein et al. 1985[16]	13	Placebo-controlled, crossover	Atenolol, 100 mg OD	9 + 2	11 + 2	0.0015	127 + 17	93 + 16	0.0015
Bassan et al. 1987[17]	10	Double-blind, crossover	Propranolol, 80–120 mg/day	283 + 26 s	274 + 25 s	NS	151 + 6	115 + 5	<0.01
Misra et al. 1989[18]	43	Open-label, crossover	Atenolol, 100 mg OD	12.1 + 4.6	13.5 + 4.1	NS	180 + 29.6	127.7 + 20.3	<0.01
			Verapamil, 80 mg TID	12.1 + 4.6	13.9 + 5.2	NS	180 + 29.6	162.2 + 20.5	<0.05
Ahuja et al. 1989[22]	10	Open-label, crossover	Digoxin, 0.25 mg BD	6.7 + 1.8	8.1 + 2.4	NS	153.7 + 21.5	141.6 + 14.3	NS
			Metoprolol, 100 mg BD	6.7 + 1.8	11.4 + 2.7	<0.01	153.7 + 21.5	126.8 + 11.3	<0.01
			Verapamil, 80 mg TID	6.7 + 1.8	9.0 + 2.7	<0.05	153.7 + 21.5	147.7 + 7.7	<0.05
Patel et al. 1995[19]	19	Double-blind, crossover	Atenolol 100 mg od/Acebutolol 400 mg od	9.2 + 1.8	8.8 + 1.7	NS	171 + 12	135 + 22	<0.01
Mardikar et al. 1995[23]	50	Placebo-controlled, crossover	Atenolol, 100 mg OD	5.0 + 1.41	8.8 + 1.49	<0.001	138 + 11	108 + 12	<0.01
Stoll et al. 1995[20]	15	Double-blind, crossover	Atenolol, 50 mg OD	12.0 + 4.3	10.8 + 4.0	NS	144 + 15	113 + 23	<0.01
			Atenolol, 100 mg OD	12.0 + 4.3	11.3 + 4.4	NS	144 + 15	103 + 21	<0.01
Alan et al. 2002[21]	40	Diltiazem vs. atenolol, randomized	Diltiazem, 60 mg TID	534 + 120 s	570 + 126 s	NS	172.9 + 5.5	167.07 + 14.8	NS
	40		Metoprolol, 50 mg BD	452 + 120 s	520 + 90 s	<0.05	173 + 216.4	161 + 19	<0.05

[a] Time in minutes (unless specified).

Table 11.4 Studies comparing β-blockers versus ivabradine in mitral stenosis and sinus rhythm

Study	N	Study design	Drug	Exercise time/capacity[a]			Maximum HR (beats/min)		
				Baseline	Drug	p value	Baseline	Drug	p value
Parakh et al. (2012)[24]	50	Open-label, randomized, crossover	Atenolol, 50 mg OD;	410 ± 115 s	464 ± 113 s	0.001	170 ± 20	156 ± 22	0.001
			ivabradine 5 mg BD	410 ± 115 s	501 ± 100 s	0.001	170 ± 20	149 ± 17	0.001
			Atenolol vs. ivabradine			0.0009			0.04
Saggu et al. (2015)[27]	34	Open-label, crossover	Metoprolol, 100 mg BD	7.9 ± 1.6 min	10.3 ± 1.7 min	0.001	172 ± 23	130 ± 24	0.001
			Ivabradine 10 mg BD	7.9 ± 1.6 min	10.6 ± 1.6 min	0.002	172 ± 23	133 ± 24	0.001
			Atenolol vs. ivabradine			NS			NS
Rajesh et al. (2016)[26]	82	Open-label, randomized	Atenolol, 50 mg OD	290 ± 92 s	339 ± 100 s	0.0001	153 ± 14	163 ± 10	0.001
			Ivabradine 5 mg BD	298 ± 99 s	349 ± 103 s	0.0001	155 ± 11	163 ± 10	0.001
			Ivabradine vs. atenolol			NS			NS
Agrawal et al. (2016)[25]	97	Open-label, randomized	Metoprolol, 50 or 100 mg OD or BD	6.94 ± 0.79 METS	7.55 ± 0.84 METS	0.001	184 ± 11	152 ± 7	0.001
			Ivabradine 5–7.5 mg BD	6.69 ± 0.84 METS	8.09 ± 0.72 METS	0.001	186 ± 8	147 ± 7	0.001
			Metoprolol vs. ivabradine			0.001			0.001

[a] Exercise time in minutes or seconds, or exercise capacity in METS.

MS and normal sinus rhythm is not well established; these are sometimes used if β-blockers are not effective or contraindicated. Digoxin is useful when resting rates are high, while β-blockers are more effective in blunting the exercise-associated increase in heart rate. Digoxin may be more useful in patients with AF compared to sinus rhythm especially because of its vagotonic effect on the AV node. Digoxin potentiates the effect of β-blockers and this combination is useful in some patients of resistant AF wherein rate control is essential. Alternatively, one could use cardioversion to get sinus rhythm in a patient troubled with AF and fast rates. Slow pathway modification using radiofrequency ablation has been attempted by some investigators, but in general the success rates have been limited, especially on follow-up.

ENDOCARDITIS/INFLUENZA/PNEUMOCOCCAL PROPHYLAXIS

Antibiotic prophylaxis for infective endocarditis (IE) prevention is recommended for high-risk procedures in high-risk patients, such as patients with prosthetic heart valves or prosthetic material used for valve repair, or in patients with previous endocarditis. MS by itself (without MR or AR) is among the low-risk valvular heart disease for IE and antibiotic prophylaxis is not recommended except for those with prosthetic heart valve replacement for MS or previous endocarditis.[1] Maintenance of good oral hygiene and asepsis during invasive procedures should be reinforced. Influenza and pneumococcal vaccination may be used for severe cases.

DISEASE MODIFICATION

A retrospective analysis of 315 patients with rheumatic MS showed a significantly slower progression of MS in 35 patients treated with statins (0.027 cm^2/year) compared with 280 patients not taking statins (0.067 cm^2/year). These findings could have an important impact in the early medical therapy of patients with rheumatic heart disease.[2] Disease modification for MS or RHD needs further research. ACE inhibitors have been tried in patients with mitral stenosis and heart failure with some (unproven) benefit[28] Digoxin may be beneficial in patients in sinus rhythm who have associated right-sided heart failure.[29]

CONCLUSIONS

MS is essentially a mechanical problem requiring intervention in the advanced stages of disease. In patients in the early stages and those waiting for intervention, medical therapy with β-blockers may be helpful. Diuretics should not be prescribed as a routine, but given to only those patients who are significantly symptomatic. Secondary prevention for rheumatic fever is an essential component of rheumatic MS. IE prophylaxis is reserved for high-risk patients. Disease-modifying therapies, especially those with statins, need further studies.

REFERENCES

1. Boon NA, Bloomfield P. The medical management of valvar heart disease. *Heart* 2002;87:395–400.
2. Antonini Canterin F, Moura LM, Enache R, Leiballi E, Pavan D, Piazza R. Effect of hydroxymethylglutaryl coenzyme A reductase inhibitors on the long term progression of rheumatic mitral valve disease. *Circulation* 2010;121:2130–6.
3. El-Dosouky II, Meshrif AM. Role of the mitral valve resistance in evaluation of mitral stenosis severity. *J Med Diagn Meth* 2016;5:202.
4. Nishimura RA, Otto CM, Bonow RO et al. 2014 AHA/ACC Guideline for the management of patients with valvular heart disease: A report of the American College of Cardiology/American Heart Association task force on practice guidelines. *Circulation* 2014;129:521–643.
5. Sorajja P, Borlaug BA. Severe heart failure in the setting of relatively mild mitral stenosis: The role of invasive hemodynamic assessment. *Catheter Cardiovasc Interv* 2008;72:739–48.
6. Picano E, Pibarot P, Lancellotti P, Monin JL, Bonow RO. The emerging role of exercise testing and stress echocardiography in valvular heart disease. *J Am Coll Cardiol* 2009;54:2251–60.
7. Gorlin R. The mechanism of the signs and symptoms of mitral valve disease. *Br Heart J* 1954;16:375–80.
8. Kasalicky J, Huryck J, Widimsky R, Dejdar R, Metys R, Stanek V. Left heart haemodynamics

at rest and during exercise in patients with mitral stenosis. *Br Heart J* 1969;30:188–95.

9. Manyemba J, Mayosi BM. Penicillin for secondary prevention of rheumatic fever. *Cochrane Database Syst Rev* 2002; (3):CD002227.

10. Saxena A, Kumar RK, Gera RP, Radhakrishnan S, Mishra S, Ahmed Z. Working Group on Pediatric Acute Rheumatic Fever and Cardiology Chapter of Indian Academy of Pediatrics. Consensus guidelines on pediatric acute rheumatic fever and rheumatic heart disease. *Indian Pediatr* 2008;45:565–73.

11. Gorlin R, Haynes FW, Goodale WT, Sawyer CG, Dow JW, Dexter L. Studies of the circulatory dynamics in mitral stenosis. II. Altered dynamics at rest. *Am Heart J* 1951;41:30–45.

12. Gorlin R, Sawyer CG, Haynes FW, Goodale WT, Dexter L. Effects of exercise on circulatory dynamics in mitral stenosis. III. *Am Heart J* 1951;41:192–203.

13. Gorlin R, Lewis BM, Haynes FW, Spigel RJ, Dexter L. Factors regulating pulmonary capillary pressure in mitral stenosis. IV. *Am Heart J* 1951;41:834–54.

14. Bhatia ML, Shrivastava S, Roy SB. Immediate haemodynamic effects of a β-adrenergic blocking agent—propranolol—in mitral stenosis at fixed heart rates. *Br Heart J* 1972;34:638–44.

15. Kumar R, Saran RK, Dwivedi SK et al. Beneficial effects of long-term metoprolol therapy on cardiac haemodynamics in patients with mitral stenosis in sinus rhythm—A randomised clinical trial. *Indian Heart J* 1994;46:297–301.

16. Klein HO, Sareli P, Schamroth CL, Carim Y, Epstein M, Marcus B. Effects of atenolol on exercise capacity in patients with mitral stenosis with sinus rhythm. *Am J Cardiol* 1985;56:598–601.

17. Bassan MM, Michaeli J, Shalev O. Failure of propranolol to improve exercise tolerance in patients with mitral stenosis in sinus rhythm. *Br Heart J* 1987;58:254–8.

18. Misra M, Bhandari K, Thakur R, Puri VK. Failure of oral atenolol and verapamil to increase the capacity and duration of exercise in patients in sinus rhythm with mitral stenosis. *Int J Cardiol* 1989;23:37–41.

19. Patel JJ, Dyer RB, Mitha AS. β-adrenergic blockade does not improve effort tolerance in patients with mitral stenosis in sinus rhythm. *Eur Heart J* 1995;16:1264–8.

20. Stoll BC, Ashcom TL, Johns JP, Johnson JE, Rubal BJ. Effects of atenolol on rest and exercise hemodynamics in patients with mitral stenosis. *Am J Cardiol* 1995;75:482–4.

21. Alan S, Ulgen MS, Ozdemir K, Keles T, Toprak N. Reliability and efficacy of metoprolol and diltiazem in patients having mild to moderate mitral stenosis with sinus rhythm. *Angiology* 2002;53:575–81.

22. Ahuja RC, Sinha N, Saran RK, Jain AK, Hasan M. Digoxin or verapamil or metoprolol for HR control in patients with mitral stenosis— A randomised cross-over study. *Int J Cardiol* 1989;25:325–31.

23. Mardikar HM, Sahasrabhojaney VS, Jalgaonkar PD, Mahorkar UM, Mardikar MH, Waghmare BG. Long term effects of atenolol in patients of mitral stenosis & normal sinus rhythm. *Indian J Med Res* 1995;101:25–7.

24. Parakh N, Chaturvedi V, Kurian S, Tyagi S. Effect of ivabradine vs atenolol on HR and effort tolerance in patients with mild to moderate mitral stenosis and normal sinus rhythm. *J Card Fail* 2012;18:282–8.

25. Agrawal V, Kumar N, Lohiya B et al. Metoprolol vs ivabradine in patients with mitral stenosis in sinus rhythm. *Int J Cardiol* 2016;221:562–6;27420578.

26. Rajesh GN, Sajeer K, Sajeev CG et al. A comparative study of ivabradine and atenolol in patients with moderate mitral stenosis in sinus rhythm. *Indian Heart J* 2016;68:311–15.

27. Saggu DK, Narain VS, Dwivedi SK et al. Effect of ivabradine on HR and duration of exercise in patients with mild-to-moderate mitral stenosis: A randomized comparison with metoprolol. *J Cardiovasc Pharmacol* 2015;65:552–4.

28. Carabello BA. Modern management of mitral stenosis. *Circulation* 2005; 112:432–7.

29. Beiser GD, Epstein SE, Stampfer M, Robinson B, Brannwald E. Studies on digitalis: XVI/I: Effects of ouabain on the hemodynamic response to exercise in patients with mitral stenosis in normal sinus rhythm. *N Engl J Med* 1968;278:131–7.

Percutaneous transvenous mitral commissurotomy: Techniques and hardware

NEERAJ PARAKH AND RAVI S. MATH

INTRODUCTION

Percutaneous transvenous mitral commissurotomy (PTMC) is the current standard of care for rheumatic mitral stenosis (MS). It has also been termed "balloon mitral valvotomy," "percutaneous mitral valvotomy," or "percutaneous balloon mitral valvotomy." Various techniques for the percutaneous therapy of MS have evolved over the time but, currently, Inoue's technique is almost exclusively used the world over. The indications for PTMC have been covered in Chapter 10. Left-atrial (LA) thrombus, more than 2/4 mitral regurgitation (MR) and severe bicommissural calcification are the only absolute contraindications for PTMC. Other valvular diseases or coronary artery disease requiring surgery are also contraindications for PTMC. Relative contraindications include left-atrial appendage (LAA) thrombus, grade 2/4 MR, calcific valve, commissural calcification, significant subvalvular disease (SVD), and distorted anatomy. For the same degree of MR, a central jet of MR is more favorable for performing PTMC than an eccentric jet of MR. In this chapter, technical details and hardware used in routine PTMC will be discussed. Difficult scenarios will be dealt with in Chapter 13.

TECHNIQUES

Inoue's technique has gained popularity because of its safety and efficacy. This technique will be covered in detail whereas the basic principles of other techniques will be dealt in brief.[1]

Retrograde nontransseptal approach

Retrograde nontransseptal balloon mitral valvuloplasty was described by Stefanadis et al.[2] This involved the use of a specially designed, externally steerable LA guiding catheter by means of which entry into the LA is achieved retrogradely via the aorta and left ventricle (LV). Subsequently, a stiff 0.038″ exchange length J-tip wire was placed in the LA and stabilized by either forming loops in the LA or by introducing into a pulmonary vein. Mitral valvuloplasty was performed using a single or double (Mansfield) balloon over this wire. The disadvantages of this technique were the use of a large arterial sheath that can increase access site complications, risk of LV/LA perforation, and the risk of subchordal entanglement with resultant damage. As a result, this technique is rarely used today.[3]

Metallic commissurotomy

Metallic commissurotomy was developed on the principles of Tubb's dilator, used in closed mitral commissurotomy (CMV) by surgeons. This device can be used multiple times after sterilization and offers a low-cost percutaneous treatment for MS (Figure 12.1). Various studies have reported comparable acute and long-term results with this device.[4] However, the procedure is very demanding and there is a steeper learning curve for this device. One area of concern is the higher risk of LV perforation and pericardial tamponade.[5] At present, only a few operators/centers use this device.

Double balloon technique

The double balloon technique requires crossing the LV with two wires and then simultaneous inflation of two balloons over these wires for mitral valve (MV) dilatation. The premise of this technique is that two balloons will exert more focused pressure on the mitral valve commissures than a single balloon. This technique is more cumbersome and time-consuming than Inoue's technique and chances of

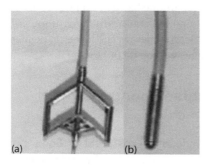

Figure 12.1 Metallic commissurotome in open **(a)** and closed **(b)** position.

LV perforation by the two wires or the balloon tip is a possibility. A multi-track system variant was devised by Bonhoeffer et al. to simplify the double-balloon valvuloplasty technique. With this system, one of the balloons is a rapid-exchange balloon, while the other has a conventional design, enabling both to be aligned in the mitral valve orifice over a single guidewire. The complexities involved with this system makes it a less preferred technique.[6]

INOUE'S TECHNIQUE

The Japanese surgeon Kanji Inoue developed a new dumbbell-shaped balloon in 1982 and successfully performed PTMC. Because of its safety, efficacy, and ease of technique, it is the most popular method used to perform percutaneous mitral valvotomy in the present era.[1]

Hardware

BALLOON

The original Inoue balloon was designed in 1982 and upgraded to a less compliant balloon in 1989. Subsequently, many Inoue-like balloons have entered the market. They work on the same basic principle as the original Inoue balloon but have minor variations in their design and manufacturing. These are less expensive than the Inoue balloon. The various balloons available are:

1. *Inoue*: Toray International, Tokyo, Japan
2. *Accura*: Vascular Concepts Ltd, Bengaluru, India
3. *SYM PBMV balloon*: Lifetech Scientific, China
4. *Synergy*: Advance Life Sciences Pvt Ltd, Delhi, India

The Inoue balloon is a dumbbell-shaped balloon that self-positions itself in the mitral valve because of its unique physical properties and mode of inflation. It has two latex layers with a nylon mesh in between, giving the balloon its unique shape and inflation characteristics. The shaft of the balloon is a 12F coaxial double-lumen catheter made up of polyvinyl chloride. The inner lumen of the catheter is used for the insertion of a metal tube, a guide wire (up to 0.032″) or a stylet and also for pressure measurements. The outer lumen connects proximally with a two-way stopcock and a vent (three proximal ports). These are used to connect the balloon to an inflation/deflation syringe. The vent also helps in deairing the balloon prior to use and serves as a safety mechanism in the event of deflation failure. In addition, there are two small holes in the balloon that allow slow seepage of contrast in case of deflation failure. The uninflated, unstreched balloon is 25 mm in length and it inflates in three sequential stages because of the specially designed synthetic mesh in the balloon. The distal end of the balloon inflates first, followed by the proximal half, with a constriction remaining in the middle to facilitate positioning across the mitral valve. Finally, at full inflation, the constriction disappears and the balloon assumes a more barrel-like shape with a maximal length of 45 mm. Several balloon sizes are available (20, 22, 24, 26, 28, and 30 mm in diameter), and each can be inflated in a 4-mm diameter zone. At the therapeutic level of inflation, the intra-balloon pressure ranges from 1 to 4 atmospheres depending on the size and degree of inflation of balloon. While performing stepwise balloon dilatation, it is important to understand the pressure zone of balloon inflation. The balloon pressure is in the low-pressure zone if the inflated balloon diameter is less than 2 mm of nominal balloon size, while it is in the high-pressure zone when the balloon diameter is within 2 mm of nominal balloon size. Intra-balloon pressure is in the range of 2–3 atmospheres in the low-pressure zone while it is around four atmospheres in the high-pressure zone. The Accura balloon provides higher and stable balloon pressure but the range of low-pressure dilatation is more with the Inoue balloon.[7] Inflations in the low-pressure zone result in

less mitral regurgitation than inflations in the high-pressure zone using a smaller-sized balloon. For example, a 26-mm balloon inflated to a diameter of 24 mm is in the low-pressure zone, whereas a 24-mm balloon inflated to 24 mm is in the high-pressure zone. For calcified and tough fibrotic valves and those with subvalvular deformity, high-pressure-zone inflation may be required. The balloon size for such patients should be one less than the calculated nominal size, which should then be inflated to its high-pressure-zone diameter. The Accura balloon, although manufactured on similar principles, has an 11F shaft (the Inoue balloon's is 12 F) and measures 80 cm in length. The Accura balloon lacks the additional vent and thus has only two proximal ports. There are no holes on the outer surface of the Accura balloon. Finally, the range of dilatation is 3 mm for the Accura balloon. The coiled-tip guide-wire and J-tipped stylet provided with the Accura balloon are less stiff than that of the Inoue balloon and provide lesser support (Figure 12.2).

BALLOON ACCESSORIES

- 80-cm balloon-stretching metal tube (0.032″ maximum inner lumen, silver color)
- 70-cm, 14F polyethylene dilator (black with tapering tip)
- 180-cm, 0.025″ stainless steel guide-wire with coiled floppy tip
- 80-cm, 0.038″ J-tipped spring wire stylet
- 30-mL plastic syringe and connecting tube
- Caliper for measuring balloon size

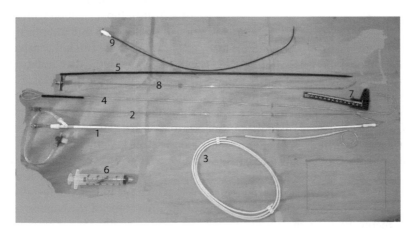

Figure 12.2 Accura PTMC balloon with accessories and septal puncture instruments. (1) Accura balloon; (2) balloon stretching stellate; (3) coiled wire; (4) J-tipped wire stylet; (5) septal dilator; (6) 30-mL syringe; (7) caliper; (8) Brockenbrough needle; (9) Mullin's dilator (without outer sheath).

SEPTAL PUNCTURE ACCESSORIES

- Brockenbrough needle
- 7F or 8F dilator catheter (Mullin's)
- Outer sheath catheter (optional)
- 0.032" hydrophilic or ordinary wire (preferably "J"-tipped)
- Pigtail catheter

Details and usage of accessories are discussed in the steps of PTMC.

Preprocedural evaluation

Prior to the PTMC procedure, the operator should personally review the echocardiogram. This helps to assess the MV anatomy, commissural fusion, valve thickness, calcification, submitral apparatus, degree of MR, presence of LA/LAA clot, and involvement of other valves. Further, the profile of the interatrial septum (IAS) (i.e., its orientation, bulge, thickness, aneurysm) and the relative size of the right and left atria should be evaluated. The operator can form a mental echocardiographic picture to anticipate potential difficulties in the performance of PTMC and take appropriate measures beforehand. The presence of an echocardiogram machine during the PTMC procedure is essential. It not only helps in the evaluation of success and complications of the PTMC procedure but guides the procedure as well. Even if echocardiogram has been done a few days prior, an on-table, preprocedure transthoracic or transesophageal echocardiogram is a must to rule out LA/LAA clot, which may form in the intervening period.

Patient preparation

The patient should be fasting overnight or for eight hours prior to operation; the fasting time should be shorter for children. Oral anticoagulation should be stopped three to four days prior to the procedure and INR on the day of procedure should be <1.5. Intravenous heparin infusion or low-molecular-weight heparin as per body weight is recommended during this period for patients with high thromboembolic risk. Many experienced operators have switched to performing PTMC without stopping anticoagulation (as in AF ablation). Other medications, such as β-blockers, calcium channel blockers, digoxin, and diuretics, may be continued. Patients with a fast ventricular rate require rate control with intravenous calcium channel blockers or beta blockers. Antibiotic prophylaxis is ideally not required. However, given the fact that most centers reuse the PTMC balloon, this is often practiced. The procedure is performed under local anesthesia and sedation is usually avoided. Although this may cause some patient discomfort, it facilitates neurological evaluation and early detection of stroke during the procedure. For uncooperative patients and children, sedation or even general anesthesia may be required. For very sick patients, who are unable to lie supine due to pulmonary edema and heart failure, elective endotracheal intubation is necessary.

Procedure

BALLOON PREPARATION

Diluted contrast (one part contrast and four parts saline) is used to prepare the Inoue balloon. Some centers use a dilution ratio of up to 1:9 (especially with the Accura balloon and ionic contrast agents) to avoid any deflation failure. The central lumen and side vent should be flushed to de-air the balloon. The balloon reference size is calculated on the basis of Hung's formula[8]:

$$\text{Balloon reference size (mm)} =$$
$$\frac{\text{Height (cm; rounded to nearest zero)}}{10} + 10$$

For example, if the patient's height is 152 cm, then the maximum balloon size that can be used is 150/10 + 10 = 25 mm. So, in this patient, we would use a 26-mm Inoue balloon with a maximum inflation diameter of 25 mm (the starting balloon diameter is usually less. This is discussed later in stepwise balloon dilatation). After inflating and measuring the balloon up to the desired size, the excess diluted contrast in the syringe is discarded (Figure 12.3). The balloon is then deflated with the contrast filled syringe attached to the inflation vent. Next, the balloon is stretched and slenderized using the 80-cm balloon stretching tube. The first step after inserting the metal tube into the central lumen of the balloon is to attach the hub of the metallic tube to the hub of the inner tube of the balloon (remember, "gold" and "silver" go together). This assembly should now be pushed further to be attached to the outer plastic balloon hub and rotated into the locked position (Figure 12.4). Coiled stainless steel wire should be

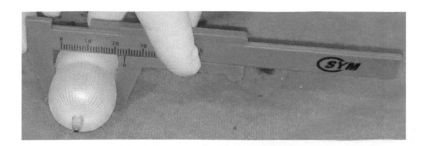

Figure 12.3 Measuring balloon size.

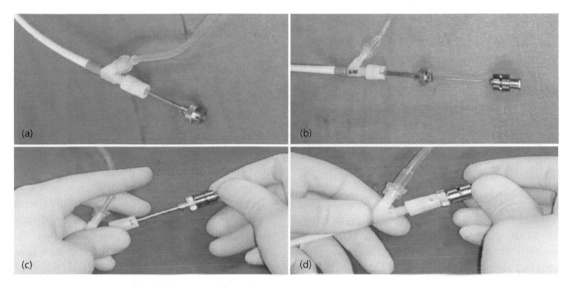

Figure 12.4 Tube stretching. **(a)** Balloon without inner stretching tube; **(b)** balloon with inner tube inserted; **(c)** inner tube attached to balloon tube hub; **(d)** gold-silver assembly attached to plastic balloon hub.

handled carefully as it is very long and stiff and may injure the operators or move out of the sterile area. The coiled end should be kept carefully in the insertion tool provided with the wire. Alternatively, the dilator of the vascular access sheath can be used as the insertion tool for the coiled wire.

VASCULAR ACCESS

The right femoral vein and artery are the preferred vascular access for PTMC. A 7F vascular sheath for the vein and a 5/6F sheath for the artery are commonly used. A long subcutaneous track can create resistance to the passage of the septal dilator/ PTMC balloon. In order to avoid this, the puncture needle should be kept more vertical than usual during the initial venous access (approximately 60° rather than 45°). In thinly built patients, the femoral vein will be superficial and hence it is best to start probing for the vein superficially rather than deep. Some operators (especially in the learning phase) take an additional left venous access for keeping a Swan-Ganz catheter in the pulmonary capillary wedge (PCW) position. This provides continuous hemodynamic monitoring during the procedure, an extra portal of venous access, and an anatomic landmark during LV entry.

CARDIAC CATHETERIZATION

Cardiac catheterization during PTMC has largely been replaced by echocardiography but it is still performed at many centers as a part of an academic exercise. Simultaneous pulmonary capillary wedge pressure (PCWP) and LV end diastolic pressure (LVEDP) provide the pressure gradient across the mitral valve. Femoral artery and pulmonary artery (PA) saturations are recorded for calculating

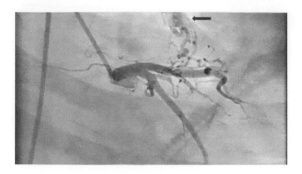

Figure 12.5 Bunch of vessels opacifying LAA clot (black arrow) during coronary angiogram.

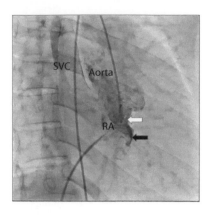

Figure 12.6 Simultaneous injection of contrast dye in aorta and SVC-RA showing relationship of various structures in RAO 30°. White arrow: non-coronary cusp; black arrow: septal tricuspid leaflet; SVC, superior vena cava, RA, right atrium.

cardiac output by Fick's principle. A preprocedure coronary angiogram may be performed in patients' aged over 40 years and those with a history of myocardial infarction or angina. If a need for emergency MVR arises, a knowledge of coronary anatomy is useful to the operating surgeon. It is not uncommon to see a bunch of small vessels opacifying a chronic LA/LAA clot (Figure 12.5).

SEPTAL PUNCTURE

Transseptal puncture (TSP) is the most critical step in the performance of a successful PTMC. A correctly executed TSP not only avoids complications but also ensures successful LV entry.

Anatomy of the interatrial septum

A detailed knowledge of the anatomy of the IAS and its surrounding structures is essential. The ideal site for TSP is the fossa ovalis (FO). Inferior to the FO is the inferior vena cava (IVC) with the coronary sinus (CS) at the antero-inferior border. The septal part of the tricuspid annulus is located anteriorly. The superior vena cava (SVC) is located superiorly with the non-coronary sinus of the aorta forming the antero-superior component (Figure 12.6). The ridge around the superoposterior aspect of the FO is the limbus, which represents the infolding of the atrial roof comprising two muscular layers, and an inner adipose layer. Puncture through this infolding would lead to stitch phenomenon and pericardial effusion involving both the atria. The operator should form a mental picture of all these structures while performing TSP. The most important structure to be avoided during TSP is the aortic root. A pigtail positioned at the non-coronary sinus provides the landmark for safe puncture.

Instruments

The first TSP was performed by Ross, Braunwald, and Morrow in 1959 as a diagnostic technique for obtaining accurate left-heart hemodynamic and angiographic information.[9] Their technique was further improvized in 1962 by Brockenbrough, who designed the Brockenbrough needle.[10] Subsequently, Mullins introduced the combined catheter and dilator set designed to precisely fit over the Brockenbrough needle (Figure 12.2; Table 12.1).[11] The proximal end of the needle has a flange with an arrow that points towards the needle tip. The terms "Brockenbrough needle" and "Mullins sheath" are often used generically when referring to transseptal needles and sheaths, respectively. Care must be taken to ensure that the needle, dilator, and sheath are all compatible. BRK needles from St. Jude Medical are also available for TSP. A plain BRK needle is suitable for routine TSP. A BRK-1 needle has a 51° angle and is used for TSP with very large RA. Unlike Brockenbrough needles, BRK needles have a stop valve at the proximal end. Many operators and centers use Mullin's dilator alone (without the outer sheath) for TSP as the feel of septal pulsation and control on the needle is better without the sheath. However, use of the sheath is recommended, for two reasons: (1) to avoid the rare occurrence of inadvertent perforation of the dilator catheter by the needle during its insertion; (2) to prevent LA perforation during the entry of the catheter/needle assembly into the LA as the tip of the sheath acts as a safety mechanism at the septum.

Table 12.1 Types and specifications of septal puncture hardware

Mullins sheath				
Type	Outer diameter	Maximum diameter (lumen)	Dilator length (cm)	Sheath length (cm)
Adult	8F	0.032"	67	59
Pediatric	6F/8F	0.025"	52	42
Septal puncture needle				
Type	Shaft diameter	Tip diameter	Length (cm)	Other
Brokenbrough (Medtronic Inc)				
Adult	18G	21G	71	
Pediatric	19G	22G	56	
BRK (St. Jude Medical) (four curves), BRK, BRK 1, BRK 2, BRK-XS	18G, 19G (in 56-cm length only)		56, 71, 89, 98	BRK have 19° curve, while BRK-1 have 51° curve (for large RA), have a stop valve at proximal end

Catheter/needle fitting and handling

When completely inserted in the Mullin's sheath, the Brockenbrough needle projects out of the tip of the sheath. The needle should be withdrawn further until its tip is concealed slightly (2–3 mm) within the catheter tip. The needle hub is connected to a 2- or 5-mL contrast-filled syringe. Alternatively, the needle hub may be connected to the pressure transducer so as to monitor the change of pressure waveforms from RA to LA during septal puncture. The operator should fix his/her right index finger between the catheter hub and the direction indicator of the needle to prevent the needle from moving forward and protruding from the catheter tip. The right middle finger and the thumb on the needle are kept along either side of the direction indicator. Thus, during in vivo manipulation of the catheter/needle, it is easier to rotate the needle (Figure 12.7).

Positioning of the needle (Figure 12.8)

A pigtail catheter is placed in the noncoronary sinus of the aortic root. Its position can be confirmed by injecting a small amount of contrast dye. A 0.032" wire is positioned in the superior vena cava (SVC) and the Mullins sheath is advanced over the wire. This assembly can be pushed further into the left brachiocephalic vein so that when it is withdrawn

its lie is along the medial border of SVC. The 0.032" wire is removed and the Brockenbrough needle is inserted into the Mullins dilator. While the needle is advanced within the Mullins dilator/sheath, care must be taken not to perforate the sheath and subsequently the IVC. Some resistance may be encountered at the level of posterior inferior iliac spine in females, which can be circumvented by moving the needle-sheath assembly together at this point. Sometimes, a stylet in the needle keeps the tip of the needle from catching on the body of the Mullin's dilator as the needle is advanced. The stylet must be withdrawn from the needle before the needle gets too close to the tip. The needle tip should be positioned 2–3 mm within the tip of the Mullins' sheath/dilator as discussed above. The patient must be lying straight without any rotation of the spine, as this may distort the septal anatomy and fluoroscopic landmarks. The whole assembly (needle and sheath/dilator) is then withdrawn smoothly towards the patient's feet while observing the catheter movement on fluoroscopy. The needle should be held with the right hand with the index finger interposed between the dilators' hub and needle. The left hand is used to withdraw the assembly. The arrow at the proximal end of the needle should be at "3 o'clock" (when viewed from the foot end of the patient) to begin with and should be rotated to

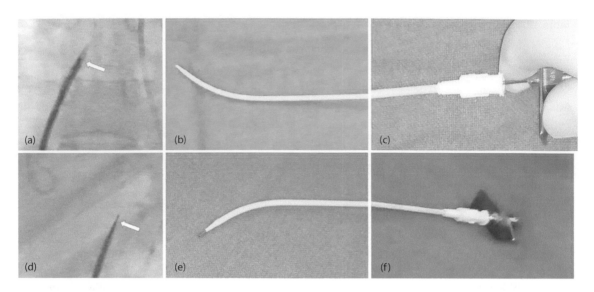

Figure 12.7 Upper panel showing needle-in position in Brokenbrough-Mullins assembly. **(a)** Fluoroscopic image with arrow pointing towards needle tip; **(b)** Mullins tip with needle in; **(c)** Mullins and needle hub with index finger wedged in between the two. Lower panel shows needle-out position. **(d)** Fluoroscopic image with arrow pointing towards needle tip; **(e)** Mullins tip with needle out; **(f)** needle hub completely inserted in the Mullins dilator.

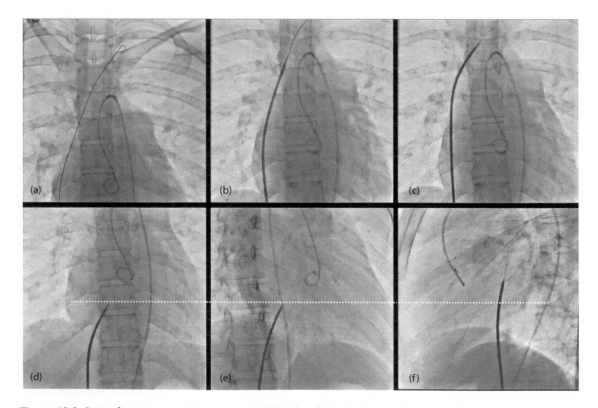

Figure 12.8 Steps for transseptal puncture. **(a)** Pigtail catheter in the aortic root and 0.032″ wire in superior vena cava; **(b)** Mullins dilator over the wire; **(c)** Brockenbrough needle in the dilator with tip in the dilator; **(d)** needle position in AP view; **(e)** needle position in RAO 30° view; **(f)** lateral view after transseptal puncture with contrast injection in LA. Dotted line represents the level of septal puncture. (See Videos 12.1 and 12.2.)

"4 o'clock" when the tip reaches the SVC-RA junction. With further descent, two movements will be seen: (1) The catheter falling into the RA from the SVC; and (2) The catheter falls from the thicker muscular IAS into the fossa ovalis. The assembly should then be gently advanced and if in the correct position it may catch on the lip of the fossa and the needle should be fixed here. (Figure 12.8c; Video 12.1)

Septal puncture techniques

A number of techniques based on angiographic and fluoroscopic landmarks/lines have been described. With experience, operators tend to perform TSP without calculating these imaginary lines and rely more on the movement and feel of the needle and fluoroscopic landmarks.

1. Inoue's angiographic method. The crux of this method is a midline that supposedly divides the IAS into anterior and posterior halves. This line is defined based on the landmarks obtained from RA angiography (with levophase filling LA) during normal respiration in the frontal plane. On a stop-frame of the RA angiographic image, the upper end of the tricuspid valve at systole is assumed to be the anterior limit of the atrial septum, termed as the "T" point. This "T" point is translated to a stop-frame LA image (in levophase). On the LA image, an imaginary horizontal line is drawn from point "T" until point "L," where the line intersects the lateral border of the atrium encountered first (remember the double atrial shadow). Point "L" is assumed to be the posterior limit of the IAS because the lateral border of the RA is lateral to that of the LA, and there is no IAS beyond the LA border. A vertical line, the "midline," is drawn to cross at the midpoint (point M) between "T" and "L." The puncture site is on the "midline" at about two-thirds of a vertebral body height above point where the "midline" intersects with the caudal edge of the left atrium. Inoue's angiographic method is suited for operators inexperienced with the TSP technique, cases in which atrial silhouettes are not well visualized under fluoroscopy and in extremely difficult cases of TSP, e.g., in the presence of a giant left atrium or severe kyphoscoliosis.
2. Hung's modified fluoroscopic method is the most commonly used technique. In most of the cases of MS, the LA silhouette is visible under fluoroscopy, so fluoroscopy can be used as a landmark. In this method, a pigtail catheter is placed in the noncoronary cusp of the aortic valve. The tip of the pigtail catheter serves as the landmark for the upper end of the tricuspid valve because the two valves are in close proximity to each other. Midway between the pigtail and the right lateral edge of the left atrium, a vertical line is drawn and its intersection with the caudal edge of the left atrium is noted. The puncture site is determined on the "midline" at a point about a vertebral body height above the intersection with the caudal edge of the LA. In AP view, the tip is roughly two-thirds to one vertebral height caudal to the tip of the pigtail catheter. Various views may be used to perform TSP (AP, LAO 45°, Lateral 90°, RAO 30°) depending on the operator's preference (Figure 12.8d, e, f; Video 12.2). However, it is essential to verify in at least two views before the needle is advanced. In the RAO view, check that the needle tip is away from the aorta and coronary sinus. Fluoroscopically, the IAS is *en face* in this view and the needle tip is just lateral to the lateral border of the spine. In the LAO/lateral view the needle tip should be away from the aorta and in the inferoposterior third. It should be remembered that the inferior limit of IAS is best seen in AP view. Other fluoroscopic landmarks and structures that need to be avoided are the right atrial wall, medial to midline, inferior LA border, and lateral LA border. When viewed from the foot end of the patient, with the patient lying supine, the plane of the atrial septum runs from "1 o'clock" to "7 o'clock." Fluoroscopically, the FO is posterior and caudal to the aortic root, anterior to the free wall of the RA, superior and posterior to the ostium of the CS, and well posterior of the TA and RA appendage. These anatomic relations need to be maintained while positioning the tip of the needle at FO. FO is approximately 2 cm in diameter and is bounded superiorly by the thick edge of the limbus. The needle tip should engage the caudal edge of the limbus while performing TSP. In MS, the IAS buldges into the RA due to high LA pressure and this results in shifting of the FO, inferiorly. Rather than lying at the junction of the lower and middle thirds of IAS, the FO tends to lie lower (inferiorly) in MS, and in severe disease the limbic ledge is found in the

lower third of IAS. It means that IAS becomes more horizontal and tends to bow into RA as the LA pressure rises. The septal bulge displaces the FO and paraseptal gutters. This distortion of anatomy interferes with the mobility of the puncture needle set in RA and creates difficulty in probing the FO. At the author's institution, TSP is usually performed in lateral 90°. Some gentle manipulation and probing may be required to locate the ideal puncture site. Once in FO, a slight cranial move of the needle tip will engage the limbus and help in stabilizing the needle tip. Appreciation of pulsation from the tense LA confirms that the needle tip is in the thinner part of the IAS (true fossa ovalis). The lateral view serves to confirm the appropriate posterior direction of the needle/catheter assembly. The atrial septal outline and orientation by the septal flush/stain is best appreciated in the lateral view (Figure 12.9). The septal flush method involves continuous flushing of the posteromedially directed dilator/needle with contrast medium as it is withdrawn caudally (Videos 12.3 and 12.4). This maneuver outlines the RA aspect of the septum and its orientation, thus a high (cranially) septal puncture can be avoided. It also facilitates TSP in cases of difficult/distorted anatomy such as septal aneurysm. Sometimes a push for the TSP is made but no blood is aspirated. This could be a case of dissection of the high septum by the needle or entanglement of the needle in the thick part of the septum. Septal staining helps to differentiate between the two. When the high septum is dissected, it appears stained in a more vertical fashion.

In this situation, the catheter/needle should be withdrawn and a septal puncture made at a lower site.

Once the site is confirmed and satisfied, the needle/dilator assembly is pushed against the septum. The feeling of good septal pulsation due to the tense LA reinforces the fact that the needle is at the ideal puncture site. The assembly should be kept stable and firmly pressed against the septum to prevent any slippage. Next, the stopper index finger is removed and only the needle is advanced to puncture the IAS. As the needle enters the LA, a feeling of giveaway is appreciated. Inadvertent slipping of the needle into atrial gutters may happen and should be visible fluoroscopically. In that case, the entire series of steps is reinitiated with descent from the SVC to reengage the FO. Persistence of resistance suggests that the needle is stuck in the thick muscular septum. It is important to recognize an inappropriate puncture at the earliest and withdraw the needle. The chance of tamponade due to needle puncture alone is extremely low. Most of the time, tamponade will manifest after the insertion of the Mullins' dilator or more commonly after the dilatation of the septum with 14F dilator.

3. Another useful technique is to probe the FO so that TSP can be performed without actual needle puncture (Videos 12.5 through 12.8). This was first described by Albridge in 1964[12] and further elucidated by Bloomfield and Sinclair-Smith in 1965.[13] The anatomical basis for this is as follows. In 20%–25% of adult patients, the FO is probe-patent and may not require

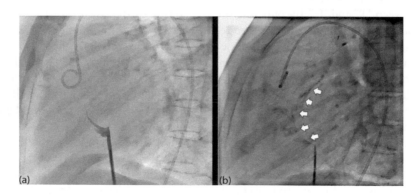

(a)   (b)

Figure 12.9 **(a)** Septum stain in lateral view; **(b)** septal flush in lateral view (arrows point towards septum) (see Videos 12.3 and 12.4).

needle puncture. In two-thirds of patients, the FO is paper-thin, and the catheter can be passed into the LA with gentle pressure and rotation of the dilator. Puncture is associated with a tactile feeling of the septum giving way. In our experience, the technique is successful in approximately 80% of cases. Other authors have reported success rates of more than 90%.[14] In the AP view, the needle/dilator assembly is brought down from the SVC. as described earlier. As the assembly passes in to the RA, observe for the two jumps as described earlier. Next, we go to RAO 30° view. In this view, the septum is *en face* and the tip of the needle/catheter assembly should be midway between pigtail in the aorta and the medial border of the double atrial shadow. This view is essential as sometimes, the second jump may actually be due to the catheter jumping into one of the atrial gutters. The assembly should then be repositioned by either clockwise or anticlockwise rotation to be at the center of IAS. Subsequently, the view is changed to LAO 45° or lateral. The Brockenbrough needle is not brought out of the Mullins sheath but is kept approximately 0.5 cm within the tip of the dilator (Figure 12.7). This stiffens the tip of the needle-sheath assembly. With a gentle, firm pressure, the assembly is pushed in the direction of the left shoulder. If the FO is correctly engaged, the needle-sheath assembly pops in to the LA without using the needle for actual needle puncture. In the words of Bloomfield

and Sinclair-Smith,[13] "this greatly enhanced the safety, the sureness, and the speed of left heart catheterization." Advantages of this needleless technique are: (1) since no needle is used for TSP, risk of tamponade is almost eliminated; (2) septal dilatation with the 14F dilator is easy and smooth; (3) LV entry with a PTMC balloon is technically less demanding.

4. Venous-only TSP (Figure 12.10; Videos 12.9 through 12.13). All the manipulation for the actual performance of PTMC occurs through the venous access. The arterial access serves primarily to guide TSP (pigtail) and for hemodynamic monitoring (arterial BP and calculation of valve area). With the ubiquitous availability of echocardiography within the cath lab, the success and complications of PTMC are being assessed more often by TTE rather than by hemodynamic calculations. Electrophysiologists performing atrial fibrillation ablation do not prefer to take arterial access (to place a pigtail in the NCC) for performing TSP. Rather, they use a totally venous approach for TSP using either a His bundle catheter or a CS catheter for guidance. With this background, some highly experienced operators have moved to a totally venous approach for PTMC as well. The TSP remains the critical step. Two techniques may be used. First, the needle-less TSP technique as described earlier may be used. If actual needle puncture needs to be performed, the following landmarks are chosen. Vertically, as the needle is brought down from the SVC, one needs to

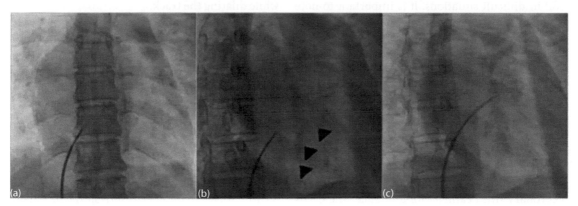

Figure 12.10 Venous only transseptal puncture. (a) Vertically, the TSP needle is one vertebral space above the caudal margin of the LA. (b) RAO 30° view: the needle is positioned midway between the AV groove anteriorly (arrow heads, seen as a radiolucent area on fluoroscopy) and the spine, posteriorly; (c) transseptal puncture performed. (Courtesy of DR CM Nagesh SJICS & R, Bangalore, India.) (See Videos 12.9 through 12.13.)

observe for the same two jumps, as described earlier. Usually, this is one vertebral space above the caudal margin of the LA. Next, in the RAO view, the needle should be midway between the AV groove anteriorly and the vertebral spine posteriorly. The AV groove is seen as a semi-circular radiolucent area that is better seen on dynamic fluoroscopic/cine images, rather than still images (here the AV groove replaces the CS catheter). At this point, TSP is performed. The rest of the PTMC steps are similar. As mentioned earlier, this technique is being used only by highly experienced operators and is not routinely recommended.

Confirmation of LA entry. LA entry is confirmed by: (1) aspiration of bright-red LA blood from the needle; (2) checking pressure; and (3) contrast injection. Once LA entry is confirmed, and there is no or little resistance, the catheter/needle is advanced forward into the LA. Then, the catheter alone is advanced while the needle is being withdrawn. Following TSP, it is always advisable to perform an echo if the operator is a beginner or the puncture site was doubtful so as to ensure that there is no effusion and to document an appropriate puncture site. A simultaneous LA-LV gradient should be taken by advancing the pigtail into the LV.

Various imaging modalities, such as transthoracic echocardiogram (TTE), transoesophageal echocardiogram (TEE), intracardiac echocardiogram (ICE), and so on, may be used to assist TSP in difficult situations. It is important to note that while using echocardiography for assisting TSP, tenting of the septum by the needle/dilator is the only reliable sign of the location of the needle tip. The simple presence of the catheter shadow across the septum may be deceptive due to acoustic effects. Another useful modality is to visualize the LA and the IAS in the levophase of a pulmonary angiogram in the RAO and LAO view. Electrophysiologists perform TSP by using EP catheter landmarks, such as a His catheter, as surrogate markers for the non-coronary cusp and a coronary sinus catheter for guidance. The CS os defines the anteroinferior margin of the FO. Using the CS catheter, the puncture site is superior and posterior to the CS catheter with the needle running parallel to the CS catheter in the RAO view. In the LAO view, the puncture site is superior to

the CS catheter. CT image integration with fluoroscopic image also facilitates TSP. A dedicated NRG needle (Baylis medical) for radiofrequency ablation of fossa ovalis and LA entry is also available.

SEPTAL DILATATION

Following TSP and passage of the Mullin's sheath/dilator into the LA, the Brockenbrough needle is withdrawn. Free aspiration of blood from the Mullin's dilator should be present and any air bubble must be removed by aspiration alone. It is extremely important never to flush saline into the LA to avoid air embolism. The specially designed 0.025" stainless steel guidewire (with coiled tip) is advanced into the LA (Figure 12.11). An insertion tool is provided with the wire to facilitate the insertion of coiled wire into the dilator. Alternatively, the coiled end of the wire can be inserted with the help of the dilator of a 6F/7F vascular sheath. Once the coiled wire is placed in the LA, the Mullins sheath/dilator system is removed.

Two maneuvers may be performed to facilitate the subsequent passage of the septal dilator/PTMC balloon. First, a small nick may be given to the skin using a narrow scalpel with the bevel pointing upwards to the ceiling (to avoid inadvertent incision on the vein). This is especially useful in thin individuals where the fatless skin tends to snugly hold onto the dilator. Second, using an artery forceps, the short subcutaneous track may be dilated along the guide wire. This may not be needed in thinly built individuals. Needless to say, one should be careful not to injure the femoral vein while dilating the track.

The septal dilator is passed over the wire for adequate dilatation of the septal puncture site (Video 12.14). If resistance is felt at the groin, then the same dilator can be used to dilate the groin puncture site. It is important to keep a watch on the systemic pressure and other hemodynamics at this time as cardiac tamponade due to inappropriate septal puncture usually manifests at this time. Systemic anticoagulation is given after the septal puncture to prevent the formation of the thrombi on the wires and catheters. Some operators prefer to anticoagulate after insertion of the balloon into the LA as the time taken between the septal puncture and balloon insertion is not much and, in case of tamponade due to inappropriate septal puncture, anticoagulation can be withheld. On the other hand, there are operators who give heparin

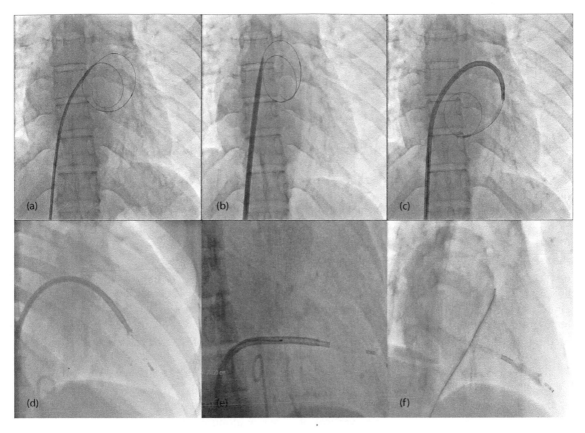

Figure 12.11 Steps after transseptal puncture. **(a)** Coiled wire in LA; **(b)** septal dilatation; **(c)** balloon in LA; **(d, e, f)** direct, horizontal, and reverse-loop method of crossing the mitral valve, respectively (see Videos 12.14 through 12.18).

at the start of the PTMC procedure (before TSP) as the time required for TSP may be unpredictable and there are chances of thrombus formation on the catheters (further compounded by the fact that the catheters are reused). We use a standard dose of 2500–3500 U of unfractionated heparin. Additional doses of heparin are given if there is difficulty in entering the LA or LV and procedure time is prolonged. For pediatric PTMC, 50–100 U/kg of heparin is used. The current dose of heparin used at most of the experienced centers is much less than what was recommended earlier as the procedure time following TSP is much shorter. Moreover, cardiac tamponade is a much more common problem than stroke due to thrombus formation on wires/ balloon.

LEFT-VENTRICULAR ENTRY

After dilating the septum and groin, the previously prepared, measured, and slenderized PTMC balloon is tracked over the coiled wire (Figure 12.11).

Sometimes, a more vertical angulation at the groin facilitates balloon entry at the groin site if a shallower angle of entry fails. Entry into the LA through IAS is usually easy if the TSP is at the thin part of the FO/IAS. In case of TSP through the thicker part of the IAS, balloon entry into the LA may be difficult. Rotating the balloon assembly in a screwdriver fashion facilitates the entry of the balloon into the LA. Following entry of the slenderized portion of the balloon into the LA, the inner metal tube is withdrawn first. This will deslenderize the balloon. As the inner metal tube is withdrawn, the PTMC balloon is advanced further into the LA to form a generous loop in the LA. This will enable subsequent LV entry and prevent flipping of the balloon in the LAA (this may inadvertently dislodge a previously missed LAA thrombus). Next, the balloon tube is unlocked and withdrawn. One should take care to avoid entrapment of the balloon in the IAS or pulmonary vein. The preformed J-tip wire is then introduced into the balloon.

During the exchange of hardware, slight inflation of the balloon tip prevents the balloon from inadvertently slipping back into RA. The stylet has a preformed J-shaped tip with a waist length of about 4.5 cm. The curve may be increased or decreased depending on the size of the LA and the site of puncture (greater diameter for larger LA and vice versa, smaller curve for low puncture). Giving the stylet tip an anterior curve will direct the balloon towards the anteriorly placed MV orifice. LV entry is done in RAO 30° view as the LV long axis is displayed in profile. In difficult cases, an additional lateral view or the use of biplane labs is useful for confirming anterior angulation of the balloon tip. The right hand is used to maneuver/rotate the J-curve wire and the left hand is used to pull or push the balloon. The J-curved wire is rotated anticlockwise so that the balloon tip starts to point anteriorly towards the LV and, simultaneously, the balloon is gradually withdrawn. Traditionally, four methods have been described for LV entry.[15]

1. The vertical method (withdrawing the stylet only). With further withdrawal of the balloon (as the loop of the balloon catheter in the LA opens and the balloon tip becomes vertical) it may fall into the LV during diastole and come back into the LA in systole. Occurrence of VPCs will confirm entry into the LV. Now the operator should carefully withdraw the stylet at the onset of diastole so that the balloon may slide into the LV. If the balloon is still vertical and is not aligned with the long axis of the LV, it should be partially withdrawn so as to align with the long axis of the LV. To prevent the PTMC balloon from popping out of the LV, the distal half of the balloon should be inflated as soon as the balloon falls into the LV.
2. The direct method (withdrawing the stylet, advancing the catheter). If the vertical method does not succeed in crossing the mitral valve (not an uncommon scenario), the balloon is further withdrawn so as to align the balloon with the long axis of the LV. Some rotatory adjustments with the stylet may need to be done so as to point the balloon tip towards the mitral orifice. As soon as the balloon tip approaches the mitral orifice, to-and-fro movement of the balloon tip will occur ("woodpecking" sign), marking the site of LV entry (Video 12.15). While carefully observing the movements of

the catheter, the stylet is withdrawn with simultaneous advancement of the balloon into the LV. This movement should start with the onset of diastole, which is marked by the beginning of the movement of the balloon tip towards the LV. Hand-eye coordination is very important at this step. The presence of AF or a fast ventricular rate may make this step more challenging. However, with experience, this method is the most successful one and is a commonly used method of LV entry. If the balloon tip is not well aligned to the MV orifice or the balloon is pushed during systole then it will not enter the LV and will bend back into the LA. In that case, all the steps, starting from making a loop in LA, need to be repeated.

3. The horizontal sliding method (advancing the catheter only). This method is useful if the previous two techniques fail. It is also helpful in cases of caudal septal puncture and horizontal orientation of LV. The catheter is further pulled and the stylet is slightly withdrawn so that the orientation of the balloon becomes more horizontal. The balloon tip is slightly inflated so as to facilitate entry into the LV during diastole along with blood flow. As the balloon tip approaches across the mitral orifice it will show jerky to-and-fro movement. The balloon is then gently pushed into the LV at the onset of diastole with the operator carefully watching the to-and-fro movement. Vigorous balloon movements should be avoided as the balloon may slip into the LAA. There are high chances of the balloon slipping out into the RA as the balloon length in the LA is much shorter.
4. The reverse (posterior) loop method. This method is useful in the presence of a very large LA or if the puncture is too anterior or too caudal in relation to the MV. The PTMC balloon is inserted deep into the LA in the vicinity of the MV. The stylet is withdrawn 2–3 cm. The stylet is then rotated clockwise (instead of the usual anticlockwise rotation). This will lead to the catheter of the balloon forming a loop after bouncing off the posterior LA wall. The balloon points anteriorly and to the left, i.e., towards the MV orifice. With the stylet kept fixed, the balloon is advanced across the MV orifice. Some anticlockwise twisting of the stylet may be required to position the balloon. Once the balloon enters the LV, the distal half of the balloon

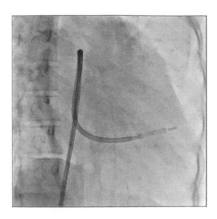

Figure 12.12 Half-reverse-loop method of crossing the mitral valve. cf. Figure 12.11 F-loop is only half-formed.

is inflated and the catheter is gently pulled to undo the loop. The balloon is now gently aligned with the long axis of the LV with the help of the stylet. Subsequently, the proximal and middle portions of the balloon are inflated. A modification of this technique is the half-reverse loop method, which is useful with a relatively smaller LA and caudal septal puncture (Figure 12.12). Rather than forming a full loop, only a half-loop is formed so that the balloon tip faces towards the mitral orifice. If loop formation using the stylet fails, then the 0.025″ coiled guidewire can be used to form the loop. By keeping the coils of the wire lying on the right side of the PTMC balloon, a loop can be formed.

Accordion maneuver (Video 12.19). After crossing the mitral valve, the balloon should not pass through the chordae and should be able to reach freely up to the LV tip. To confirm this, the accordion maneuver is performed. This involves sliding the partially inflated distal balloon back and forth by simultaneously pulling and pushing the balloon catheter and stylet in opposite directions. This is to ensure that the catheter has not strayed into the chordal apparatus. This accordion maneuver is an essential component of proper LV entry and, unless the operator has completed this maneuver, valve dilatation should not be done. Dilating a balloon that has passed through the chordae will result in chordal tear and mitral regurgitation. In case the balloon is stuck within the chordae, the balloon should be withdrawn up to the mitral annulus and, with the help of the stylet, re-advanced in a different direction so as to reach up to the LV apex. Dilating a balloon that is stuck in the chordae will cause distal balloon to deform. Early recognition of this can avert further balloon dilatation and thus injury to the mitral apparatus (Figure 12.13).

Subvalvular trapping of the balloon. Severe subvalvular disease may create problems in LV entry and may appear as one of the following three signs: (1) balloon compression sign: gross indentation of the inflated distal balloon by severe subvalvular disease; (2) balloon impasse: failure of the deflated and properly aligned balloon to cross the mitral valve/subvalvular apparatus as the balloon gets stuck/entrapped by severe subvalvular stenosis (Figure 12.14, Video 12.20). In-situ inflation reveals compression of the distal half of the balloon by subvalvular structures and inflation of the proximal half. This sign signifies an extremely high risk for the creation of MR; (3) cogwheel

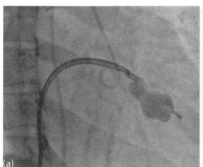
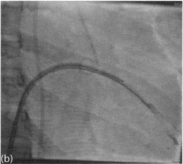
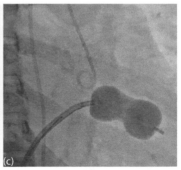

Figure 12.13 **(a)** Attempted inflation of balloon showing deformed distal part due to crossing of balloon through chordae; **(b)** performing appropriate accordion maneuver (balloon tip can be seen reaching up to apex) (see Video 12.19); **(c)** inflation of balloon after accordion results in proper inflation without any deformity.

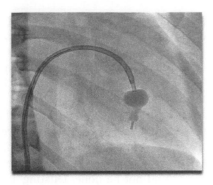

Figure 12.14 Balloon impasse as distal part is stuck in the subvalvular deformity (see Video 12.20).

resistance: while withdrawing the partially inflated balloon to anchor it at the mitral valve, cogwheel resistance may be encountered due to the presence of subvalvular disease.

BALLOON DILATATION

After entering the LV and completing the accordion maneuver, the next and most vital step of the procedure is balloon dilatation (Figure 12.15, Video 12.21). The distal portion of the balloon is fully inflated and the catheter is pulled back until it fits snugly across the MV. At this stage, the balloon is inflated further so that the proximal half inflates and locks the valve between the proximal and distal portions of the balloon. In the final stage of inflation, the middle waist portion expands, which dilates the valve orifice to the corresponding preset balloon size. A small sudden jerky expansion of the balloon waist in the final stage of dilatation usually indicates splitting of the commissure and successful valve dilatation.

Otherwise, the valve may merely get stretched without optimal opening. The balloon is rapidly deflated and quickly withdrawn into the LA so as to minimize the amount of time during which no blood flows from the LA to the LV. Systemic pressure will fall during balloon inflation and return to normal or even higher after balloon deflation, indicating successful PTMC. The pigtail catheter is advanced into the LV and the mitral valve gradient is measured to assess the success of the procedure. LA waveforms, mean LA pressure, and TTE are assessed for the appearance/increase of MR. An increase in LA "V" wave and mean LA pressure indicates MR and can be confirmed on TTE. If there is no increase in MR or no appearance of new MR, but the transmitral gradient is suboptimal, then stepwise dilatation of the MV is performed. Stepwise dilatation minimizes the risk of PTMC-related acute MR. Depending upon the valve anatomy, the beginning balloon diameter should be 2–3 mm smaller than the calculated maximum reference diameter. In the presence of calcific valves, subvalvular deformity, commissural fusion, irregular valve leaflet thickness, and more than mild regurgitation, the initial balloon size should be 2–3 mm less than the reference size and then increased in 1-mm (approximately 1 mL contrast to be added) steps after each dilatation until the optimal result or maximum reference size is achieved or there is increase/appearance of MR. For pliable valves with good anatomy, the initial balloon size should be 1–2 mm less than the reference size. For females and patients with low body mass, a smaller size (by 0.5 to 1 mm) is good enough for optimal results. Balloon inflation

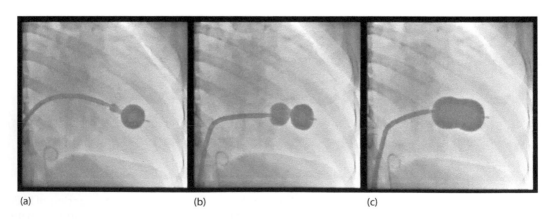

(a) (b) (c)

Figure 12.15 Three stages of balloon inflation. (a) Distal inflation; (b) proximal inflation; (c) complete inflation with inflation of middle part (see Video 12.21).

of more than the reference diameter is not recommended. In our experience, balloon dilatation up to the maximum reference diameter is required only in a minority of cases. During repeat dilatation, it is not uncommon for the balloon to slip out in the LA through a partially dilated MV. In such circumstances, the tug of force on the balloon after inflation of the distal balloon should be decreased so that the balloon remains at the MV. The proximal and middle portions of the balloon are then gradually inflated, keeping the balloon stable at the MV annulus. It must also be remembered that the balloon "popping" into the LA with fully inflated distal half indicates wide splitting of commissures (Video 12.22). Successful PTMC is often associated with a reduction in heart rate and a rise in the systemic BP as compared to pre-PTMC levels. In addition, the appearance of respiratory variation in the LA pressure trace is another indicator of successful PTMC.

Some operators will push the PTMC balloon after deflation into the LV (instead of pulling it in LA) for measuring LVED pressure and LV-LA pullback pressure. An acute rise in LVED pressure will indicate MR and pullback will indicate the transmitral gradient. Re-dilatation is done if LVED pressure has not increased and there is presence of a transmitral gradient. This technique is useful when a pigtail is not used for septal puncture and the procedure is done through venous access only.

Sometimes, the balloon may get stuck at the IAS during manipulation. Partial inflation of the distal half of the balloon to prevent it from slipping into the RA and reinsertion of the coiled wire and inner metal tube will help in tracking the balloon back into the LA. Quite often, maneuvering with the stylet (clockwise rotation) itself helps in disengaging the balloon from the septum into the LA.

Sudden bradycardia, significant hypotension, and even asystole may sometimes occur during or just after balloon dilatation and may not recover immediately. Intravenous atropine, IV mephentermine, and temporary pacing leads should be ready and used immediately for recovery.

Mechanism of PTMC. Successful PTMC is a result of the splitting of mitral commissures. Echocardiographic and pathological studies have validated this mechanism. Mere stretching of the mitral valve without commissural splitting may result in some immediate gain in MVA but recoil of the valve nullifies the benefit. In case of

a fixed and calcified mitral valve, balloon dilatation results in increased pliability and mobility of the valve by fracturing the calcium deposits. This explains the decrease or disappearance of fixed-orifice MR after successful PTMC. Leaflet tear may occur at the point of maximum leaflet weakness, especially if commissures are fused and do not give way.

TERMINATION OF THE PROCEDURE

A successful PTMC is defined as more than or equal to a 50% improvement in valve area with a final MVA greater than 1.5 cm^2 (>1 cm^2/m^2 BSA), in the absence of any major complication. It is an indication for the completion of procedure. The splitting of at least one commissure or a decrease in valve gradient by 50% are other parameters that are considered as successful PTMC. In some cases, a single commissure is split during one of the first balloon inflations. This is often the result of asymmetric commissural fusion or calcification. The splitting of a single commissure often makes it difficult to split the second commissure, since the inflated balloon will be displaced into the already-opened side of the valve. This typically results in an adequate rather than an excellent postprocedure valve area. Acceptance of suboptimal results in unsuitable valves decreases the chance of MR. Mitral regurgitation of more than Grade 2/4 has been considered a suboptimal result by many studies but it is important to look at the overall picture, including the site of origin of MR (commissural vs. cuspal), overall mitral valve area, and transmitral gradient. Commissural MR tends to regress over time. Appearance or increment of MR by more than Grade 1/4 warrants termination of the procedure as further dilatation may lead to severe MR.

REMOVAL OF BALLOON ASSEMBLY

Following the completion of PTMC, the stainless-steel guidewire-metal tube assembly is reinserted through the balloon. The balloon is reslenderized by inserting the metal tube. During reslenderization the sequence of joining is as follows. First, the hub of the metallic tube is attached to the hub of the inner tube of the balloon (once again, gold and silver go together). Then, the final elongation is done by pulling the plastic balloon hub into the metallic hub, which is held firmly. This is to ensure that it should not injure the roof of the atria during slenderization. The coiled guidewire is pulled enough to leave only part of the soft coiled end beyond the balloon tip. Subsequently, the balloon and wire assembly is pulled in to the RA. Finally, the balloon is pulled out, leaving the coiled guidewire in the RA. If everything is under control, then an 8F vascular sheath is inserted into the femoral vein over the wire and the coiled wire is removed. Post-procedure, hemodynamic study is completed and vascular sheaths removed. Post-procedure echocardiogram for the confirmation of absence of any pericardial effusion, MR, etc., may be done.

Post-procedure care

Patients need to be monitored overnight in a step-down unit and can be discharged the next day. Usual care for sheaths is required. Evaluation of MVA using pressure half-time is not reliable immediately after PTMC due to changes in the LA compliance, and planimetry may overestimate the MVA on day one. It is better to assess the MVA two to three days after PTMC.

Follow-up

Immediately after PTMC, there is an increase in MVA, cardiac output, and systemic pressure, while the transmitral gradient, LA pressure, PA pressure, and PCWP decrease. Hypertensive TR also regresses, especially in younger patients. The regression of TR is less common, with organic TV disease and in older patients. Pre-load-dependent LV dysfunction also improves after PTMC. Left-atrium size and volume decreases after PTMC in about 90% of cases. This effect is less pronounced in the presence of AF as compared to those in NSR.[16]

Complications

Approximately 1% of procedures are abandoned due to failure to cross the IAS. Complications occur in 1%–5% of patients, the most common being acute MR and inadvertent puncture into the pericardial space (see Table 10.4). The predictors of complications/mortality are:

- Echocardiographic score of >8
- Increasing age
- Prior surgical valvotomy
- NYHA functional class IV

- Higher post-procedural PA pressure
- Preprocedural mitral regurgitation ≥2+
- Postprocedural mitral regurgitation ≥3+

Mortality in experienced hands is rare (<1%). Cardiac tamponade rates are around 1%. Severe MR remains the dreaded complication; reported rates range from 2%–10% with a need for urgent MVR in up to 5% of cases (<1% in experienced centers).[17] It is mainly seen in those with unfavorable morphology. It may be due to leaflet or chordal tears but sometimes may also be commissural. Atrial septal defect (ASD) following PTMC is common (66% by TEE) but most of these are small (mean diameter 4 mm).[18] Only 1%–2% have a significant ASD. Most of the ASDs close spontaneously by six months. A residual ASD may remain for up to three months and persists longer in 3%–16% of PTMC cases. Very rarely, Qp/Qs can be >2, requiring intervention for the residual defect.

Reuse of hardware

PTMC balloons are recommended by the manufacturers for only single use. However, PTMC hardware is routinely re-used in order to keep the cost of procedures low in resource-limited countries. Recommendation as a single-use device implies that it can be used safely and reliably only once. It does not, however, imply that it cannot be used safely and reliably more than once, if appropriately reprocessed. There are limited guidelines/legislations as to how often a device can be reused. An expert group in India has recommended a maximum of up to three instances of reuse of a PTMC balloon.[19] We strongly recommend that operators should follow the local rules, laws, and guidelines for reusing PTMC hardware. For reuse, the balloon and accessories should be thoroughly cleaned and should be free from any organic residue. The balloons should be resterilized using ethylene oxide and use of glutaraldehyde is strongly discouraged. The holes on the outer surface of an Inoue balloon allow the blood to enter between the two layers of latex. Therefore, cleaning of an Inoue balloon is more tedious and time-consuming. Putting a few drops of heparin in the cleaning bowl and multiple inflation-deflation cycles during balloon cleaning helps to remove the blood trapped between the two latex layers. In this respect, the Accura balloon is easier to clean.

VIDEOS

Video 12.1 (Corresponding Figure 12.8c) Descent of needle and Mullin's dilator assembly from superior vena cava to interatrial septum. Note the two movements: (1) The catheter falls into the right atrium from the superior vena cava and (2) the catheter falls from the thicker muscular interatrial septum into the fossa ovalis. https://youtu.be/4RNpo-e97Dw

Video 12.2 (Corresponding to Figure 12.8f) Septal puncture in the lateral view. Appreciate the giveaway movement at the time of entry into the left atrium. https://youtu.be/jOV780jypBI

Video 12.3 and 12.4 (Corresponding to Figure 12.9b) Septal flush done by continuously injecting contrast with the Mullin's dilator while pulling it down from the superior vena cava—shows interatrial septum in anteroposterior (12.3) and lateral view (12.4). https://youtu.be/LhsJhupDiQw and https://youtu.be/GMZaDnTdZpE

Video 12.5 Needleless septal puncture (probing for the fossa ovalis). The Brockenbrough needle/ Mullin sheath assembly is brought down from the superior vena cava into right atrium. The two jumps are noted, namely, the assembly dropping from superior vena cava to right atrium and then subsequently into the fossa ovalis. https://youtu.be/0uQXAx-YR-I

Video 12.6 Needleless septal puncture (probing for the fossa ovalis). In the RAO 30° view, the tip of the catheter is midway between pigtail in the aorta and the medial border of the double atrial shadow. https://youtu.be/CG1iix30JRQ

Video 12.7 Needleless septal puncture (probing for the fossa ovalis). In the LAO view, with the Brockenbrough needle 0.5 cm within the tip of the Mullins sheath. https://youtu.be/25NCoV-oSuM

Video 12.8 Needleless septal puncture (probing for the fossa ovalis). A firm, gentle pressure is applied towards the left shoulder. The assembly pops into the LA without actual needle puncture. https://youtu.be/T-XIhY0tEAw

Video 12.9 (Corresponding to Figure 12.10) Venous-only PTMC (Courtesy Dr. Nagesh C.M.). The Brockenbrough needle/Mullin sheath assembly is brought down from the superior vena cava into right atrium. The two jumps are noted, namely, the assembly dropping from superior vena cava to right atrium and then subsequently into the fossa ovalis. Note the absence of arterial access (no pigtail catheter in the aortic root). https://youtu.be/TnypaDx60_M

Video 12.10 (Corresponding to Figure 12.10) Venous-only PTMC (Courtesy Dr. Nagesh C.M.). In the AP view, the tip of the assembly is one vertebral space above the caudal margin of the LA. https://youtu.be/_9meAaykjLg

Video 12.11 (Corresponding to Figure 12.10) Venous-only PTMC (Courtesy Dr. Nagesh C.M.). In the RAO 30° view, the assembly is midway between atrioventricular groove anteriorly and the vertebral spine posteriorly. The atrioventricular groove is seen as a semicircular radiolucent area. https://youtu.be/w12PrWOWiqE

Video 12.12 (Corresponding to Figure 12.10) Venous-only PTMC (Courtesy Dr. Nagesh C.M.). Trans-septal puncture is performed in RAO 30°. https://youtu.be/xa_FE3tZqS0

Video 12.13 (Corresponding to Figure 12.10) Venous-only PTMC (Courtesy Dr. Nagesh C.M.). Left atrial entry is confirmed by contrast injection. https://youtu.be/f0n0DJj_vSc

Video 12.14 (Corresponding to Figure 12.11b) Dilatation of interatrial septum over the coiled wire. https://youtu.be/X7SASXvCnik

Video 12.15 Woodpecker movement of the balloon suggesting tip at the mitral orifice followed by the entry of balloon into the left ventricle. https://youtu.be/cSmy5Qu8Dfk

Video 12.16 (Corresponding to Figure 12.11e) Methods of crossing mitral valve—direct entry. (https://youtu.be/kArgOtMpA7s)

Video 12.17 (Corresponding to Figure 12.11f) Methods of crossing mitral valve—horizontal entry. (https://youtu.be/oyzXiAIlJJ0)

Video 12.18 (Corresponding to Figure 12.11g) Methods of crossing mitral valve—reverse loop entry. (https://youtu.be/pc-B2kFliUM).

Video 12.19 (Corresponding to Figure 12.13b) Accordion manoeuvre https://youtu.be/4zF41SEaN3Q

Video 12.20 (Corresponding to Figure 12.14) Balloon impasse sign. In situ inflation of a properly aligned deflated PTMC balloon leads to inflation of proximal half and compression of distal half indicating that balloon is trapped in subvalvular apparatus. https://youtu.be/UIkNkSdbPAQ

Video 12.21 (Corresponding to Figure 12.15) Balloon dilatation. https://youtu.be/ycKUEKsywjw

Video 12.22 Balloon popping out sign. With fully inflated distal half, the PTMC balloon prolapsing into the left atrium while being pulled back from left ventricle indicates wide splitting of commissures. https://youtu.be/hlupnZj_wwk

REFERENCES

1. Inoue K, Owaki T, Nakamura T et al. Clinical application of transvenous mitral commissurotomy by a new balloon catheter. *J Thorac Cardiovasc Surg* 1984;87:394–402.
2. Stefanadis C, Kourouklis C, Stratos C et al. Percutaneous balloon mitral valvuloplasty by retrograde left atrial catheterization. *Am J Cardiol* 199065:650–4.
3. Bahl VK, Juneja R, Thatai D et al. Retrograde nontransseptal balloon mitral valvuloplasty for rheumatic mitral stenosis. *Cathet Cardiovasc Diagn* 1994;33:331–4.
4. Cribier A, Rath PC, Letac B. Percutaneous mitral valvotomy with a metal dilator. *Lancet* 1997;349:1667–8.
5. El-Sayed MA, Anwar AM. Comparative study between various methods of percutaneous transvenous mitral commissurotomy: Metallic valvulotome, Inoue balloon, double-balloon techniques. *J Interven Cardiol* 2000;13:357–64.
6. Bonhoeffer P, Esteves C, Casal U et al. Percutaneous mitral valve dilatation with the Multi-Track System. *Catheter Cardiovasc Interv* 1999;48:178–83.
7. Nair KK, Pillai HS, Thajudeen A. Comparative study on safety, efficacy, and midterm results of balloon mitral valvotomy performed with triple lumen and double lumen mitral valvotomy catheters. *Catheter Cardiovasc Interv* 2012;80:978–86.
8. Lau KW, Hung JS. A simple balloon-sizing method in Inoue balloon percutaneous transvenous mitral commissurotomy. *Cathet Cardiovasc Diagn* 1994;33:120–9.
9. Ross Jr J, Braunwald E, Morrow AG. Left heart catheterization by the transseptal route: A description of the technique and its applications. *Circulation* 1960;22:927e934.
10. Brockenbrough EC, Braunwald E, Ross Jr J. Transseptal left heart catheterization. A review of 450 studies and description of an improved technic. *Circulation* 1962;25:15e21.
11. Mullins CE. Transseptal left heart catheterization: Experience with a new technique in 520 pediatric and adult patients. *Pediatr Cardiol* 1983;4:239e245.
12. Aldridge HE. Transseptal left heart catheterization without needle puncture of the interatrial septum. *Am J Cardiol* 1964;13:239–42.
13. Bloomfield DA, Sinclair-smith BC. The limbic ledge. A landmark for transseptal left heart catheterization. *Circulation* 1965;31:103–7.
14. Krishnamoorthy KM, Dash PK. Transseptal catheterization without needle puncture. *Scand Cardiovasc J* 2001;35:199–200.
15. Hung JS, Lau KW. Pitfalls and tips in Inoue-balloon mitral commissurotomy. *Cathet Cardiovasc Diagn* 1996;37:188–99.
16. Fawzy ME. Percutaneous mitral balloon valvotomy. *Catheter Cardiovasc Interv* 2007;69:313–21.
17. Hung JS, Lau KW, Lo PH, Chern MS, Wu JJ. Complications of Inoue balloon mitral commissurotomy: Impact of operator experience and evolving technique. *Am Heart J* 1999;138:114–21.
18. Manjunath CN, Panneerselvam A, Srinivasa KH et al. Incidence and predictors of atrial septal defect after percutaneous transvenous mitral commissurotomy—A transesophageal echocardiographic study of 209 cases. *Echocardiography* 2013;30:127–30.
19. Kapoor A, Vora A, Nataraj G, Mishra S, Kerkar P, Manjunath CN. Guidance on reuse of cardio-vascular catheters and devices in India: A consensus document. *Indian Heart J* 2017;69:357–63.

13

Challenges in percutaneous transvenous mitral commissurotomy

RAVI S. MATH AND CHOLENAHALLY NANJAPPA MANJUNATH

INTRODUCTION

Percutaneous transvenous mitral commissurotomy (PTMC) is the preferred treatment for symptomatic patients with moderate to severe mitral stenosis (MS). It is usually performed using dumbbell (hourglass)-shaped balloons (i.e., either the Inoue or Accura balloon). Both balloons have been shown to be similar with respect to safety and efficacy.[1,2] The technique of PTMC has a steep learning curve. Even after having acquired expertise in the technique, difficulties may be encountered at various steps. This chapter will deal with techniques that can be used to overcome difficulties during PTMC. At the authors' institution, more than 1000 PTMCs are being performed every year. Difficulties in PTMC may be encountered at various anatomical levels as well as in certain special subsets of patients.

DIFFICULTIES AT THE ANATOMICAL LEVEL

Technical difficulties may arise at the groin level, at the interatrial septum (IAS) level, or at the level of the mitral valve (MV) (Table 13.1).

Table 13.1 Technically difficult situations

At the Groin

Venous access

Passage of septal dilator/PTMC balloon

At the Level of Transseptal Puncture

Bulging of IAS

Giant RA

Dilated coronary sinus

Thick septum

Septal aneurysm

Cardiac malpositions

IVC Anomaly

At the Level of Crossing the Mitral Valve

Critical MS <0.5 cm^2

Giant LA

Small LA

Inadequate septal puncture site

Severe submitral disease

Abnormal mitral valve orientation

Abbreviations: PTMC, percutaneous transvenous mitral commissurotomy; IAS, interatrial septum; RA, right atrium; LA, left atrium; MS, mitral stenosis.

Groin

PTMC is essentially a procedure performed via the femoral vein (some experienced operators have even stopped taking arterial access, making PTMC an exclusive venous intervention). Often, femoral venous access and insertion of the septal dilator or the PTMC balloon is a smooth procedure. At times, difficulties may be encountered. Sometimes it may be difficult to get access to the femoral vein. This may happen if patients have been fasting for long or if they have been vigorously treated with diuretics causing the IVC and femoral veins to collapse. Further, many of these patients are thin and cachectic, resulting in the absence of groin fat that normally acts as a support/cushion for the femoral vein. Finally, groin scarring from previous PTMC procedures and femoral vein thrombosis may be additional causes for difficult femoral access. There are no standard procedures in such a scenario. Use of the femoral head as a fluoroscopic landmark is helpful. It may be more useful to take the arterial puncture first and then use the arterial puncture site as a guide for the venous access (normally, we take venous access before arterial puncture).

It is important to remember that in thin and cachetic patients, the femoral vein is often very superficial. So going deep with the puncture needle will be unsuccessful. After repeated failed attempts a change of hands is advised (even with a junior colleague!). In the case of scarred groin/femoral vein thrombosis, the contralateral unaffected groin may be used.

If recurrent attempts to pass the septal dilator through the groin fail, one should consider the possibility that the venous puncture has been through, rather than under, the inguinal ligament. In such a scenario, repeat puncture of the femoral vein at a lower level should be performed. If passage of the septal dilator has been smooth, but there are difficulties in maneuvering the PTMC balloon, the following steps may be taken. Keeping the guidewire taut (which is held by the assistant), firm pressure is applied to the skin cephalad to the puncture site to stretch it. The PTMC balloon is advanced parallel to the skin using a slight side-to-side rotational motion. Too much twisting should be avoided as it may cause the internal metal tube to bend. This may also lacerate the femoral vein. If this is unsuccessful, the PTMC balloon is advanced at a more obtuse angle of 90 degrees until it touches the posterior venous wall.[3] Subsequently, it is tilted more horizontally and then further advanced over the guidewire. In both the above described maneuvers, excessive force should be avoided. If these maneuvers are unsuccessful, the femoral vein and subcutaneous track should be redilated using the 14F septal dilator. Finally, if all measures fail, a 14F vascular sheath should be inserted through which the 11–12F PTMC balloon can be easily passed.

Interatrial septum

Hung's fluoroscopic method[4] is the commonly used technique for transseptal puncture (TSP). The appreciation of septal bounce, the septal stain, and septal flush technique can further aid the TSP. A detailed description of the TSP technique has been provided in the previous chapter. Various imaging modalities, such as transthoracic echocardiogram (TTE) (Figure 13.1), transesophageal echocardiogram (TEE), intracardiac echocardiogram (ICE), etc., may be used to assist TSP in difficult situations. A useful modality that is readily available in the catheterization lab is to visualize the left atrium (LA) and the IAS in the levophase of a pulmonary angiogram in the right anterior oblique (RAO) and left anterior oblique (LAO) view. A recently described technique of TSP in difficult septal anatomy is to ask the patient to take a deep

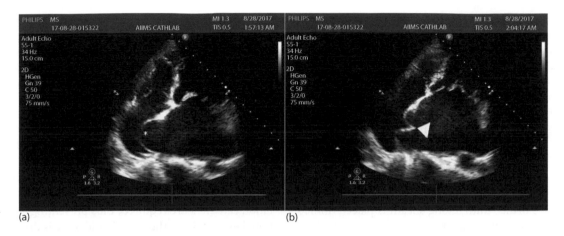

Figure 13.1 TTE guided transseptal puncture (TSP) in a case of IAS aneurysm. **(a)** IAS aneurysm (*); **(b)** TSP needle abutting the IAS aneurysm (arrowhead). IAS, interatrial septum; TTE, transthoracic echocardiography.

breath and hold during TSP.[5] During deep inspiration, the IAS moves towards the right, enabling successful TSP. This technique was useful in the presence of IAS aneurysm, thick IAS, and excessively mobile IAS where the conventional TSP had failed.

TSP via the left groin is more difficult than from the right. The procedure is essentially the same. As the course of the left iliac vein is more tortuous, it may be difficult to advance the Brockenbrough needle. There may be traction on the inferior vena cava during the passage of the needle through the Mullins sheath/dilator and this may lead to lower abdominal pain. To overcome these hurdles, it is best to allow the needle to rotate freely as it is advanced through the Mullins sheath/dilator in the iliopelvic region.[6] Another option is to advance the Mullins sheath/dilator along with the needle as a whole, keeping a watch on the dilator tip in the SVC. The angle of the tip of the needle with the IAS is less when TSP is performed via the left groin. A larger curve has to be given to the Brockenbrough needle so as to engage the IAS or else the tip will slide over the IAS.[7] Another maneuver that can aid in engaging the IAS is to bend the patient's shoulders and chest to the right. This will make the IAS more perpendicular to the needle tip.[6] This maneuver can also be used to aid the advancement of the needle/sheath/dilator in the iliac veins and IVC as it will straighten the course of the needle.[8]

Left ventricle entry

Traditionally, four methods have been described for left ventricle (LV) entry, namely: (1) the direct method (withdraw stylet, advance catheter); (2) the vertical method (withdraw stylet only); (3) the horizontal (sliding) method (advance catheter only); and (4) the loop method. These have been described in the previous chapter. Sometimes, these traditional methods fail and recourse may be taken to more advanced techniques (Table 13.2).

Over-the-wire technique. The over-the-wire (OTW) technique relies on the placement of a stiff wire directly into the LV and then threading the PTMC balloon over the stiff wire. This method was first described by Meier.[9] His initial description involved the following steps: (a) over the 0.025″ pigtail guidewire, a diagnostic right Judkins catheter was placed in the LA; (b) through the Judkins catheter, a 0.020″ back-up wire with a steerable J-tip wire was placed in the LV; (c) the Judkins catheter was then advanced over the 0.020″ wire into the LV; (d) subsequently, the 0.025″ pigtail guidewire was

Table 13.2 Methods of crossing the MV in difficult situations

1. Inoue method
   - Changing stylets
   - Push-pull technique
   - Loop method
2. Meier's technique
3. Mehan and Meier's technique (Swan-Ganz balloon assistance)
5. Manjunath's modified over-the-wire technique
6. Predilatation with a small peripheral balloon

advanced into the LV; and (e) introduction of the Inoue balloon over the wire into the LV. The second method advocated by Mehan and Meier[10] involved: (a) crossing the mitral valve with a balloon floatation catheter (Swan-Ganz); (b) maneuvering the balloon catheter into the aorta; (c) the positioning of a 0.021″-long "back-up" valvuloplasty guide wire through this catheter in the descending aorta; and (d) introduction of the Inoue balloon over the wire (Figure 13.2, Video 13.1). One drawback of this method is that the balloon floatation catheter may just float within a large LA and not find the mitral valve orifice until a long sheath is placed immediately in front of the MV.

Manjunath and colleagues modified the above technique and simplified the steps (Figure 13.3, Videos 13.2 through 13.7).[11] The steps involved are: (1) placing the 0.025″ pigtail guidewire in the LA; (2) reintroducing the Mullin sheath with dilator into the LA over the pigtail guidewire and withdrawing the coiled portion of the guide wire into the sheath; (3) positioning the Mullins sheath/dilator near the MV orifice (Figure 13.3a) and placing a pigtail guidewire directly into the LV (Figure 13.3b). This step may initially appear to be difficult because of the pigtail tip. However, with some perseverance and practice it can be easily achieved; (4) this is followed by further advancement of the Mullin sheath/dilator into the LV cavity (Figure 13.3c) for obtaining optimal coiling of the pigtail guidewire (at least two to three coils; Figure 13.3d); and (5) threading the PTMC balloon over the wire into the LV cavity. The PTMC balloon should not be deslenderized until at least two-thirds of the balloon has

crossed the IAS (Figure 13.3e and 13.3f) keeping a sustained forward push on the pigtail guidewire. After crossing the mitral valve, the PTMC balloon is positioned across the valve and the dilation performed in the usual way (Figure 13.3g and 13.3h). While removing the pigtail guidewire from the LV, it is essential that the wire be withdrawn into the PTMC balloon when it is still placed in the LV so as to avoid slicing of the submitral apparatus. Only then (Figure 13.3i) should the entire assembly be withdrawn into LA. No additional accessories like back up guidewires, right Judkins catheter, or floatation catheters are required, thus preventing additional expenses. As the pigtail guidewire is directly introduced into the LV, multiple exchange involved in other conventional OTW techniques are avoided, resulting in lesser fluoroscopic procedural time and a high success rate. Since the technique is associated with frequent ventricular ectopics and short runs of non-sustained ventricular tachycardia, it has been felt that this may make the patient hemodynamically unstable. An analogy may be drawn to balloon aortic valvuloplasty, where during the placement of the extrastiff wire into the LV, similar ectopy is noted. However, once the wire has a stable position the rhythm stabilizes. Similar findings are noted in the OTW technique. Once optimum coiling of the pigtail guidewire is obtained, the ectopy disappears. Another concern has been that the 0.025″ pigtail guidewire may not provide adequate support to the PTMC balloon, resulting in prolapse of the balloon into LA. The trick here is that the PTMC balloon should not be deslenderized until at least two-thirds of the balloon has crossed the IAS. Further,

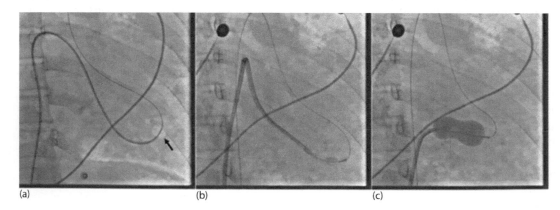

(a)   (b)   (c)

Figure 13.2 Swan-Ganz Assistance: **(a)** Crossing the mitral valve with a Swan-Ganz catheter (arrow) and 0.032″ wire **(b)**, **(c)** PTMC balloon threaded over wire with successful PTMC. PTMC, percutaneous transvenous mitral commissurotomy (see Video 13.1).

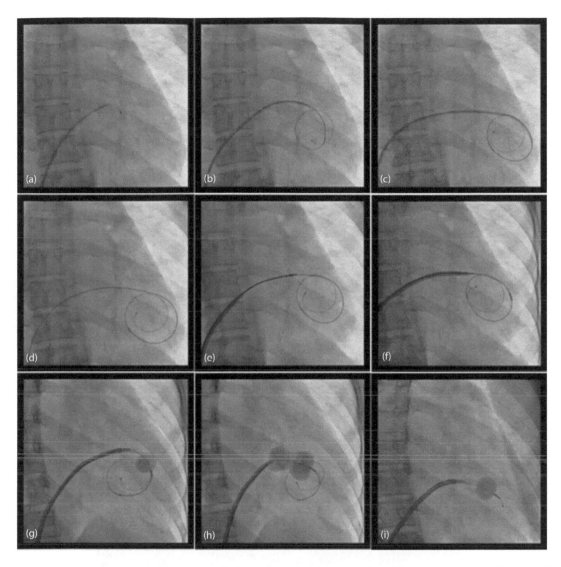

Figure 13.3 Modified over-the-wire technique described by Manjunath and colleagues.[11] **(a)** Mullins sheath positioned near the mitral orifice; **(b)** pigtail guidewire passed directly into the LV; **(c)** Mullins sheath advanced into the LV cavity; **(d)** optimal coiling of the pigtail guidewire (at least two to three coils); **(e–f)** PTMC balloon catheter being introduced over the pigtail guidewire into the LV cavity; **(g)** distal half of PTMC balloon inflated; **(h)** PTMC balloon withdrawn up to the mitral valve and approximately half inflated; **(i)** pigtail guidewire withdrawn into the PTMC balloon before withdrawing entire assembly. PTMC, percutaneous transvenous mitral commissurotomy (see Videos 13.2 through 13.7).

concern has been expressed that the guidewire may get inserted between the chordate tendineae, which may get damaged during balloon inflation, leading to severe mitral regurgitation.[12] In our experience, we have not found this to be a concern over the past 15 years. When two to three optimal coils of the pigtail guidewire are made in the LV, the possibility of entering the subvalvular apparatus is precluded due to the large diameter of the coils.[13] Identifying the "balloon impasse" or "balloon compression" signs will prevent inadvertent inflation of the balloon in the subvalvular apparatus. More recently, we reported the use of the OTW technique in transjugular PTMC as well.[14] In the event of a low puncture, LV entry was difficult in one of the four cases of transjugular PTMC. The OTW technique was successfully used to enter the LV and the PTMC was successfully performed.

Finally, Deora and colleagues[15] used a 0.035″, 260 cm, hydrophilic glidewire over a 4F Amplatz right-1 diagnostic coronary catheter to enter the LV. The hydrophilic wire was then exchanged with a 0.035″ Amplatz super-stiff guidewire, which was coiled in vitro to make extra loops of its floppy portion. The Inoue PTMC catheter was slenderized directly over this super-stiff wire without its metal stylet and gradually negotiated to park across the stenotic mitral valve orifice.

In the event the OTW technique fails to provide sufficient support to the PTMC balloon for LV entry, the establishment of a venoarterial loop (Babic technique) has been found to be helpful. Such a scenario may arise in the presence of severe submitral disease wherein advancement of the PTMC balloon may be difficult.[16] In such a scenario, through the Mullins sheath placed in the LV, an exchange length 0.032″/0.035″ hydrophilic wire is advanced into the descending aorta from where it is snared using a gooseneck snare inserted through the femoral artery. Using the venoarterial loop as a railroad, the PTMC balloon is tracked over the loop (Figure 13.4, Videos 13.8 and 13.9). Since the 0.032″ wire is unsheathed within the LV, traction during the establishment of the AV loop can transect the MV apparatus leading to mitral regurgitation. In order to avoid this, it is essential to maintain the curve of the wire in the LV (avoiding the immediate direct route from MV to aortic valve) by pushing and pulling simultaneously at the venous and arterial ends. No force should be applied. A safer alternative is to first pass a balloon floatation catheter into the LV and aorta and then advance the 0.032″ wire over the balloon floatation catheter before being snared from the femoral artery. Needless to say, all manipulations should be gentle.

For all OTW techniques, with wire positioned in the LV, direct measurement of LA pressure is not possible (except if the PTMC balloon is exchanged for a multitrack catheter). The success (or otherwise) of the procedure has to be monitored with TTE. Mitral regurgitation may be overestimated due to the wire interfering with leaflet coaptation.

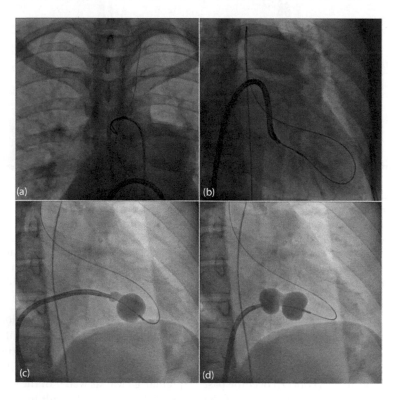

Figure 13.4 Venoarterial loop. **(a)** A 0.035″ glidewire (Terumo wire) is passed through the LV into the aorta where it is snared using a gooseneck snare; **(b)** a PTMC balloon threaded over the 0.035″ glidewire maintaining the loop in the LV **(c)** and **(d)** PTMC completed. PTMC, percutaneous transvenous mitral commissurotomy. (Courtesy of Prof. S. Shankar, SJICS&R, Bangalore-India [See Videos 13.8 and 13.9].)

The OTW technique is useful in a number of situations, such as giant LA, low septal puncture, thick IAS, LA/LA appendage clot, critical MS (see Videos 13.10 through 13.13), dextrocardia/malposed cardia, jugular PTMC, etc. It forms an important armamentarium in the cases of difficult LV entry.

Retrograde nontransseptal mitral valvotomy has been described using a coronary catheter (LIMA catheter, EBU guide catheter) to cross the mitral valve (passed via femoral artery, aorta, and LV into LA[17]; this is similar to passing a radiofrequency ablation catheter retrograde). This is followed by the placement of an exchange- length extrastiff wire in the LA and the passage of a valvuloplasty balloon (e.g., Tyshak balloon). It is essential to confirm that the passage of the coronary catheter and the wire is not through the submitral apparatus.

SPECIFIC SUBSETS

Left-atrial/left-atrial appendage clot

Left-atrial thrombus occurs in 3%–13% of patients with MS and its presence is generally considered a contraindication for PTMC due to the risk of systemic embolization with potentially devastating complications. There have been few studies of successful PTMC in the presence of an LA/LAA clot. In most of these studies, the clot was restricted to the LA appendage. In one such study, during balloon catheter manipulation (RAO 30°), the catheter in the LA was always kept to the left of the pigtail catheter preplaced in the LV, in order to avoid the LAA region.[18]

We have classified LA thrombus, based on their location, extension, and mobility as assessed by TTE/TEE as follows (Figure 13.5; Table 13.3):[19] patients were considered for PTMC if they had type Ia, type Ib, and type IIa LA clots. Patients were anticoagulated (INR 2.0–3.0) for 8–12 weeks. A deliberate low-IAS puncture is performed. The modified OTW as described earlier is used (Figure 13.4). By adopting this technique, the LA is virtually excluded from the track of septal dilator and balloon catheter exchanges and hence the possibility of disturbing the thrombus is negligible. In a prospective study of 108 patients[19] with LA thrombus at our institute, there were no thromboembolic episodes during the procedure. However, there was one case of transient ischemic attack, which occurred six hours after a successful PTMC. There

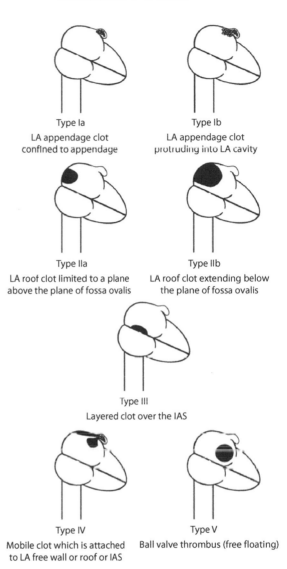

Type Ia
LA appendage clot
confined to appendage

Type Ib
LA appendage clot
protruding into LA cavity

Type IIa
LA roof clot limited to a plane
above the plane of fossa ovalis

Type IIb
LA roof clot extending below
the plane of fossa ovalis

Type III
Layered clot over the IAS

Type IV
Mobile clot which is attached
to LA free wall or roof or IAS

Type V
Ball valve thrombus (free floating)

Figure 13.5 LA/LAA clot classification. LA: left atrium; LAA: left-atrial appendage; IAS: interatrial septum. (Reproduced from Manjunath CN et al., *Catheter Cardiovasc Interv* 2009;74(4):653–61. With permission.)

was significant and comparable improvement in the mitral valve area, mitral valve gradient, LA mean, and pulmonary artery systolic pressure following the procedure. All these procedures were performed by experienced operators who had performed more than 500 PTMCs.

Giant atrium

Encountering a giant LA is not uncommon in PTMC. It poses unique challenges for TSP and LV

Table 13.3 LA/LAA clot classification

Type Ia:	LA appendage clot confined to appendage
Type Ib:	LA appendage clot protruding into LA cavity
Type IIa:	LA roof clot limited to a plane above the plane of fossa ovalis
Type IIb:	LA roof clot extending below the plane of fossa ovalis
Type III:	Layered clot over the interatrial septum (IAS)
Type IV:	Mobile clot which is attached to LA free wall or roof or IAS
Type V:	Ball valve thrombus (free-floating)

Abbreviations: IAS: interatrial septum; LA: left atrium.

entry. The IAS bulges toward the RA and the fossa ovalis is displaced downwards. Sometimes, the IAS is close to the RA wall, leaving only a narrow space between the two. This makes manipulation of the TSP needle difficult. Further, the RA border may be medial to the LA border and it is the RA border that is the posterior limit of the IAS. Assistance with TTE, TEE, or ICE may be helpful in TSP. Right-atrial angiography or the levophase of the pulmonary angiogram can serve to delineate the IAS (Figure 13.6a, Videos 13.14 through 13.16). Further, as the catheter-needle assembly is withdrawn, flushing with contrast medium helps in demarcating the IAS (Figure 13.6b, Videos 13.14 through 13.16). TSP is done at a site more caudal than usual. The IAS bulge makes it difficult to align the catheter tip with the midline and perpendicular to the IAS. For

this, the curve of the needle should be straightened somewhat. During the clockwise rotation maneuvers, the catheter flips over the IAS bulge into the posterior or anterior recess.[10] This is best appreciated in the RAO view, where the septum is *en face*. Inadvertent puncture at these sites will lead to cardiac tamponade. The needle indicator should be rotated to the "6–7 o'clock" position (rather than the "5 o'clock" position), keeping slight pressure against the IAS. Another useful technique is the needleless septal puncture technique, as described earlier to probe the fossa ovalis (FO). As mentioned earlier, the fossa is displaced inferiorly in a giant LA. LV entry is also difficult in patients with giant LA. It is advisable to do a low puncture as this will aid subsequent LV entry. We have found the OTW technique[11] extremely useful for LV entry. Another useful maneuver is the reverse-loop technique.

In patients with giant RA, the IAS bulge is towards the LA. The tip of the transseptal needle may not engage the IAS. For this, the needle should be bent to make a more acute curve. During TSP, the needle indicator should point to the "4 o'clock" position.

Small left atrium

A small LA may be encountered in children. This condition leads to a unique set of problems since the PTMC balloons are primarily designed for adult use. The length of the slenderized balloon is 4.5 cm and the stylet has a preformed J-shaped tip with a waist length of about 4.5 cm. Negotiating a small-sized LA with this hardware becomes difficult.

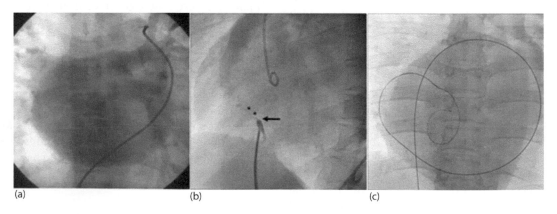

(a)   (b)   (c)

Figure 13.6 Giant left atrium. **(a)** levophase of pulmonary angiogram; **(b)** septal stain (*) and tenting (arrow); **(c)** 0.025″ coilwire outlining giant LA. (Courtesy of Prof. S. Shankar (a) and Prof. T. R. Raghu (b, and c), SJICS&R, Bangalore-India [Videos 13.14 through 13.16].)

In their paper, Trehan and colleagues[20] described these problems in detail. Since the length of the stretched balloon was more than the vertical LA dimension (2.8 cm) of their eight-year-old patient, they could not advance the stretched balloon into the LA. To overcome this, the stretcher was partially advanced so that the length of the partly stretched slightly lower-profile balloon was almost equal to the vertical dimension of the LA. Next, the small size of the LA resulted in repeated entrapment of the balloon at the septal puncture site, preventing LV entry despite being able to advance the 0.025″ pigtail wire into the LV. To free the balloon from the IAS, a double loop of the Inoue balloon was made over the coil wire in LA. After completing one full circle in excess of the usual lie of the Inoue balloon catheter, the tip of the Inoue balloon was now pointing at the mitral valve orifice. The coiled wire was passed into the LV and the Inoue balloon catheter was then easily advanced into the LV. This maneuver was possible because of the small height of the patient, with enough length of the balloon shaft lying outside the body.

Moderate mitral regurgitation

While associated MR of grade ≥3 is a contraindication for PTMC, PTMC may be successfully performed in patients with Grade 2 MR. The prerequisites for this are as follows: the MR should be central and not commissural, there should be no commissural calcification, and the LA should be large. More often, in the above scenario, it is a fixed-orifice MR due to non-coaptation of leaflets. Following a successful PTMC, MR will regress (Figure 13.7). It is advisable to use a stepwise dilatation technique starting initially with the recommended size (RS) minus 4 mm (RS-4). Following each inflation, the echo should be reassessed to determine the degree of MR and splitting of commissures. If no worsening of MR occurs, the balloon may be upsized and PTMC performed again.

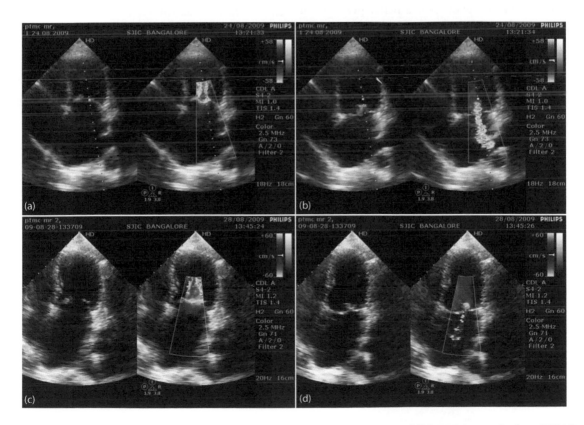

Figure 13.7 TTE images of PTMC in presence of moderate MR. **(a)** and **(b)** TTE image before PTMC revealing severe MS and moderate central MR; **(c)** and **(d)** TTE images after PTMC showing successful PTMC and mild MR.

Calcific mitral stenosis

Patients with calcific MS are older, more commonly have AF, have a higher Wilkin's score, more severe MR, and lower MV area than those with noncalcific MS. MV calcification has been shown to be a predictor of poor outcomes following PTMC both in the immediate and long-term follow-up. Complication rates are higher, namely, mitral regurgitation from leaflet tear and embolization of calcific material. Previous studies have reported success rates of as low as 52% for PTMC in calcific valves.[21] As the degree of fluoroscopic calcification increased, the success rate dropped dramatically (33% for Grade 4 calcification). Studies have differed in the method of assessment of valve calcification. Older studies used fluoroscopy, whereas the later ones used echocardiography. Fluoroscopy does not localize the site of calcification. Echocardiography is more sensitive and can assess not only the extent of calcification but also the site. As the mechanism of PTMC is commissural splitting, assessment of commissural morphology is a better predictor of outcome. Commissural calcification is a simple but strong predictor of PTMC outcome. Patients without commissural calcification can safely undergo PTMC irrespective of the degree of calcification elsewhere (i.e., leaflets, annulus) (Figure 13.8, Video 13.17). However, bicommissural calcification is an absolute contraindication for PTMC. PTMC can be attempted in those with unicommissural calcification. It is advisable to start with a balloon of RS-4 size. Subsequently, a stepwise graded approach is recommended. As the Inoue balloon is inflated the calcified commissure will not yield, whereas the non-calcified commissure gives way on serial graded, guided inflations[22] (Figure 13.9, Video 13.18). Using this technique, immediate success rates of 80%–85% have been reported for calcific MS.[23,24] However, the long-term survival at 20 years was 50% for calcified valves vs. 81% for non-calcified valves with good functional result noted in only 12% and 38%, respectively.[24] This poor survival in calcific MS was mainly restricted to patients above 50 years. For patients below 50 years, the 20-year survival for calcific and non-calcific valves was similar (89% vs. 85%, respectively).[24] Thus, while PTMC is associated with

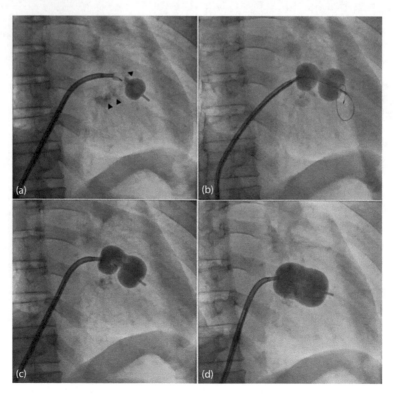

Figure 13.8 See Video 13.17. **(a)** Heavy annular calcification (arrowheads); **(b)** PTMC ballon with waist; **(c)** lateral commissure split, followed by; **(d)** medial commissure.

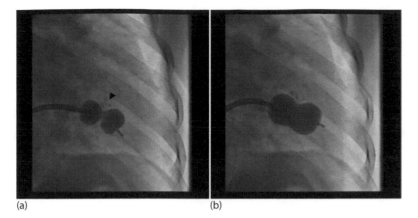

(a)   (b)

Figure 13.9 Calcification of mitral valve. **(a)** calcified mitral valve; **(b)** dense calcification confined to the lateral commissure (arrowhead); the medial commissure is free of calcium. The calcified lateral commissure does not yield, the non-calcified medial commissure splits on serial graded, guided inflation. (Courtesy of Prof. B. C. Srinivas, SJICS&R, Bangalore-India [see Video 13.18]).

acceptable immediate outcomes in patients with calcific MS, these patients need careful follow-up with greater need for mitral valve replacement (MVR). Predictors of immediate poor outcome with PTMC in calcific MS include extent of calcification, older age, lower MV area, and use of single/double-balloon technique (as opposed to an Inoue balloon). Predictors of poor long-term outcomes after good immediate results were severe valve calcification, older age, higher NYHA class, AF, and higher mean gradient after PTMC. Thus, younger patients in sinus rhythm with lower NYHA class derived greater long-term benefits with PTMC.

Severe subvalvular disease (SVD)

Severe submitral disease is a predictor of adverse outcomes after PTMC. It is a strong independent risk factor for the development of severe mitral regurgitation after PTMC.[25] It is also a predictor for failure of PTMC procedure (unsuccessful dilatation). In severe SVD, the valve leaflets get pulled down to form a funnel, as a result of which the narrowest portion is at the chordal level (rather than at leaflet tips) well into the LV.[26] The fibrosed leaflets contain columns of fused chordae. In severe cases, there may only be a single column. An in vitro study of balloon dilatation of surgically excised intact rheumatic valves found that extensive involvement of subvalvular apparatus was associated with increased risk of leaflet tearing, thereby explaining the increased risk of MR.[27] It was noted that leaflet tears originated in the apex of

spaces between the fused chordal columns and then extended upwards towards the annulus. Sometimes, fortuitously, the tear may be along the commissural plane, leading to successful PTMC.

While the Wilkin's score does take into consideration subvalvular thickening, it does not take chordal or papillary muscle fusion into consideration. A newly described score classifies SVD as mild, moderate, or severe[25] (to mild-multiple, thickened, discrete chordae; moderate-thickened, and fused chordae form two identifiable thick chords; severe-fused chordae appear as a single, thick chord). Indicators of SVD include disproportionately high LA and PA pressure despite only moderate MS as assessed by MV area. During PTMC, SVD can be recognized by the balloon compression sign, the balloon-impasse sign,[28] and repeated popping out of the balloon into LA.[29] In order to avoid the complication of severe MR, one should abort balloon dilation whenever the balloon compression or balloon impasse is seen. It has been recommended to use a smaller 18- or 20-mm Inoue balloon in the presence of SVD. Only a smaller balloon may stretch the subvalvular apparatus without tearing it. If further dilatations are needed, a catheter one size larger is used. While this will minimize MR, it does not ensure total prevention. As 18/20-mm balloons are not easily commercially available, a peripheral balloon may be used. When repeated attempts fail to reduce the gradient, the procedure should be abandoned.

Failure of the PTMC balloon to reach the LV apex is another important sign of SVD. In such a

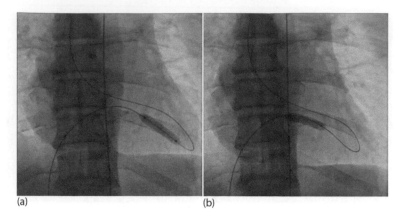

(a)　　　　　　　(b)

Figure 13.10 Serial dilatation of subvalvular apparatus with peripheral balloon after establisihing arteriovenous loop (see Videos 13.19 and 13.20).

scenario, a smaller peripheral balloon is used to dilate the submitral apparatus followed by PTMC balloon (Figure 13.10, Videos 13.19 and 13.20). In one such case,[26] we faced marked difficulty in advancing the PTMC balloon due to severe subvalvular disease (mitral valve orifice area of 1.0 cm^2 at cusp level and 0.4 cm^2 at chordal level). With the support of a Judkins right catheter, a 0.035″ Terumo wire (Terumo Corporation) was introduced into the LV and then advanced into the aorta and the right subclavian artery. An 8 × 20-mm Opta-Pro PTA balloon (Cordis Corporation) was passed over the Terumo wire and the submitral apparatus was serially dilated. The Terumo wire was then exchanged for the coiled guidewire and the procedure was completed with a PTMC balloon catheter. The medial commissure was split and the submitral stenosis was released.

The presence of SVD is not an absolute contraindication for PTMC. However, its presence should lead to a strong consideration for MVR especially in the presence of other unfavorable factors for PTMC (e.g., severe TR needing annuloplasty, repeat PTMC, etc.).

Anomalies of inferior vena cava

The transfemoral approach to PTMC is not possible in acquired or congenital interruption of the inferior vena cava (IVC). In such cases, PTMC may be performed from the transjugular route. In the transjugular approach, the critical step is the performance of TSP. There are two issues here. First is the selection of needle for septal puncture and second is the optimal puncture site. The adult

Brockenbrough needle is too long and unwieldy for transjugular PTMC (71 cm). If used for transjugular TSP, the curve of the adult Brockenbrough needle has to be increased. We have used the 56-cm pediatric Brockenbrough needle as it provides easy maneuverability from the neck.[14] The needle has to be manually bent at the tip. This creates a more acute angle that prevents the needle from slipping down the septum. Others have used the Endry's transseptal puncture needle for TSP. The second issue is that of the optimal puncture site. A high puncture site is preferable in the transjugular approach as it aids LV entry. However, unlike the transfemoral route, there are no standard landmarks for TSP in the transjugular approach. The limbic edge cannot be relied upon in the transjugular approach. Recourse needs to be taken to delineation of the IAS by angiography. We performed a PA angiogram in the LAO 45° and RAO 30° view.[14] The LA opacification in the levophase demarcates the septum and acts as a roadmap. During TSP, the needle indicator should point to the "7–8 o'clock" position, unlike the conventional "5 o'clock" position. We chose a site midway between the pigtail catheter (placed in the non-coronary sinus) and the vertebral border, a little below the level of the pigtail. TSP was performed in the LAO view. After TSP, the IAS was dilated using the septal dilator. Subsequent LV entry required the stylet to be rotated in a clockwise manner, unlike the anticlockwise rotation in the femoral approach. Reshaping the stylet in an S-shaped configuration helps LV entry. The LV entry is hampered by the lack of fulcrum-like support that the IAS provides during the rotation maneuvers, as in the transfemoral route. A low septal puncture (e.g., fossa ovalis) makes LV entry even more difficult. In such cases, the OTW technique is very useful. Thus, with the help of conventional PTMC hardware, transjugular PTMC can be successfully preformed. We have also successfully performed repeat PTMC via the jugular route (first and second PTMC via jugular route [Figures 13.11 and 13.12, Videos 13.20 through 13.28]). As the operator works from the head end, radiation exposure is greater.

Joseph and colleagues have the largest series in transjugular PTMC.[30] They used a different approach. TSP was performed using the Endry's pediatric transseptal set. The Endry's needle is even shorter (30 cm). They performed the PA angiogram in the 45° RAO view. TSP was performed 2 cm below the roof of the LA (one vertebral body height), midway between the aorta and anterior border of the spine. Further steps were modified and included the positioning of a 20 cm-long, 14F, J-shaped Cook sheath directly into the LA, the use of a balloon floatation catheter to assist LV entry, and the use of a JOMIVA balloon for MV dilatation.

Other percutaneous options for patients with interrupted IVC are retrograde nontransseptal balloon mitral commissurotomy and percutaneous transhepatic mitral commissurotomy.

Dextrocardia

Cardiac malposition leads to difficulties in TSP and LV entry. In situs inversus with dextrocardia, the procedure should be performed from the left groin to reduce the angulation of the puncture needle at the confluence of the iliac veins to the left-sided IVC.[31] For operator comfort, the fluoroscopic image may be reversed (fluoroscopic imaging inversion).[31,32] When the images are flipped, the dextrocardia appears as the usual levocardia simulating normal anatomy. Thus, with the C arm in the LAO 30° view or RAO 45° view, a pseudo-RAO 30° view or pseudo-LAO 45° view is obtained respectively (Figure 13.13, Videos 13.29 through 13.32). After passage of the Brockenbrough needle into the left-sided SVC, the Mullins sheath-Brockenbrough

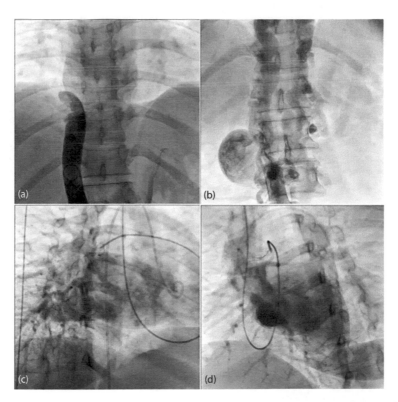

Figure 13.11 Redo-transjugular PTMC. A 30-year-old female had CMV in 2009 followed by transjugular PTMC in 2011 and redo-transjugular PTMC in 2017. **(a)** IVC obstruction; **(b)** azygous and hemiazygous continuation; **(c)** pulmonary artery angiogram in RAO 30°; and **(d)** pulmonary artery angiogram in LAO 45° to delineate the left atrium and the interatrial septum in the levophase; see Videos 13.21 through 13.28.

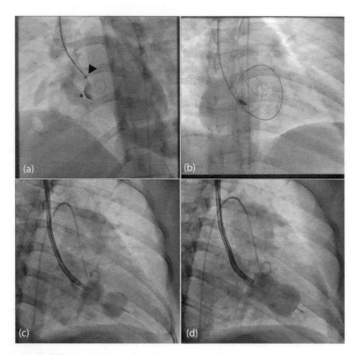

Figure 13.12 Continuation of Figure 13.11. **(a)** Septal puncture done in the left anterior oblique view at the level of pigtail, midway between the pigtail and the spine (arrowhead denotes the site of TSP, * denotes contrast persistence in noncoronary sinus after failed attempt at TSP); **(b)** 0.025″ pigtail guide-wire passed into LA; **(c,d)** PTMC completed with conventional technique.

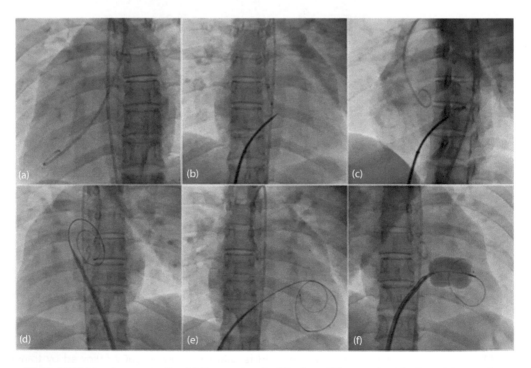

Figure 13.13 PTCM in dextrocardia: **(a)** Dextrocardia PA view; **(b)** pseudo-AP view; **(c)** septal puncture in pseudo-left lateral view; **(d)** septal dilation in PA view; **(e)** and **(f)** OTW technique Accura balloon in Pseudo-RAO 30°. (Courtesy of Prof. K. H. Srinivas, SJICS&R, Bangalore-India.)

needle assembly is withdrawn, keeping the needle oriented to the "9 o'clock" position. Subsequently, for septal puncture the needle pointer is oriented to the "7 o'clock" position rather than the "4 o'clock" position in the pseudo-LAO view (i.e., RAO 45°). If possible, probing for the PFO may be attempted. If there are difficulties in TSP, the levophase of the pulmonary angiogram is useful to delineate the septum and its relationship to the pigtail in the noncoronary aortic sinus. Septal staining and use of echo guidance can further aid TSP in such cases. LV entry is done with clockwise rotation rather than anticlockwise rotation in pseudo-RAO view (i.e., LAO 30°). In cases of difficult LV entry, we have used the OTW technique, while others have used the reverse-loop technique. In more complex cases, it may be necessary to establish a venoarterial loop for LV entry.

Previous commissurotomy

Reappearance of symptoms after commissurotomy (surgical or percutaneous) may be due to: (1) inadequate relief of the stenosis; (2) development of MR; (3) progression of aortic or tricuspid disease; (4) mitral restenosis.[33] Mitral restenosis is responsible for the majority of patients (97% in one study) for late deterioration.[34] The mechanism of mitral restenosis is important in deciding further intervention. Restenosis may be due to commissural fusion, progressive sclerosis and rigidity of leaflets, and fusion of chordae (chordae of each cusp are matted together, chordae of one cusp fuse with that of the other cusp across the valve).[33,35] Often, there is a combination of these mechanisms. Repeat PTMC can be performed in the presence of bilateral commissural fusion.[36] On the other hand, if one or both commissures remain open, the restenosis is presumed to be due to a valvular and/or subvalvular pathology and PTMC is not attempted.[36,37] In addition, patients with bicommissural or massive calcification, MR > Grade 2, or associated coronary or aortic valve disease are best treated by surgery. PTMC gives good results in appropriately selected patients with previous commissurotomy. Among patients who have previously undergone PTMC, repeat PTMC is feasible in one out of four patients with restenosis, thereby postponing the need for surgery. In these patients, immediate success rates of 77%–94% have been reported.[38,39] Among patients with prior surgical commissurotomy, PTMC in appropriately selected patients has immediate success rates of 82%.[40]

Rarely, patients have presented with mitral stenosis following surgical mitral valve repair for rheumatic MR or combined MS/MR. In one series, three patients (out of 818) developed severe MS after valve repair.[41] All three patients were in NYHA Class 4 and underwent reoperation. We have performed PTMC in this group of patients using the above-mentioned criteria for PTMC (i.e., PTMC for bicommissural fusion).[42] While the overall technique remains the same, challenges were encountered during TSP and LV entry (Figure 13.14, Videos 13.33–13.38). TSP was difficult due to the enlarged LA (from previous MR now converted to MS). TSP was performed in the RAO 30° view, as the IAS is en face. Further, LV entry was difficult due to the abnormal orientation of the repaired valve. In one such case, we could not achieve LV entry despite repeated attempts. Subsequently, the OTW technique (as described earlier) was attempted. Attempts to position the coil wire into the LV over the Mullins sheath failed. Use of a right Judkin's catheter to enter the LV was unsuccessful, too. Finally, we achieved LV entry using a cobra catheter. Through the cobra catheter, the pigtail guidewire was passed into the LV and the PTMC procedure was completed using an Accura balloon. It is likely that the annuloplasty ring used for MV repair may protect against annular tear during balloon inflation.

Kyphoscoliosis

The presence of kyphoscoliosis and severe MS is a particularly challenging scenario.[43-45] These patients are at high risk for surgery on account of their spine deformity given the abnormal cardiovascular and pulmonary function. On the other hand, severe kyphoscoliosis was a contraindication for TSP (a prerequisite for PTMC) in the past. This was because kyphoscoliosis distorts the relative positions of the cardiac structures, making the traditional landmarks for TSP unreliable. The risk of cardiac perforation and tamponade is higher. In addition, on account of the kyphoscoliosis, patients may not be able to lie flat during the PTMC procedure, adding to the complexity.[44] However, with suitable modifications, PTMC has been performed successfully.

The TSP is the most crucial step. Depending on the convexity of the spine and the degree of LA enlargement, the anatomy of the IAS would be randomly distorted. As such, the best method is to delineate the IAS by means of angiography

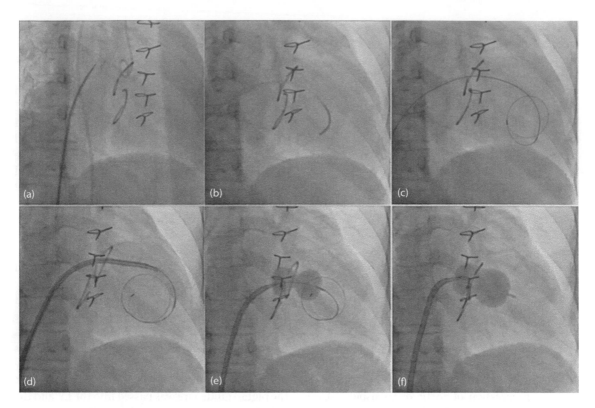

Figure 13.14 Post-MV repair status. A 37-year-old female had undergone MV repair and TV annulo-plasty one year previously. She presented with severe MS in AF with a fast ventricular rate in cardio-genic shock. After stabilization, PTMC was performed. **(a)** Mitral and tricuspid annuloplasty rings seen. TSP was performed in RAO 30° view. LV entry was difficult. Success was achieved with a cobra catheter and glidewire passed through a Mullins sheath; **(b)** a Mullins sheath was advanced over the cobra cath-eter into the LV and subsequently the 0.025" pigtail guidewire was placed in the LV; **(c–f)** PTMC was completed using OTW technique (see Videos 13.33 through 13.38).

in two orthogonal views. In the first report, a biplane right-atrial angiogram was performed in the frontal and lateral view until the aorta was visualized.[43] In addition, the septal flush and stain technique was also used to delineate the septum. Often, the puncture site may not be at an optimal site and this may hamper LV entry. In such a case, the reverse loop may be used for LV entry. We have utilized the levophase of a PA angiogram in the RAO 30° and LAO 45° to aid TSP. In addition, for difficult LV entry, the OTW technique was found to be useful (Figure 13.15, Videos 13.39 and 13.40). The use of ICE and TEE for TSP guidance has been recommended in the presence of severe kyphosco-liosis. TEE must be performed with caution given tortuosity in the esophagus.

Finally, if the kyphoscoliosis is mainly restricted to the lower spine, then the transjugular technique can be used as it provides a short and direct route

to the IAS.[45] TSP is performed using a pediatric Brockenbrough needle using the levophase of PA angiogram.

Dilated coronary sinus

A dilated coronary sinus (CS) may pose challenges to PTMC. A mildly dilated CS is often encountered in patients in congestive cardiac failure and is of little consequence in the performance of PTMC. A markedly dilated CS is encountered in the pres-ence of a persistent left superior vena cava (PLSVC). When this is combined with absence of the right superior vena cava, the CS becomes aneurysmally dilated[46] (Figure 13.16). This distorts the cardiac anatomy leading to technical difficulties in PTMC. In the absence of RSVC, the usual technique of withdrawing the Brockenbrough needle from the RSVC and observing for the two jumps during

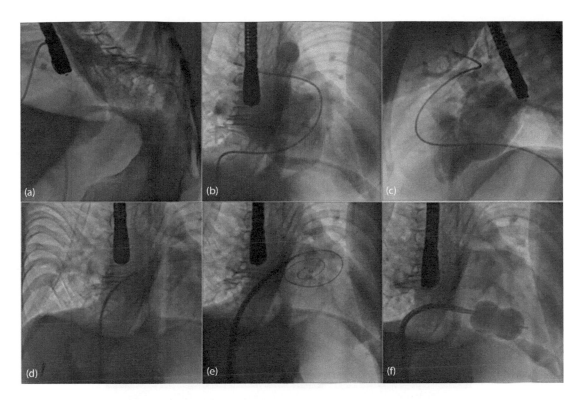

Figure 13.15 Kyphoscoliosis. **(a)** PTMC performed under TEE guidance; **(b)** levophase of PA angiogram used to delineate the IAS in the RAO 30° **(b)** and LAO 45° **(c)** view; **(d)** TSP performed in RAO 30° view; **(e)** septal dilator passed; **(f)** PTMC completed. (Courtesy of Dr. Harsha Basappa, SJICS&R, Mysore India [see Videos 13.39 and 13.40].)

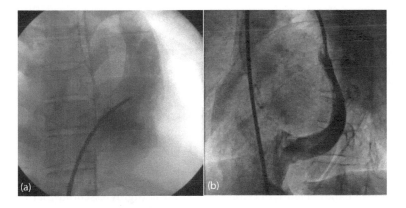

Figure 13.16 Dilated CS. **(a)** Aneurysmally dilated CS in absent right SVC and persistent left SVC; **(b)** markedly dilated CS in persistent left SVC with right SVC (catheter course right SVC to connecting vein to left SVC to CS). CS, Coronary sinus; SVC, Superior vena cava. (Courtesy Prof. B. C. Srinivas (a) and Prof. K. H. Srinivasa (b), SJICS&R, Bangalore-India.)

TSP is not possible. The aneurysmal CS pushes the IAS upwards. Each time TSP is attempted, the Brockenbrough needle–Mullins sheath will slip and fall into the aneurysmal CS, leading to a risk of CS perforation. This is compounded by the fact that the IAS bulge towards the RA due to high LA pressure in severe MS. In such cases, the margins of the CS os can be delineated by contrast injection into the CS (Figure 13.17, Videos 13.41 through 13.44). In the RAO view, the IAS is viewed *en face* with the

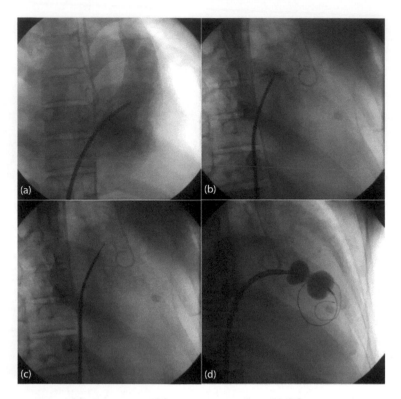

Figure 13.17 PTMC in dilated coronary sinus. **(a)** RAO view with contrast injection into CS through Mullins sheath and dilator; **(b)** septal staining to localize correct site of septal puncture, just above the lower end of the pigtail, midway between spine and pigtail; **(c)** TSP performed; **(d)** PTMC completed using OTW. (Courtesy of Prof. B. C. Srinivas, SJICS&R, Bangalore-India [see Videos 13.41 through 13.44].)

CS os located anteroinferiorly with respect to the fossa ovalis. As usual, the TSP site should be posterior to the noncoronary aortic cusp. However, the puncture site is higher than the usual site when the CS is dilated. The site is just above the lower end of the pigtail in the posterosuperior aspect of the FO in the RAO view midway between the pigtail and spine[46] (Figure 13.19c). The correct site can further be confirmed by septal staining (Figure 13.19b) and by TTE. As the TSP site is higher, difficulties may be encountered during LV entry. As such, the OTW technique may come in handy (Figure 13.19d).

PTMC in pregnant women, in children, and in Lutembacher syndrome are discussed in their respective chapters. A short synopsis is presented here.

Pregnant women

Ideally, the best time for PTMC during pregnancy is the second trimester (24–26 weeks) as: (1) fetal organogenesis is complete; (2) the fetal thyroid is still not active (avoiding the risk of hypothyroidism

due to the iodine contrast medium); (3) the uterus is small and more distant from the mother's chest, thereby being exposed to lesser radiation. PTMC should be performed by experienced operators. To limit radiation exposure, the patient's abdomen is circumferentially wrapped from the subcostal margin to the symphysis pubis with a lead apron (Figure 13.18, Videos 13.45 and 13.46). However, it must be remembered that the radiation that the fetus receives is not the direct radiation but the scatter radiation (from mother's internal organs). So, it is highly essential that fluoroscopy be used only when absolutely essential. Avoid cineangiography and use fluoroscopy-saved images. Avoid angulated views and reduce the frame rate. Avoid right-heart study and LV angiogram. As far as possible, all hemodynamic data should be obtained by TTE. A stepwise dilation technique is advisable. In advanced stages of pregnancy, the large gravid uterus compresses the IVC, making the movements of the balloon and dilator painful. As such, balloon and dilator exchanges should be done slowly and

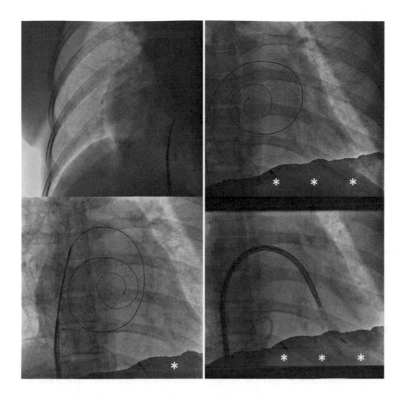

Figure 13.18 PTMC in a 22-year-old pregnant female. See Videos 13.45 and 13.46 (fluoroscopic images; note the lead shield [*]).

gently or the patient may need to be tilted towards the left position. The usual fluoroscopy time for PTMC in pregnant females is two to five minutes.

Juvenile mitral stenosis

In juvenile MS (<20 years of age) the valves are more fibrotic and rubbery with severe subvalvular disease. Technically speaking, the steps are the same with the exception that we may need a pediatric set.[47] Second, it is always better to undersize the balloon due to the risk of MR. Kothari and colleagues[16] started dilation in children (<12 years of age) using an initial balloon sized at 2–4 mm less than what would be the maximum recommended diameter based on adult nomograms (RBS = height in cm/10 + 10). The objective in children should be to create a MV area >1 cm^2/m^2 body surface area (BSA) and/or percentage increase in MV area of >50%.

Lutembacher's syndrome

Traditionally, Lutembacher's syndrome has been treated by open heart surgery. With the advent of percutaneous therapies for the treatment of MS and atrial septal defect (ASD), a definitive percutaneous therapy is now possible for Lutembacher's syndrome as well.[48,49] The choice between PTMC (with device closure of ASD when suitable) versus surgical closure of ASD with open mitral valvotomy (OMV)/MVR has its pros and cons. A primary percutaneous therapy avoids a sternotomy, leaving an option for a future first surgery at lower risk in the event of mitral restenosis. The percutaneous approach may, however, preclude future repeat PTMC following the placement of an ASD device. A TSP may be attempted through the native septum around the ASD device, if available. In addition, TSP through an amplatzer septal occluder device (with placement of 11F sheath) has been reported in patients undergoing AF ablation. This study was performed with ICE guidance and did not report any device embolization.[50] As of now, we are not aware of any reported case of PTMC in the presence of an ASD device. In such cases, a retrograde approach is still feasible.

For open heart surgery, the options are surgical closure of ASD along with CMV/OMV or MVR. MVR entails a prosthetic valve with its attendant complications and is best avoided in a young patient. CMV/OMV have the same or higher risk of restenosis as PTMC, which will need a repeat procedure in the future. Redo surgery poses a higher risk to the patient. Redo PTMC for mitral restenosis in such cases has its own challenges. TSP in a patient who has undergone surgical closure of ASD may damage the site of repair. TSP is challenging due to altered anatomical landmarks and the obliteration of the fossa ovalis. Despite this, TSP has been shown to be safe and efficacious when the ASD had been closed by means of stitch, pericardial patch and even Dacron patch.[51] However, if a Gore-tex patch has been used, TSP cannot be performed as the material is harder to penetrate.[51]

Last, not all the ASDs are suitable for device closure and open-heart surgery is the only option for such patients. However, quite often, Lutembacher syndrome patients are critically ill with deranged hepatic and renal parameters where surgery carries a higher risk of mortality. In such patients, PTMC is extremely useful as it restores hemodynamics and significantly improves symptoms and metabolic parameters. After a few weeks, surgical ASD closure can be done electively, if needed. It may appear that the presence of an ASD in Lutembacher syndrome may simplify the PTMC procedure by precluding the need for TSP. On the contrary, the large defect in the septum makes the PTMC balloon catheter unstable, due to the lack of anchoring support by the IAS, making its passage into the LV difficult.[52] The balloon repeatedly prolapses into the RA. In such situations, the OTW technique is very useful in enabling direct placement of the PTMC balloon into the LV. If the pigtail guidewire does not provide adequate support, a stiffer wire (e.g., Amplatzer extra-stiff wire) can be used. Another option is to perform a separate septal puncture in the anterior IAS, if sufficient rim of IAS is available. When suitable, an ASD device closure is best attempted two to three days after PTMC, after proper assessment of the PTMC outcome.[49] In the event of a suboptimal result or the presence of moderate MR, the ASD device should be deferred and the patient referred for surgery.

MANAGEMENT OF COMPLICATIONS

Cardiac tamponade

Cardiac tamponade is a potentially lethal complication of PTMC accounting for the most

procedure-related deaths. This may occur during TSP or LV entry. The most common cause of cardiac tamponade during PTMC is TSP. It is a good practice to perform a TTE immediately after TSP (before advancing the 14F dilator). TTE will not only document the site of TSP but also the appearance of new pericardial effusion. In such a scenario, the TSP needle should be withdrawn. Pericardial effusion developing after needle puncture can usually be managed by needle withdrawal without the need for pericardiocentesis as the rent is usually very small and will close spontaneously.

The mechanism of tamponade after TSP may be due to puncture of the following structures: (1) anterosuperiorly, aortic root perforation; (2) inferiorly, at the IVC-RA junction; (3) posteriorly, RA free wall; (4) anteroinferiorly, coronary sinus; and (5) rarely, LA roof or posterior wall.

Aortic root perforation

Aortic root perforation occurs due to puncture of RA at its junction with SVC adjacent to the aortic root.[53] To prevent this complication, the needle should be directed posteriorly and inferior to the plane of the aorta in the lateral/LAO view and to the left of the aorta in the RAO view. Further, the transseptal set should not be allowed to slip superiorly over the "limbic ledge."[54] Aortic puncture by TSP needle can be recognized early by contrast injection or by recording aortic pressure. Needle puncture of aorta is usually not of consequence unless a sheath or septal dilator has been passed. If a sheath/dilator has been passed and tamponade develops, then surgical correction is needed. There have been a few case reports of percutaneous closure of aortic puncture using Amplatzer ductal occluder[55] and Amplatzer septal occluder.[56] It is essential that the guidewire be retained in the aorta.

Right lateral wall and IVC perforation

Anatomically, the "true" IAS is a small area of the septum that can be removed without exiting from the cardiac cavities. This is restricted to the floor of the fossa ovalis and its oval immediate margin. There is no true septum beyond or near the right lateral and inferior border of the LA in the frontal view (there is infolding of the adjacent right- and left-atrial walls with extracardiac adipose tissue in between).[4] Puncture at these sites will lead to perforation of the RA wall followed by entry into the pericardial space and then re-entry into the LA, leading to the stitch phenomenon. Depending on the puncture site, there may be an RA-LA stitch (right lateral wall)[4] or a RA/IVC junction-LA stitch.[57] In such a scenario, as a LA pressure recording is obtained (along with aspiration of bright-red blood and contrast injection visualizing LA), it is thought that the TSP is performed at the correct site. Once the septal dilator is passed and withdrawn after dilation, massive cardiac tamponade ensues. In such a situation, the 14F septal dilator should be repositioned across the false track to seal the rent temporarily. Simultaneously, pericardiocentesis and completion of PTMC through another venous puncture is performed (see later). Technically, it is possible to close the stitch percutaneously by means of an atrial septal occluder. Two devices are needed, one between the LA and pericardial space and the second between the RA (or IVC-RA junction) and pericardial space.

Cardiac tamponade following LV entry is uncommon with the Inoue technique. It was earlier seen with the single/double balloon technique.[53,58] The mechanism included: (1) LV perforation by the stiff guidewires; (2) LV perforation by straight-tipped balloon catheters; or (3) "watermelon seeding" in the double-balloon technique, where one balloon advances rapidly to the LV apex during balloon inflation. LV perforation with the Inoue technique is uncommon due to: (1) the absence of guidewires in LV; (2) short balloon length; and (3) the dumbbell shape preventing migration of the balloon towards the LV apex during inflation. However, vigorous attempts at LV entry may sometimes damage the LAA or the pulmonary vein and lead to tamponade with the Inoue technique as well. Inadvertent inflation of the balloon in the left lower pulmonary vein (believing it to be the LV) is another possibility. Last, the greater use of the over-the-wire technique may lead to an increase in LV perforation. As mentioned earlier, the use of the pigtail guidewire may protect against this as it coils up in the LV.

Any drop in blood pressure should be viewed suspiciously and a TTE should be performed immediately to exclude pericardial effusion. Subtle signs such as yawning may be a pointer to the development of pericardial effusion. Another important clue is the observation of reduced pulsations of the left cardiac border on fluoroscopy. It must be remembered that even a small pericardial effusion can lead to tamponade.

The development of cardiac tamponade warrants immediate pericardiocentesis. Anticoagulation should be reversed with protamine if no further procedure is contemplated (we do not immediately reverse the anticoagulation until the PTMC is completed). Autotransfusion should be initiated as it is likely that the collection will reappear repeatedly, leading to the loss of a considerable volume of blood. The surgical team should be mobilized. The aspiration of bright-red blood indicates that the rent is in the LA while dark-red blood indicates an RA rent. The former will almost always need surgical intervention while the latter may seal off with conservative management. If the pericardial effusion has developed after dilation of the IAS with the 14F dilator, the dilator should be left in place as it will serve to occlude the rent. Removal of the dilator will lead to a dramatic increase in pericardial effusion and hemodynamic deterioration. The development of tamponade does not mandate that the PTMC procedure be aborted. Through a contralateral venous access, the procedure can be completed, preferably by a more experienced operator. The IAS is repunctured and the PTMC completed while another team continues the pericardial aspiration. We have successfully completed the PTMC in 78% of cases with tamponade (Figure 13.19, Videos 13.47 through 13.52). A successful PTMC in this scenario has three advantages. First, relief of the MS will reduce the elevated LA pressure thereby reducing the pericardial effusion. The tachycardia associated with tamponade will raise the LA pressure and transmitral gradient predisposing to the development of pulmonary edema. Second, relief of MS enables fluid resuscitation for tamponade to proceed unhindered. Third, if the tamponade warrants a surgical correction, the surgeon only needs to seal the rent, without the need for MVR. This will reduce the cardiopulmonary bypass time as well as postoperative complications. However, there is a risk of development of severe MR with PTMC, which can worsen the already compromised hemodynamics of cardiac tamponade. Once the PTMC is completed, an activated clotting time (ACT) is performed. If the ACT is elevated, anticoagulation is reversed. Recurrent appearance of pericardial effusion after pericardiocentesis is an indicator for surgery.

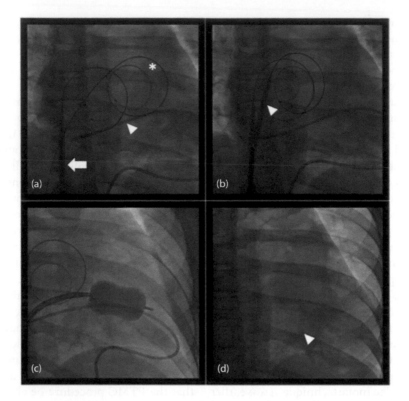

Figure 13.19 Pericardial tamponade. **(a)** One septal dilator with two pigtail guidewires in the LA. The passage of the first septal dilator (arrowhead) was followed by tamponade. The septal dilator was placed across the IAS and a fresh TSP was performed and a second pigtail guidewire (*) was placed in the LA. A pigtail is seen in the pericardial cavity (arrowhead); **(b)** two septal dilators and two pigtail guidewires in the LA. Repeat septal dilatation with the second septal dilator (arrowhead); **(c)** PTMC completed; **(d)** vascular sheath (arrowhead) in the pericardial cavity. After successful PTMC, continuous pericardiocentesis was carried out. Subsequently, pericardial accumulation stopped. The first septal dilator was slowly removed with pigtail guidewire in-situ. No further fluid accumulation was seen. The pigtail guidewire was removed and so was the pigtail in the pericardial cavity. A vascular sheath was left in the pericardial space for any delayed fluid accumulation (see Videos 13.47 through 13.52).

Severe mitral regurgitation

Severe MR develops in approximately 3% of cases and severe MR needing urgent surgery is seen in 1% of cases. The mechanism of MR includes leaflet tear, chordal rupture, annular tear, and commissural splitting. In an individual patient, no scoring system can reliably predict the development of severe MR or the lack of it since the balloon inflation is not a controlled one. A perfectly pliable, noncalcified valve can develop severe MR, whereas a heavily calcified valve with severe submitral disease may have a perfect PTMC result. The selection of an appropriately sized balloon, the use of a stepwise dilatation technique, and the performance of a TTE before the next balloon dilatation will help in reducing the incidence of severe MR. The appearance of new tall "v" waves on the LA pressure trace accompanied by a failure to fall or an increase in LA pressure is an important clue to the development of significant MR. This can easily be confirmed by performing a color Doppler echo. It must be remembered that some of these MR jets are eccentric and may not be easily picked in the supine position (as it is difficult to turn the patient on the table). A high index of suspicion needs to be maintained. The development of MR is an indicator to abort PTMC. Patients respond variably to the development of severe MR. Some are asymptomatic and hemodynamically stable, especially if the MS has also been relieved. Patients who become symptomatic for severe MR need emergency or urgent surgery. A common misconception is that symptomatic patients will develop pulmonary edema following development of severe MR. The large, dilated LA can accommodate the regurgitant volume and prevents pulmonary edema. The usual presentation is the development of hypotension due to reduced forward output. Among 50 patients who underwent MVR following the development of severe MR after PTMC, hypotension was seen in 72% of cases and pulmonary edema in only 12% of cases.[59] Operative mortality was greater in those in whom surgery was delayed beyond 24 hours compared to those who underwent MVR within 24 hours ($p < 0.001$). This is important since the absence of pulmonary edema may lead to a false impression that the patient is stable while the BP drops with a delay in surgery. The surgical team should be informed immediately. Hypotensive patients will need inotropic support and insertion of an intra-aortic balloon pump. Those in pulmonary edema need intravenous diuretics, morphine, and ventilatory support (noninvasive/invasive) as they await surgery. Leaflet, chordal, or annular tear almost always needs valve replacement. Severe commissural MR can be safely monitored conservatively if the patients are asymptomatic and hemodynamically stable. Subsequently, the criteria for MVR are the same as that for chronic, asymptomatic, severe MR. Commissural MR tends to regress over time.

Embolic stroke

The third important complication of PTMC is the occurrence of an embolic stroke. Embolic material may be clot (old, organized or freshly formed), air, or calcified valve material.[60] Treatment depends on early recognition. Once a stroke has been recognized on the table, a cerebral angiogram should be immediately performed in anteroposterior and lateral view to localize the site of occlusion (Figure 13.20, Videos 13.53 through 13.56). Ideally, cerebral imaging should be performed to rule out an intracerebral bleed. Intravenous or intraarterial thrombolytic therapy is recommended for cardioembolic ischemic stroke.[61] Intraarterial thrombolytic therapy may be preferred over intravenous thrombolysis as the former enables a higher concentration of thrombolytic agents to be delivered to the site of occlusion at lower doses with greater rates of recanalization. In addition, intrarterial thrombolysis can

be given in those where the INR is >1.7 (wherein IV thrombolytics are contraindicated) and up to six hours after a stroke (IV thrombolysis up to three hours after stroke onset).[61] Finally, given the presence of arterial and venous access, the larger IV dosage can lead to greater access site complications. Agents that have been used for intra-arterial thrombolysis are urokinase, tPA, reteplase, and tenecteplase.[62-64] Only urokinase has been evaluated in a randomized clinical trial (MELT trial) for ischemic stroke via the intrarterial route.[63] However, none of the agents have US FDA approval for intraarterial use. There are no standard regimens. Various studies have used various doses for varying durations. Common to all regimens is that the thrombolytic agent is given in small incremental doses followed by a cerebral angiogram every 10–15 minutes until complete recanalization is achieved or the maximum dose of the thrombolytic agent has been given or suspicion of extravasation of contrast material arises. Doses that have been studied are as follows: urokinase 50,000–100,000 units every 10 minutes up to 600,000 units; tPA-2–4 mg up to a total of 22 mg; reteplase 1 IU up to a total of 6–8 IU; tenecteplase 1 mg up to a total of 10 mg. Recently, many trials have shown the superiority of mechanical thrombectomy (using stent retrievers) over intravenous thrombolytic therapy for ischemic stroke.[65] They have the added advantage that they may be used in those with contraindications for fibrinolytic therapy (e.g., oral anticoagulants) up to 6–24 hours after stroke. They have better recanalization rates than IV tPA. Mechanical thrombectomy using stent retrievers is the indicated option in those in whom thrombolysis is contraindicated or has failed. This is also an option when the embolus is an organized clot or calcific material wherein thrombolytic therapy is ineffective.

Finally, the question arises as to when to imitate anticoagulation in a patient who has had an ischemic stroke. The early use of heparin (within 72 hours) is associated with a 15%–25% chance of converting a non-hemorrhagic stroke into a hemorrhagic stroke. Hence, anticoagulation should be withheld for the first 72 hours. If a computed tomography scan at that time reveals little or no hemorrhage, heparin should be administered along with warfarin until the desired INR is achieved. If the CT scan demonstrates significant hemorrhage, antithrombotic therapy should be withheld until the bleed is treated or has stabilized.

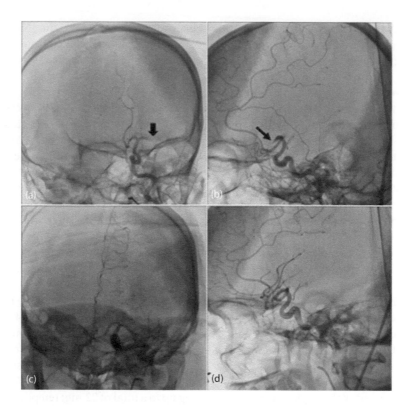

Figure 13.20 Embolic stroke. A 36-year-old female underwent redo-PTMC for restenosis. Preop TEE did not reveal LA/LAA clot. After two balloon inflations, the patient became nonresponsive and had developed right hemiplegia. Immediate cerebral angiogram in AP **(a, arrow)** and lateral view **(b, arrow)** revealed thrombotic occlusion of left middle cerebral artery. Intrarterial urokinase at a dose of 1 lakh unit was given every five minutes to a total of 3 lakh units. Within 15 minutes, patient started talking coherently and her power in the left upper and lower limbs had become Grade 3. Repeat cerebral angiogram showed marked improvement in cerebral flow in the MCA territory **(c)** and **(d)**. Within 24 hours, the power had returned to Grade 5. Repeat CT scan showed a small infarct in the MCA territory without hemorrhagic transformation (see Videos 13.53 through 13.56).

Complications associated with reused hardware

The PTMC hardware is routinely reused to keep the cost of procedure low in resource-limited countries. There are no guidelines as to how often a PTMC device can be reused. It has been shown that the Accura balloon can be safely reused six times and the Inoue balloon five times.[1,2] In practice, the usage far exceeds these figures. Repeated handling and sterilization can lead to malfunctioning of the device. Three commonly encountered scenarios are fracture of the pigtail guidewire, failure of deflation of the PTMC balloon, and failure to slenderize the PTMC balloon.

Fracture of pigtail guidewire. The 180-cm, stainless steel 0.025″ pigtail guidewire has a floppy coiled tip that is soldered to the stiffer, straight portion.[66] The junction between the floppy and straight portion is the site where fracture may occur. Factors that may lead to fracture include reuse, abnormal angulation between guidewire and dilator during septal dilatation, advancing the balloon or dilator with the soldered portion at the IAS (rather than deep into the LA), use of the over-the-wire technique, and, rarely, manufacturing defects.[66] Often, a combination of factors is at play.

It is good practice to examine the guidewire outside the body for any kinks or excessive undulations. Such wires should be discarded. If a kink develops after the guidewire has been introduced into the LA, it is best to withdraw the guidewire (over a Mullins sheath to maintain LA access) rather than proceeding with the PTMC procedure. Once a guidewire has fractured, it can be retrieved percutaneously. Often, the fractured wire will be floating in the LA, sometimes in the LV (during OTW techniques), and, rarely, in the RA. Various techniques have been described. It is important to remember that the fractured wire has a large loop. As such the retrieval device also needs to be large enough to accommodate the loop. A 10-mm goose neck snare can successfully be used to snare a fractured guidewire.[67] Sometimes, the appropriate hardware or the appropriate size may not be available. We devised an indigenous snare for this purpose.[66] A 300-cm exchange-length 0.014″ PTCA guidewire was made into a large loop and introduced into a 6F multipurpose catheter to form a snare unit (Figure 13.21, Videos 13.57 through 13.64). The loop could be increased or decreased by fixing one free end and pushing or pulling the other free end into the multipurpose catheter. The snare unit was deployed into the LA through the Mullins sheath. The broken pigtail guidewire could be snared within minutes as the loop formed by the snare was large enough. The broken pigtail guidewire cannot be withdrawn

into the Mullins sheath. As such, the whole unit (Mullins sheath, multipurpose catheter, indigenous snare, captured pigtail guidewire) must be removed *en bloc*. There is a theoretical risk of damage to the IAS or the femoral vein, but this was not encountered. To overcome this and to maintain continued LA access, a 10F Amplatzer delivery sheath (used in ASD device closure) was reported in one case.

Finally, if a portion of the fractured pigtail guidewire is still within the Mullins sheath or the PTMC balloon, it can be successfully retrieved using a 0.014″ angioplasty wire and PTCA balloon (Figure 13.22). In one case,[68] during use of the over-the-wire technique, the pigtail guidewire got fractured, with part of the pigtail guidewire within the LV and part within the Accura balloon. A 0.014″ PTCA floppy guidewire was passed into the Accura balloon by the side of the broken wire. Over the PTCA wire, a 1.5 mm × 10 mm noncompliant PTCA balloon was advanced just beyond the broken pigtail guidewire within the Accura balloon and inflated to 15 atm.

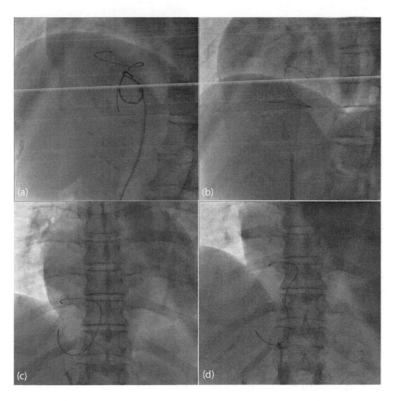

Figure 13.21 Snaring fractured pigtail guidewire by indigenous snare. **(a)** Fractured pigtail guidewire in the right atrium. The regular gooseneck snare could not snare the guidewire; **(b)** indigenous snare made from 300 cm PTCA wire. Note the large loop of the snare; **(c,d)** fracture guidewire caught by the indigenous snare and the assembly removed via femoral sheath (see Videos 13.57 through 13.64). (Courtesy of Dr. Satish Karur, SJICS&R, Bangalore-India.)

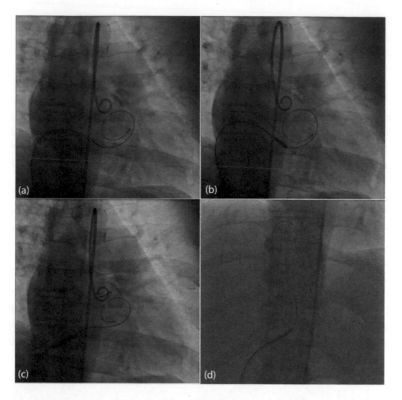

Figure 13.22 Fractured pigtail guidewire. **(a)** Fractured pigtail guidewire with some portion still within the Mullins sheath and a larger portion in the left atrium; **(b)** 0.014″ PTCA wire with 2×10 mm PTCA balloon passed by the side of the proximal part of the fractured pigtail guidewire. The PTCA balloon was inflated within the Mullins sheath, trapping the proximal portion of the fractured pigtail guidewire; **(c,d)** the entire assembly withdrawn *en masse*.

This trapped the broken pigtail guidewire between the outer wall of the inflated PTCA balloon and the inner wall of the Accura balloon. The entire assembly was then withdrawn *en masse*.

Deflation failure of the PTMC balloon. Failure of deflation of the PTMC balloon is a very rare complication. It can be catastrophic if the fully inflated balloon continues to straddle the mitral valve, obstructing forward blood flow. Fortunately, such a scenario has not been reported yet.

The PTMC balloon (Inoue or Accura) is composed of two layers of latex with a nylon mesh in between. A rent in the inner latex layer can lead to a one-way valve mechanism causing the contrast to accumulate in between the two latex layers, thereby preventing deflation of the PTMC balloon.[69] In addition, insufficient dilution of the contrast material used for balloon dilatation may cause the two latex layers to stick together. Finally, any kink in the balloon shaft (from excessive twisting) may also lead to deflation failure.

The Inoue balloon has two inbuilt safety mechanisms to prevent deflation failure. First, it has a vent tube that is meant for deairing the Inoue balloon during preparation. Opening the vent stopcock will allow contrast to flow out, enabling deflation. Second, it has two tiny holes in the outer latex layer. In the event of deflation failure, the accumulated contrast material can slowly escape, causing the balloon to collapse over time. Both these safety mechanisms are lacking in the Accura balloon.

In order to avoid deflation failure, the following steps may be followed. The dilution of contrast may be increased (nine parts saline and one part contrast, rather than fourfold if an ionic dye is used). The balloon should be checked for integrity outside the body with smooth inflation and deflation. There should be no undue resistance when the balloon is slenderized over the metal tube. Finally, while advancing the PTMC balloon into the patient, vigorous twisting movements should be avoided.

If deflation failure occurs, several steps may be considered. If the balloon is straddling the mitral valve, it should be dislodged by pushing it into LV or pulling into the LA. The latter is preferable. Continuous negative suction can be tried. A small amount of saline may be pushed into the balloon to dilute the contrast. In the case of the Inoue balloon, opening the vent tube may allow the contrast to flow out. Further, the two tiny holes provided in the Inoue balloon may allow slow seepage of contrast from the balloon. These safety measures are not present in the Accura balloon. If a kink is suspected, straightening the balloon shaft with the stainless steel pigtail guidewire can be tried. If this fails to straighten the kink, an attempt to pass the stretching tube may be tried. If these attempts fail, then it will be necessary to rupture the balloon. Two methods have been described. In the first, the hard end of the 0.025″ stainless steel pigtail guidewire was passed through the balloon inflation port and advanced up to the proximal part of the balloon (Videos 13.65 through 13.67).[70] The PTMC balloon was ruptured ensuring that the balloon was in the middle of the LA, away from the LA wall. This deflated the balloon. There would be a risk of air embolism if complete deairing had not been performed prior to balloon insertion. Theoretically, a stiff 0.014″ PTCA wire may also be tried. In the second method[71] (described for a bifoil balloon but applicable for the dumbbell PTMC balloon as well), the balloon was withdrawn against the IAS to keep the proximal end of the balloon at the IAS puncture site. Through another venous access, a Mullins catheter was advanced, through which a Brockenbrough needle was passed. After confirming in multiple views, the balloon was punctured with the needle. Attempts to overinflate the balloon have been tried, but run the risk of air and balloon material embolization. When all attempts to deflate the balloon fail, open-heart surgery is needed.

Failure to slenderize the PTMC balloon. After mitral valve dilatation, the PTMC balloon has to be withdrawn from the LA into the RA. Before withdrawal, it is necessary to slenderize the balloon in the LA. This is to avoid the creation of a larger iatrogenic ASD. Further, removal of the slenderized balloon from the femoral vein is atraumatic and smooth. Failure to slenderize the PTMC balloon may occur if the stretching tube could not be advanced over the pigtail guidewire. This often occurs if the correct sequence of stretching the balloon is not followed (the correct sequence is to lock the stainless-steel tube to the gold metal tube first, and then advance the two as a whole to lock into the plastic hub. Remember: gold and silver go together!). Further, stretching should always be done over the pigtail guidewire. If, for any reason, one is not able to slenderize the PTMC balloon in the LA, the balloon can often be pulled into the RA with a little tug (this should be done over the pigtail guidewire). Within the RA, it is much easier to slenderize the PTMC balloon as the shaft is now straightened out. Removing a PTMC balloon in the deslenderized state can damage the femoral vein, but this may be resorted to as a last option if all measures to slenderize the PTMC balloon fail.

ACKNOWLEDGMENT

We would like to sincerely thank all the faculty at SJICS&R, Bangalore, India and Mysore, India for having wholeheartedly shared their experience in challenging cases of PTMC.

VIDEOS

Video 13.1 (corresponding to Figure 13.2) Crossing the mitral valve with a Swan-Ganz catheter and 0.032″ guidewire. https://youtu.be/I6k--zzV6-k

Manjunath's modified over the wire (Videos 13.2 to 13.7 corresponding to Figure 13.3)

Video 13.2 Pigtail guidewire passed directly into the LV over Mullins sheath/dilator. https://youtu.be/kwOr9wBLHmM

Video 13.3 Mullins sheath advanced into the LV cavity to enable optimal coiling of the pigtail guidewire (at least 2–3 coils). https://youtu.be/Il3X4KNugQk

Video 13.4 PTMC balloon catheter being introduced over the pigtail guidewire from RA to LA. https://youtu.be/4fjabe6duRg

Video 13.5 PTMC balloon catheter being introduced over the pigtail guidewire from LA into the LV cavity. https://youtu.be/WBeLEx-PSb4

Video 13.6 Distal half of the PTMC balloon inflated and withdrawn up to the mitral valve followed by inflation of the proximal half. https://youtu.be/G_KymaJ0dOU

Video 13.7 PTMC successfully completed with withdrawal of the pigtail guidewire into the catheter. https://youtu.be/uq1DQXVm50I

Venoarterial loop (Videos 13.8 to 13.9 corresponding to Figure 13.4, Courtesy of Prof. S. Shankar)

Video 13.8 0.035″ hydrophilic guidewire (Terumo wire) is passed through the LV into the aorta where it is snared using a gooseneck snare to create an arteriovenous loop. https://youtu.be/McyTpcrtDA8

Video 13.9 PTMC balloon threaded over the 0.032″ hydrophilic guidewire while maintaining the loop in the LV and procedure completed. https://youtu.be/ZWbL65G2jtQ

Critical MS (Videos 13.10 to 13.13, Courtesy of Prof. B. C. Srinivas)

Video 13.10 Failure of PTMC balloon to enter LV due to critical MS. https://youtu.be/c9ZdkbORigU

Video 13.11 Dilatation of MV orifice using a peripheral balloon. https://youtu.be/63W3WQWzCbg

Video 13.12 Initial dilatation using PTMC balloon demonstrating an extremely narrow waist. https://youtu.be/PJJ2Br_jBd8

Video 13.13 Final PTMC balloon dilatation with both commissures split. https://youtu.be/d3gauiSY4iM

Giant left atrium (Videos 13.14 to 13.16 corresponding to Figure 13.6)

Video 13.14 Levophase of pulmonary angiogram demonstrating a giant left atrium (Courtesy of Prof S Shankar). https://youtu.be/8Qc71GJj9E4

Video 13.15 Septal stain and tenting to aid transseptal puncture (Courtesy of Prof T R Raghu). https://youtu.be/bUPcYnIGKpU

Video 13.16 Pigtail guidewire outlining giant LA. https://youtu.be/f5wYp_BeB7k

Calcified mitral valve—PTMC in annular calcification corresponding to Figure 13.8

Video 13.17 Initially the lateral commissure splits followed by splitting of the medial commissure. https://youtu.be/vsTWRmQilvg

Calcified mitral valve—PTMC in commisural calcification corresponding to Figure 13.9 (Courtesy of Prof. B. C. Srinivas)

Video 13.18 Dense calcification confined to the lateral commissure whereas the medial commissure is free of calcium. The calcified lateral commisure does not yield, the noncalcified medial commissure splits on serial graded, guided inflation. https://youtu.be/m-Tyc2-XXek

Subvalvular disease (Videos 13.19 to 13.20 corresponding to Figure 13.10, Courtesy of Prof. C. N. Manjunath)

Video 13.19 Failure of PTMC balloon to reach the apex despite establishing arteriovenous loop. https://youtu.be/Zz04mAd_Gjs

Video 13.20a & 13.20b Serial dilatation of subvalvular apparatus with peripheral balloon (8 × 20 mm) over the arteriovenous loop. https://youtu.be/EJb-ReEhXpA; https://youtu.be/EJb-ReEhXpA

Transjugular PTMC (Videos 13.21 to 13.28 corresponding to Figures 13.11 and 13.12)

Video 13.21 IVC angiogram demonstrating interruption of IVC. https://youtu.be/hZiZRICZlfQ

Video 13.22 IVC angiogram demonstrating azygous and hemiazygous continuation. https://youtu.be/JeqZQzPyFjk

Video 13.23 Pulmonary artery angiogram in RAO 30 degree to delineate the left atrium and the interatrial septum in the levophase. https://youtu.be/0AzVJnLp6DE

Video 13.24 Pulmonary artery angiogram in LAO 45 degrees to delineate the left atrium and the interatrial septum in the levophase. https://youtu.be/MuGycV8CJVY

Video 13.25 Septal puncture done in the LAO view at the level of pigtail midway between the pigtail and the spine. Note contrast persistence in noncoronary sinus after failed attempt at TSP. https://youtu.be/PwEOlq8jb7E

Video 13.26 Septal dilatation being performed. https://youtu.be/tIF9_m7JozY

Video 13.27 LV entry with clockwise rotation of PTMC balloon. https://youtu.be/81AcnyzlhB8

Video 13.28 Successful PTMC performed. https://youtu.be/-0e9DHC62IY

Dextrocardia (Videos 13.29 to 13.32 corresponding to Figure 13.13, Courtesy of Prof. K. H. Srinivasa)

Video 13.29 Dextrocardia PA view. https://youtu.be/ioGDcgov3DE

Video 13.30 Pseudo AP view preparing for TSP. https://youtu.be/gl8-ye3lUAs

Video 13.31 Septal puncture in pseudo LAO 45-degree view. https://youtu.be/gl8-ye3lUAs

Video 13.32 Successful PTMC using the OTW technique in true PA view. https://youtu.be/ZF28in5LnNg

Post-MV repair (Videos 13.33 to 13.38 corresponding to Figure 13.14)

Video 13.33 TSP performed in RAO 30-degree view (rather than lateral or LAO view) due to marked distortion of septal anatomy. Mitral and tricuspid annuloplasty rings seen. https://youtu.be/HNmkMQOzQPs

Video 13.34 LV entry was difficult and was achieved with a cobra catheter passed through Mullins sheath. https://youtu.be/NPaZDeVgCl0

Video 13.35 0.025″ pigtail guidewire passed through cobra catheter and placed in LV while advancing Mullins sheath. https://youtu.be/AdatkofDezw

Video 13.36 PTMC balloon advanced over the 0.025″ pigtail guidewire into LV. https://youtu.be/VbKP7mDAHck

Video 13.37 First inflation of PTMC balloon with the 0.025″ pigtail guidewire in LV. https://youtu.be/tCv7RO0gcQM

Video 13.38 Final PTMC balloon inflation. https://youtu.be/hS99MzCav0Q

Kyphoscoliosis (Videos 13.39 to 13.40 corresponding to Figure 13.15, Courtesy of Dr. Harsha Basappa)

Video 13.39 PTMC under TEE guidance with general anesthesia. Fluoroscopy shows gross kyphoscoliosis. https://youtu.be/W_XceS6GZjk

Video 13.40 Successful PTMC. https://youtu.be/68VDARlck2c

Dilated CS (Videos 13.41 to 13.44 corresponding to Figure 13.17, Courtesy of Prof. B. C. Srinivas)

Video 13.41 Giant coronary sinus due to absent right superior vena cava and persistent left superior vena cava. https://youtu.be/t4uXfhiY_V4

Video 13.42 Septal stain in RAO view to localize correct site of septal puncture. https://youtu.be/UlZTsgSXyJ0

Video 13.43 Septal puncture performed. https://youtu.be/PuV4LwZrvn8

Video 13.44 Successful PTMC performed using an OTW technique due to difficult LV entry. https://youtu.be/q6dD_ab6xEA

Pregnancy PTMC in a 22-year-old female (Videos 13.45 to 13.46 corresponding to Figure 13.18)

Video 13.45 Needleless septal puncture technique used for TSP. Fluoro-save movie. https://youtu.be/glhk1MrskKo

Video 13.46 Successful PTMC performed. Note the lead shield. Fluoro-save movie. https://youtu.be/BeTBeymNgKQ

Pericardial tamponade (Videos 13.47 to 13.52 corresponding to Figure 13.19, Courtesy of Prof. C. N. Manjunath)

Video 13.47 RAO view. A pigtail is positioned in the pericardial cavity. The first septal dilator is left in-situ and attempt at second septal puncture is being made in a more anterior portion of the IAS. Note that the first septal dilator is almost at the posterior border of the right atrium indicating that the first septal puncture was at an inappropriate site. https://youtu.be/cmKXKSN6k5Q

Video 13.48 Successful second transseptal puncture. https://youtu.be/aWStLniYowA

Video 13.49 Dilatation of IAS with second septal dilator. The first septal dilator is left in place to seal the tamponade. https://youtu.be/wHV_tl1NrWM

Video 13.50 Successful PTMC performed through second puncture. https://youtu.be/vQ2TcBruudw

Video 13.51 Once pericardial accumulation ceased, the first septal is slowly removed with the first pigtail guidewire still in-situ. https://youtu.be/FlzDKZL0WK0

Video 13.52 Once no reaccumulation was confirmed, all hardware were removed with only a vascular sheath left in the pericardial space for any delayed fluid accumulation. https://youtu.be/FppiYjLGiUw

Embolic stroke (Videos 13.53 to 13.56 corresponding to Figure 13.20)

Video 13.53 & 13.54 Cerebral angiogram in AP view and lateral view revealed thrombotic occlusion of left middle cerebral artery. https://youtu.be/ojNib38hfeol; https://youtu.be/EjTfCx4w_Yk

Video 13.55 & 13.56 Repeat cerebral angiogram in AP and lateral view after 3 lakh units of intraarterial urokinase showed marked improvement in cerebral flow in the left MCA territory. https://youtu.be/9xka8LhDdVM; https://youtu.be/KQ3swEOVsko

Fracture pigtail guidewire (Videos 13.57 to 13.64 corresponding to Figure 13.21, Courtesy of Dr. Satish K)

Video 13.57 Attempt at OTW technique. Pigtail guidewire being placed in LV using Mullins sheath. https://youtu.be/HrUof-swP8A

Video 13.58 Pigtail guidewire fractured at junction of floppy and straight portion. Part of guidewire is in left atrium.

Video 13.59 Withdrawal of Mullins sheath brings the fractured portion of guidewire in right atrium. https://youtu.be/ajYITEtDOMM

Video 13.60 Attempts to snare the fractured guidewire using a 10 mm gooseneck snare failed. https://youtu.be/TED1o_83Akl

Video 13.61 Indigenous snare made from 300 cm, 0.014" floppy PTCA guidewire being placed in right atrium. https://youtu.be/sORddD3zjfE

Video 13.62 Fractured guidewire being snared by indigenous snare. https://youtu.be/HUOxlWdcgel

Video 13.63 The entire assembly (Mullins sheath, multipurpose catheter, indigenous snare, captured pigtail catheter) removed *en bloc*. https://youtu.be/elQy5L_lm8g

Video 13.64 PTMC successfully completed through another venous puncture in same groin. https://youtu.be/eHXqen3Ok6I

Deflation failure of PTMC balloon (Videos 13.65 to 13.67, Courtesy of Prof. A. C. Nagamani)

Video 13.65 Undeflated Accura balloon withdrawn from left to right atrium. https://youtu.be/-JV4XF2hrJw

Video 13.66 Undeflated Accura balloon being punctured by hard end of 0.025" stainless steel pigtail guidewire passed through the balloon inflation port. https://youtu.be/yPlsHGfUdAQ

Video 13.67 Deflation of balloon achieved. https://youtu.be/nB9z7JBtYQ8

REFERENCES

1. Manjunath CN, Gerald Dorros, Srinivasa KH et al. The Indian experience of percutaneous transvenous mitral commissurotomy: Comparison of the triple lumen (Inoue) and double lumen (Accura) variable sized single balloon with regard to procedural outcome and cost savings. *J Interv Cardiol* 1998;11:107–12.
2. Nair KK, Pillai HS, Thajudeen A et al. Comparative study on safety, efficacy, and midterm results of balloon mitral valvotomy performed with triple lumen and double lumen mitral valvotomy catheters. *Catheter Cardiovasc Interv* 2012;80(6):978–86.
3. Hung JS, Lau KW. Pitfalls and tips in Inoue balloon mitral commissurotomy. *Cathet Cardiovasc Diagn* 1996;37(2):188–99.
4. Hung JS. Atrial septal puncture technique in percutaneous transvenous mitral commissurotomy: Mitral valvuloplasty using the Inoue balloon catheter technique. *Cathet Cardiovasc Diagn* 1992;26:275.
5. Aksu T, Guler TE, Yalin K et al. A novel deep inspiration maneuver for difficult transseptal puncture. *Am J Cardiol* 2017;119(3):428–33.
6. Mullins, CE (ed.) Transseptal Left Heart Catheterization, in *Cardiac Catheterization in Congenital Heart Disease: Pediatric and Adult.* Oxford: Blackwell Publishing; 2005.
7. Naik N. How to perform transseptal puncture. *Indian Heart J* 2015 Feb 28;67(1):70–6.
8. Ross J, Braunwald E, Morrow AG. Left heart catheterization by the transseptal route. *Circulation* 1960 Nov 1;22(5):927–34.
9. Meier B: Modified Inoue technique for difficult mitral balloon commissurotomy. *Cathet Cardiovasc Diagn* 1992; 26:316–8.
10. Mehan VK, Meier B. Impossibility to cross a stenotic mitral valve with the Inoue balloon: Success with a modified technique. *Indian Heart J* 1994;46:51–2.
11. Manjunath CN, Srinivasa KH, Patil CB, Venkatesh HV, Bhoopal TS, Dhanalakshmi C. Balloon mitral valvuloplasty: Our experience with a modified technique of crossing the mitral valve in difficult cases. *Cathet Cardiovasc Diagn* 1998;44:23–6.
12. Abhaichand RK, Joseph G. Letter to the editor: Re Manjunath et al. *Catheter Cardiovasc Interv* 1999;46:117.
13. Manjunath CN, Srinivasa KH. Reply to the letter to the editor by Abhaichand and Joseph. *Catheter Cardiovasc Interv* 1999; 46:117–8.
14. Shankarappa RK, Math RS, Chikkaswamy SB et al. Transjugular percutaneous transvenous mitral commissurotomy (PTMC) using conventional PTMC equipment in rheumatic mitral stenosis with interruption of inferior vena cava. *J Invasive Cardiol* 2012;24(12):675–8.
15. Deora S, Vyas C, Shah S. Percutaneous transvenous mitral commissurotomy—A modified over-the-wire technique for difficult left ventricle entry. *J Invasive Cardiol* 2013;25:471–3.
16. Nanjappa V, Sadanand KS, Santhosh K et al. Case series: Difficult PTMC using novel technique of veno-arterial looping. *Indian Heart J* 2017;69(2):207–10.
17. Nath RK, Soni DK. Retrograde non trans-septal balloon mitral valvotomy in mitral stenosis with interrupted inferior vena cava, left superior vena cava, and hugely dilated coronary sinus. *Catheter Cardiovasc Interv* 2015;86(7):1289–93.
18. Yeh KH, Hung JS, Wu CJ, Fu M, Chua S, Chern MS. Safety of Inoue balloon mitral commissurotomy in patients with left atrial appendage thrombi. *Am J Cardiol* 1994;75:302–4.

19. Manjunath CN, Srinivasa KH, Ravindranath KS, Manohar JS, Prabhavathi B, Dattatreya PV, Sridhar L, Dhanalakshmi C. Balloon mitral valvotomy in patients with mitral stenosis and left atrial thrombus. *Catheter Cardiovasc Interv* 2009;74(4):653–61.

20. Trehan V, Mehta V, Mukhopadhyay S et al. Difficult percutaneous transvenous mitral commissurotomy: A new technique for left atrium to left ventricular entry. *Indian Heart J* 2004;56:158–62.

21. Tuzcu EM, Block PC, Griffin B et al. Percutaneous mitral balloon valvotomy in patients with calcific mitral stenosis: Immediate and long-term outcome. *J Am Coll Cardiol* 1994;23:1604–9.

22. Khandenahally Shankarappa R, Dwarakaprasad R, Karur S, Bachahally Krishnanaik G, Panneerselvam A, Cholenahally Nanjappa M. Balloon mitral valvotomy for calcific mitral stenosis. *JACC Cardiovasc Interv* 2009;2(3):263–4.

23. Abraham KA, Chandrasekar B, Rajagopal S et al. Percutaneous transvenous mitral commissurotomy for significant calcific mitral stenosis: Utility of the stepwise balloon dilatation technique and follow-up results. *J Invasive Cardiol* 1999;11(6):345–50.

24. Bouleti C, Iung B, Himbert D et al. Relationship between valve calcification and long-term results of percutaneous mitral commissurotomy for rheumatic mitral stenosis. *Circ Cardiovas Interv* 2014;7:381–9.

25. Bhalgat P, Karlekar S, Modani S et al. Subvalvular apparatus and adverse outcome of balloon valvotomy in rheumatic mitral stenosis. *Indian Heart J* 2015;67(5):428–33.

26. Nanjappa MC, Bhat P, Panneerselvam A. Modified technique of PTMC for severe submitral stenosis. *J Invasive Cardiol* 2011;23(9):387–8.

27. Sadee AS, Becker AE. In vitro balloon dilatation of mitral valve stenosis: The importance of subvalvar involvement as a cause of mitral valve insufficiency. *Heart* 1991;65(5):277–9.

28. Lau KW, Hung JS. "Balloon impasse": A marker for severe mitral subvalvular disease and a predictor of mitral regurgitation in Inoue-balloon percutaneous transvenous mitral commissurotomy. *Catheter Cardiovasc Interv* 1995;35(4):310–9.

29. Chern MS, Hsieh IC, Wu D. Popping-out of an Inoue balloon catheter. *Jpn Circ J* 1998;62(7):549–51.

30. Joseph G, George OK, Mandalay A, Sathe S. Transjugular approach to balloon mitral valvuloplasty helps overcome impediments caused by anatomical alterations. *Catheter Cardiovasc Interv* 2002;57(3):353–62.

31. Namboodiri N, Harikrishnan SP, Ajitkumar V, Tharakan JA. Percutaneous mitral commissurotomy in a case of mirror-image dextrocardia and rheumatic mitral stenosis. *J Invasive Cardiol* 2008;20(1):E33–5.

32. Nallet O, Iung B, Cormier B, Porte JM, Garbarz E, Michel PL, Vahanian A. Specifics of technique in percutaneous mitral commissurotomy in a case of dextrocardia and situs inversus with mitral stenosis. *Catheter Cardiovasc Interv* 1996;39(1):85–8.

33. Rosenmann E, Laufer A, Milwidsky H, Stern S. Mitral restenosis; a pathological study. *Pathobiology* 1963;26(2):158–66.

34. Iung B, Garbarz E, Michaud P et al. Late results of percutaneous mitral commissurotomy in a series of 1024 patients. *Circulation* 1999;99(25):3272–8.

35. Logan A, Lowther C, Turner RD. Reoperation for mitral stenosis. *Lancet* 1962;279(7227):443–9.

36. Turgeman Y, Atar S, Suleiman K et al. Feasibility, safety, and morphologic predictors of outcome of repeat percutaneous balloon mitral commissurotomy. *Am J Cardiol* 2005;95(8):989–91.

37. Bouleti C, Iung B, Himbert D et al. Long-term efficacy of percutaneous mitral commissurotomy for restenosis after previous mitral commissurotomy. *Heart* 2013;99:1336–41.

38. Bouleti C, Iung B, Himbert D et al. Reinterventions after percutaneous mitral commissurotomy during long-term follow-up, up to 20 years: The role of repeat percutaneous mitral commissurotomy. *Eur Heart J* 2013;34(25):1923–30.

39. Chmielak Z, Klopotowski M, Kruk M et al. Repeat percutaneous mitral balloon valvuloplasty for patients with mitral valve restenosis. *Catheter Cardiovasc Interv* 2010;76(7):986–92.

40. Iung B, Garbarz E, Michaud P et al. Percutaneous mitral commissurotomy for restenosis after surgical commissurotomy: Late efficacy and implications for patient selection. *J Am Coll Cardiol* 2000;35(5):1295–302.

41. Choudhary SK, Talwar S, Dubey B et al. Mitral valve repair in a predominantly rheumatic population: Long-term results. *Tex Heart Inst J* 2001;28(1):8.

42. Devegowda L, Bhat P, Manjunath CN, Rao PS. PTMC in post-MV repair status. *Indian Heart J* 2016;68:S8–10.

43. Ramasamy D, Zambahari R, Fu M, Yeh KH, Hung JS. Percutaneous transvenous mitral commissurotomy in patients with severe kyphoscoliosis. *Catheter Cardiovasc Interv* 1993;30(1):40–4.

44. Lau KW, Ding ZP, Lee CY et al. Technically demanding Inoue-balloon mitral commissurotomy: Broadened indications for the procedure. *Singap Med J* 1996;37:34–8.

45. Joseph G, Varghese MJ, George OK. Transjugular balloon mitral valvotomy in a patient with severe kyphoscoliosis. *Indian Heart J* 2016;68:S11–4.

46. Srinivas BC, Singla V, Reddy B et al. Percutaneous transseptal mitral commissurotomy in a patient with absent right superior vena cava and aneurysmally dilated coronary sinus. *Cardiovasc Interv Ther* 2013;28(4):419–21.

47. Kothari SS, Ramakrishnan S, Kumar CK, Juneja R, Yadav R. Intermediate term results of percutaneous transvenous mitral commissurotomy in children less than 12 years of age. *Cathet Cardiovasc Interv* 2005; 64: 487–90.

48. Joseph G, Abhaichand Rajpal K, Kumar KS. Definitive percutaneous treatment of Lutembacher's syndrome. *Catheter Cardiovasc Interv* 1999;48(2):199–204.

49. Goel S, Nath R, Sharma A et al. Successful percutaneous management of Lutembacher syndrome. *Indian Heart J* 2014;66(3):355–7.

50. Santangeli P, Di Biase L, Burkhardt JD et al. Transseptal access and atrial fibrillation ablation guided by intracardiac echocardiography in patients with atrial septal closure devices. *Heart Rhythm* 2011;8(11):1669–75.

51. Lakkireddy D, Rangisetty U, Prasad S et al. Intracardiac echo-guided Radiofrequency Catheter Ablation of Atrial Fibrillation in Patients with Atrial Septal Defect or Patent Foramen Ovale Repair: A Feasibility, Safety, and Efficacy Study. *J Cardiovasc Electrophysiol* 2008;19(11):1137–42.

52. Bhambhani A, Somanath HS. Percutaneous treatment of Lutembacher syndrome in a case with difficult mitral valve crossing. *J Invasive Cardiol* 2012;24(3):E54–6.

53. Joseph G, Chandy ST, Krishnaswami S et al. Mechanisms of cardiac perforation leading to tamponade in balloon mitral valvuloplasty. *Catheter Cardiovasc Diagn* 1997;42(2):138–46.

54. Cheng TO. How to avoid cardiac tamponade during percutaneous balloon mitral valvuloplasty. *Catheter Cardiovasc Diagn* 1997;42(2):147–8.

55. Mijangos-Vázquez R, García-Montes JA, Zabal-Cerdeira C. Aortic iatrogenic perforation during transseptal puncture and successful occlusion with Amplatzer ductal occluder in a case of mitral paravalvular leak closure. *Catheter Cardiovasc Interv* 2016;88(2):312–5.

56. Webber MR, Stiles MK, Pasupati S. Percutaneous repair of aortic puncture with Amplatzer closure device during attempted transseptal puncture. *J Invasive Cardiol* 2013;25:E110–3.

57. Chino M, Satoh T, Yamane M et al. Percutaneous balloon mitral commissurotomy by the Inoue balloon resulting in fatal cardiac tamponade: Stitching phenomenon. *J Interv Cardiol* 1994;7(1):33–8.

58. Wang A, Bashore TM. Editorial comment: Cardiac perforation and tamponade: Being at the wrong place but at predictable times during balloon mitral commissurotomy. *Catheter Cardiovasc Interv* 1997;42(2):149–50.

59. Nanjappa MC, Ananthakrishna R, Setty SK et al. Acute severe mitral regurgitation following balloon mitral valvotomy: Echocardiographic features, operative findings, and outcome in 50 surgical cases. *Catheter Cardiovasc Interv* 2013;81(4):603–8.

60. Shetkar SS, Parakh N, Singh B et al. Cardio-embolic stroke due to valve tissue embolization during Percutaneous Transseptal Mitral Commissurotomy (PTMC). *Indian Heart J* 2014;66(5):546–9.

61. Jauch EC, Saver JL, Adams HP Jr et al. American Heart Association Stroke Council; Council on Cardiovascular Nursing; Council on Peripheral Vascular Disease; Council on Clinical Cardiology. Guidelines for the early management of patients with acute ischemic stroke: A guideline for healthcare professionals from the American Heart Association/American Stroke Association. *Stroke* 2013;44:870–947.

62. Lisboa RC, Jovanovic BD, Alberts MJ. Analysis of the safety and efficacy of intra-arterial thrombolytic therapy in ischemic stroke. *Stroke* 2002;33(12):2866–71.

63. Ogawa A, Mori E, Minematsu K et al. Randomized trial of intraarterial infusion of urokinase within 6 hours of middle cerebral artery stroke. *Stroke* 2007;38(10):2633–9.

64. Georgiadis AL, Memon MZ, Shah QA et al. Intra-arterial tenecteplase for treatment of acute ischemic stroke: Feasibility and comparative outcomes. *J Neuroimaging* 2012 Jul 1;22(3):249–54.

65. Powers WJ, Derdeyn CP, Biller J et al. American Heart Association Stroke Council. 2015 American Heart Association/American Stroke Association Focused Update of the 2013 Guidelines for the Early Management of Patients With Acute Ischemic Stroke Regarding Endovascular Treatment: A Guideline for Healthcare Professionals from the American Heart Association/American Stroke Association. *Stroke* 2015;46:3020–35.

66. Shankarappa RK, Panneerselvam A, Dwarakaprasad R et al. Removal of broken balloon mitral valvotomy coiled guidewire from giant left atrium using indigenous snare. *Cardiovasc Interv Ther* 2011;26(1):60–3.

67. Deora S, More D, Shah S, Patel T. Successful retrieval of broken coiled guidewire from left atrium during balloon mitral valvotomy: A rare complication. *Acute Cardiac Care* 2014;16(3):110–11.

68. Patil S, Agarwal A, Ramalingam R et al. Successful percutaneous removal of broken mitral valvuloplasty coiled tip guidewire. *Cardiovasc Interv Ther* 2013;28(4):398–402.

69. Park SJ, Kim JJ, Park SW et al. Immediate and one-year results of percutaneous mitral balloon valvuloplasty using Inoue and double-balloon techniques. *Am J Cardiol* 1993;71(11):938–43.

70. Lanjewar CP, Nathani PJ, Kerkar PG. Failure of deflation of an Inoue balloon during percutaneous balloon mitral valvuloplasty. *J Interv Cardiol* 2006;19(3):280–2.

71. Patel TM, Dani SI, Patel TK. Unsuccessful deflation of a bifoil balloon during percutaneous mitral valvuloplasty. *Catheter Cardiovasc Interv* 1996;37(3):290–2.

14

Surgical treatment

SHIV KUMAR CHOUDHARY AND AMOL BHOJE

INTRODUCTION

Acquired mitral stenosis is the most common valvular heart disease in developing countries. Rheumatic heart disease (RHD) is the most common etiology in these patients. During the healing phase of rheumatic fever, free borders of leaflets become adherent at the commissures and thus the commissures get fused (Figure 14.1). This leads to restricted valve opening. At the same time, fibrosis also involves the cusps and makes them thick, non-pliable, and stiff. In longstanding disease, the valve components may even become calcified. In advanced cases, the chordae tendineae and papillary muscles are also involved in this process. This further restricts cusp movement and impairs valve opening. Sometimes, the valve cusps remain in a fixed position, neither closing completely nor opening fully. This produces a mixed physiological lesion, i.e., both mitral stenosis and mitral regurgitation.

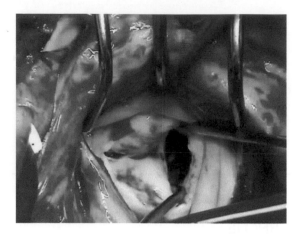

Figure 14.1 Intraoperative view, rheumatic mitral stenosis. There is severe commissural fusion, cusp thickening, and calcification.

Medical management of mitral stenosis includes diuretics, control of heart rate, and rheumatic fever prophylaxis. However, a symptomatic patient with hemodynamically significant mitral stenosis (mitral valve area <1.5 cm²) needs some catheter-based or surgical intervention. Catheter or surgical interventions aim at providing a competent and non-obstructed mitral valve. Morphology of the mitral valve, the presence or absence of left-atrial thrombus/clot, the degree of concomitant mitral regurgitation, and associated other cardiac lesions decide the type of intervention. Catheter-based balloon mitral valvotomy (BMV) or percutaneous transvenous mitral commissurotomy (PTMC) is the primary modality of choice. The surgical options include either a closed mitral valvotomy (CMV), open mitral commissurotomy (OMC), or mitral valve replacement (MVR).

This chapter describes the surgical aspects of acquired mitral stenosis, excluding congenital mitral stenosis. The etiology, pathophysiology, diagnosis, and decision-making has been discussed in separate chapters.

SURGICAL ANATOMY OF THE MITRAL VALVE

The mitral valve apparatus is composed of two leaflets (anterior or aortic, and posterior or mural), mitral annulus, subvalvular apparatus, and left ventricular wall (Figure 14.2). The anterior leaflet is semicircular or triangular in shape and is attached to two-fifths of the annular circumference. The

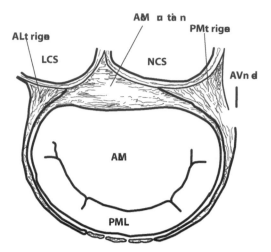

Figure 14.2 Schematic representation of surgical view of the mitral valve and neighboring structures. AL: anterolateral; AMC: aorto-mitral curtain; AML: anterior mitral leaflet; AV node: atrioventricular node; LCS: left coronary sinus; PM: posteromedial; PML: posterior mitral leaflet; NCS: non coronary sinus.

posterior or mural leaflet is quadrangular and attached to three-fifths of the annular circumference. The junctional areas of these leaflets are termed commissures: anterolateral and posteromedial. The commissural leaflet is the name given to the tissue at the commissures where these two leaflets meet. The anterior leaflet has much greater height than the posterior leaflet.

The chordae tendineae are fibrous structures connecting the leaflets with papillary muscles or the ventricular wall. Primary or marginal chordae insert on the free margins of leaflets. Secondary chordae attach to the ventricular surface of the leaflets (Figure 14.3). Tertiary chordae or basal chordae are present only in relation to the posterior leaflet. The basal chordae connect the leaflet base to the ventricular myocardium. The two papillary muscles, anterolateral and posteromedial, arise from the ventricular wall and support the chordal apparatus of the mitral valve.

The mitral annulus is a fibrous structure strongest anteriorly between the left and right fibrous trigons (Figure 14.2). In the posterior part, the annulus is very thin and prone for dilatation. The mitral annulus is attached to the left-ventricular myocardium through the interposition of a narrow membrane, which merges with the fibrous skeleton of the heart. The anterior leaflet is continuous with

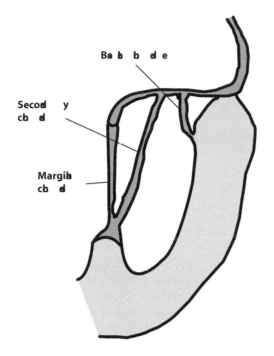

Figure 14.3 Schematic representation of different types of chordae.

the adjoining annulus of the aortic valve and the fibrous subaortic curtain, beneath the commissure between the left and noncoronary aortic sinuses. The mitral valve is surrounded by many important and vital structures (Figure 14.4). The left circumflex coronary artery traverses around the mitral annulus predominantly in the lateral part of the posterior atrioventricular groove. The coronary sinus runs in the more medial segment of the posterior atrioventricular groove. The atrioventricular node is situated close to the annulus of the anterior leaflet of the mitral valve near the posteromedial commissure. The remainder of the anterior leaflet annulus is contiguous with the aortic valve. These relationships have significant clinical implications during mitral valve surgery.

HISTORY

In 1902, Sir Lauder Brunton, for the first time, considered surgical treatment of mitral stenosis.[1] Cutler did experimental work on surgical approaches to mitral stenosis, and, in 1923, along with Levine, reported an operation via median

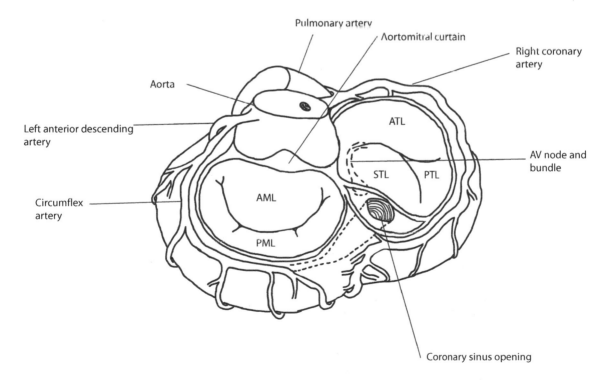

Figure 14.4 Schematic representation of the base of the heart showing relation of various structures. AML: anterior mitral leaflet; ATL: anterior tricuspid leaflet; PML: posterior mitral leaflet; PTL: posterior tricuspid leaflet; STL: septal tricuspid leaflet.

sternotomy in which a special curved knife was inserted through the left-ventricular apex to cut a stenotic mitral valve.[2] Very soon, in 1925, Souttar opened a stenotic mitral valve using a finger through the left-atrial appendage (LAA).[3] Brock in London, Harken in Boston, and Bailey in Philadelphia refined valvotomies and commissurotomies in the ensuing decades.[4-6]

Although they differed in techniques and terminology, their approaches to opening the stenotic mitral valve through the LAA were similar. Later modifications included Tubb's transventricular dilator, used with digital guide by a finger inserted through the LAA.[7]

The introduction of cardiopulmonary bypass opened the era of replacement of the diseased mitral valve. In 1960, Braunwald successfully replaced the mitral valve using a polyurethane valve.[8] In 1961, Starr and Edwards, from the University of Oregon Medical Center, first reported successful mitral valve replacement using a caged ball valve.[9] Although the Starr-Edwards valve was the "gold standard," its high thromboembolic tendency led to development of several prosthetic valves. Of these, the most successful valves were the tilting disc Bjork–Shiley prosthesis and the bileaflet St. Jude Medical valve.[10,11] The first commercially available bioprosthetic valves were developed by Hancock in the United States (1970) and Carpentier in Paris in September 1965.[12,13]

SURGERY FOR MITRAL STENOSIS

The aim of the intervention, either catheter-based or surgical, is to provide a competent and non-obstructed mitral valve. Surgical options include either a closed procedure without cardiopulmonary bypass (Closed mitral valvotomy or CMV), or an open-heart procedure requiring cardiopulmonary bypass (OMC or MVR). Morphology of the mitral valve, degree of calcification, and severity of subvalvular disease are the most important determinants of the type of intervention.

If the mitral valve is pliable, non-calcific, and without significant subvalvular disease—and if there is minimal or no mitral regurgitation, and there is no clot/thrombus in the left atrium or appendage—CMV or PTMC can be performed. In the presence of a fresh left-atrial clot, the patient is anticoagulated for 6 to 8 weeks and echocardiography is repeated. If the left atrium and its appendage are free from clot/thrombus, CMV or PTMC can be performed.

If the valve is grossly deformed with heavy calcification or severe subvalvular disease, open-heart surgical procedure in the form of OMC or MVR should be performed. The presence of significant mitral regurgitation, non-resolving left-atrial/appendicular thrombus/clot, organic tricuspid regurgitation, severe aortic valve disease, and significant coronary artery disease exclude a catheter-based or closed surgical intervention.

Closed mitral valvotomy

As mentioned above, in case of isolated, pure, non-calcific mitral stenosis with minimal or no subvalvular disease, without any atrial clot/thrombus, either PTMC or CMV can be performed. With the technological advances and widespread availability of percutaneous interventions, PTMC has taken the primary lead role, making CMV an alternate option where the facilities for PTMC are unavailable or not affordable. CMV is still an invaluable surgical option in many low-income and developing countries where advanced interventional or surgical facilities are not accessible for everyone. Current-day indications for CMV are listed in Table 14.1.

Patient evaluation and preparation

Preoperative evaluation includes a chest radiograph and echocardiography. A chest radiograph is essential for pulmonary evaluation. Transthoracic echocardiography is performed to assess the severity of disease and suitability for CMV. Other cardiac valves are also evaluated. In the presence of atrial fibrillation or when there is high probability of appendage thrombus/clot, transesophageal echocardiography is performed. The severity of subvalvular disease, leaflet thickening, pattern, and severity of mitral calcification,

Table 14.1 Indications of closed mitral valvotomy in the current era

SN	Indications
1	Facilities for PTMC not available
2	Interatrial septum could not be punctured during PTMC
3	Cardiac perforation and tamponade during PTMC

and the severity of mitral regurgitation should be assessed. Coronary evaluation should be done for age-related indication. Preoperative optimization of pulmonary function with a spirometer helps to prevent postoperative lung collapse and expedites postoperative recovery.

Surgical technique

The CMV is performed through a left fifth space anterolateral thoracotomy. The chest is entered through a curvilinear incision in the submammary fold in the fifth intercostal space. The left lung is retracted downwards and laterally. The pericardium is opened about 1 cm anterior to the phrenic nerve. An atraumatic vascular clamp is applied at the base of the LAA and a 1.5 cm-long incision is made in the body of the appendage. The cavity in the appendage is thoroughly washed to remove any clot, if present. A purse string suture is placed around the incision. The cardiac apex is gently lifted with a sponge below the heart in the pericardial cavity. A small (5 mm) purse string-controlled ventriculotomy is made at the ventricular apex. The right index finger is introduced in the LAA through a purse string suture and the mitral valve is assessed. The mitral valve orifice, subvalvular apparatus, pliability of the leaflets, and nodularity and calcification are noted. The preselected Tubb's dilator is inserted through the left-ventricular apex and guided across the mitral valve orifice-using a finger in the left atrium as a guide (Figure 14.5). This dilator is opened to split

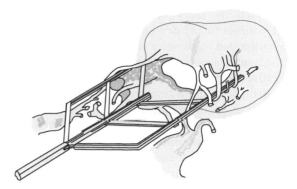

Figure 14.6 Closed mitral valvotomy. The fused commissures are fractured when the dilator is opened.

the fused commissures (Figure 14.6). The resultant opening of the mitral valve can be assessed by palpation or by intraoperative echocardiography. The index finger and Tubb's dilator are withdrawn after confirming adequate opening of the mitral valve. The atrial appendage is excised and the suture closed. The ventriculotomy is closed. The pericardium is closed with interrupted sutures. The chest is closed after inserting a large-diameter drainage tube in the pleural cavity.

Complications

Intraoperative complications like bleeding from the LAA and ventriculotomy site are uncommon and can be managed by taking extra sutures. Embolization of an undetected clot in the left atrium remains a possibility. Air embolism can also happen if airtight control is not taken over the appendage, especially when the patient becomes hypovolemic after a bleeding episode. Injury to the ventricular wall or chordal structures can occur during insertion of the dilator. Sometimes, there may be a tear in the body of a leaflet. Chordal injury or leaflet tear may cause acute mitral regurgitation. If mitral regurgitation is severe, the patient may develop low cardiac output and pulmonary edema and may require emergency mitral valve replacement.

Results

John and colleagues reported the early and long-term results of CMV in 3724 patients.[14] All survivors showed marked symptomatic improvement.

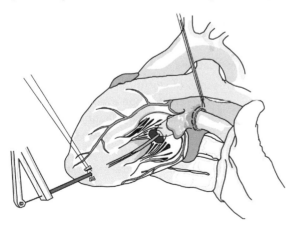

Figure 14.5 Schematic representation of closed mitral valvotomy. The metallic dilator is passed from the left ventricular apex. The guiding figure is inserted through the LAA.

Hospital mortality was 1.5%. After valvotomy, 11 patients (0.3%) developed severe mitral regurgitation that made valve replacement necessary in the immediate postoperative period. Early postoperative embolism occurred in 0.4% and 0.95% in patients with and without preoperative anticoagulation, respectively. The rate of restenosis varied from 4.2 to 11.4 per 1000 patients per year between the fifth and fifteenth year of follow-up. Repeat CMV was performed for restenosis in 130 subjects with a 6.7% mortality. Symptomatic improvement was well sustained and was evident in 86% of long-term survivors at the end of 15 years. Actuarial survival was 95%, 93.1%, 89.5%, and 84.2% at 6, 12, 18, and 24 years, respectively. Other investigators have also reported similar results.[15] By 36 years, about 44% of patients required re-operation, predominantly for restenosis. Freedom from reoperation after CMV was 81.4 +/– 1.3% at 10 years, 16.4 +/– 2.1% at 20 years, 3.1 +/– 1.2% at 30 years, and 0% at 36 years.[15]

Closed mitral valvotomy versus percutaneous transvenous mitral commissurotomy

With widespread acceptance of PTMC, comparison between PTMC and CMV is of historical significance only. In an earlier phase, several investigators[16–20] compared the immediate postoperative hemodynamic data and midterm results of CMV and PTMC. Most of the investigators[16–18] did not find any significant deference in postoperative hemodynamic data. Postoperative left-atrial pressures, transmitral gradients, and mitral valve area were comparable in both the groups.[16–18] The incidence of significant MR was also not different. There were no significant differences in both the groups regarding re-stenosis rate, re-intervention rate, and long-term survival. However, other investigators reported better outcomes with PTMC.[19,20] Farhat and colleagues[19] reported that the mitral valve area increased much more after PTMC (from 0.9 ± 0.16 to 2.2 ± 0.4 cm^2) than after CMV (from 0.9 ± 0.2 to 1.6 ± 0.4 cm^2). Residual MS (MVA <1.5 cm^2) was 0% after PTMC, and 27% after CMV. At seven-year follow-up, the mitral valve area was greater after PTMC (1.8 ± 0.4 cm^2) than after CMV (1.3 ± 0.3 cm^2; $p < 0.001$). The restenosis (MVA <1.5 cm^2)

rate was also higher after CMV. Freedom from re-intervention was 90% after PTMC, and 50% after CMV. Similar results have been reported by other investigators.[20]

OPEN-HEART SURGICAL PROCEDURES: OPEN MITRAL COMMISSUROTOMY AND MITRAL VALVE REPLACEMENT

In contrast to CMV, in open mitral commissurotomy (OMC), the procedure is performed under direct vision using cardiopulmonary bypass and cardioplegic arrest. As the procedure is performed under direct vision, there is no risk of embolization of left-atrial clot/thrombus, if present. In OMC, it is also possible to correct coexisting mitral regurgitation and moderate degree of subvalvular pathology. Co-existing tricuspid pathology and other cardiac diseases requiring cardiopulmonary bypass can also be corrected simultaneously. Table 14.2 lists the indications for open-heart surgical procedure in patients with significant mitral stenosis. If the mitral valve is pliable, and non-calcific or mildly calcific with predominant commissural fusion, OMC is performed. If the valve is badly damaged and heavily calcified, mitral valve replacement (MVR) is performed with a suitable prosthesis. Severe subvalvular disease, which is not amenable to OMC, also requires MVR.

Table 14.2 Indications for open-heart procedures in significant mitral stenosis

SN	Indications
1	Presence of clot/thrombus in the left atrium/appendage even after adequate anticoagulation
2	Significant subvalvular disease
3	Mitral valve calcification
4	Significant (>2+) mitral regurgitation
5	Failure or restenosis after closed or balloon mitral valvotomy
6	Cardiac surgical procedure is required for significant aortic valve disease, organic tricuspid regurgitation, coronary artery disease, or atrial septal defect

Surgical approaches to the heart

The heart is approached by any of the incisions shown in Figure 14.7. The most common approach is via midsternotomy (Figure 14.7a). Other minimally invasive incisions, such as upper partial sternotomy (Figure 14.7b), lower partial sternotomy (Figure 14.7c), and right anterolateral thoracotomy are becoming increasingly popular. Smaller incisions offer the advantage of rapid postoperative recovery and a shorter hospital stay.

Surgical approaches to the mitral valve

Various approaches to the stenotic mitral valve are shown in Figure 14.8a. The most common approach is via the interatrial (Waterston's) groove anterior to the junction of right-sided pulmonary veins with the left atrium (Figure 14.8b). Alternatively, if concomitant tricuspid procedure is to be performed, or if the left atrium is small, the mitral valve can be approached via a transseptal (Figure 14.8c), biatrial (Figure 14.8d), or extended transseptal approach (Figure 14.8e). These alternative approaches are helpful in cases of reoperations too.

Cardiopulmonary bypass and cardiac arrest

The essential prerequisite for open-heart surgical procedure is a bloodless and motionless surgical field. Therefore, during open-heart surgical procedure, the heart is stopped and blood is drained out of the heart. To achieve this, cardiopulmonary bypass (CPB) using a heart-lung machine temporarily substitutes the pumping and ventilatory functions of the heart and lungs. The basic components

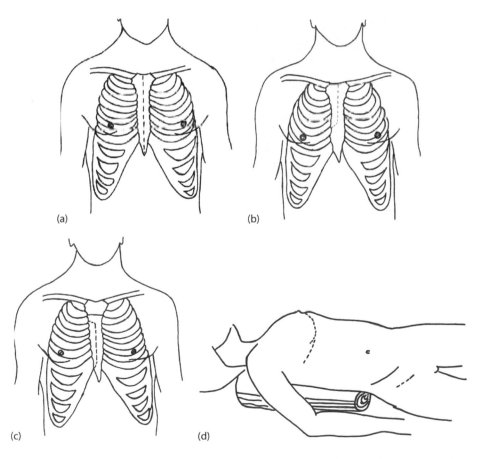

(a)   (b)   (c)   (d)

Figure 14.7 Various approaches to the heart for open-heart mitral procedures. **(a)** Midsternotomy; **(b)** upper partial sternotomy; **(c)** lower partial sternotomy; **(d)** right anterolateral thoracotomy.

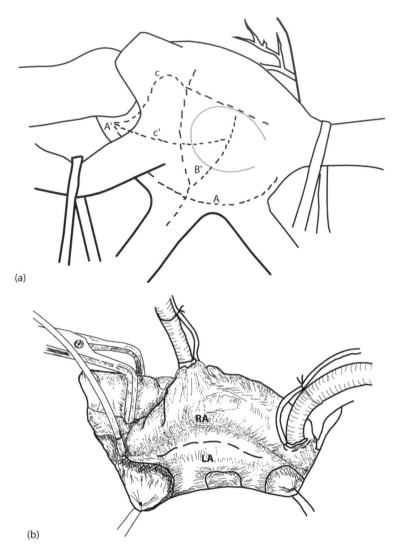

(a)

(b)

Figure 14.8 Various approaches to the mitral valve. **(a)** Incisions to expose the mitral valve (a-a': through the interatrial groove; b-b': biatrial; c: extended transseptal; c': transseptal); **(b)** approach through the interatrial groove. *(Continued)*

of the heart-lung machine include the oxygenator (for gas exchange) with integral heat exchanger (for temperature regulation) and flow pumps for whole-body perfusion, cardioplegia delivery, and suction from the operative field (Figure 14.9). Other components are one or more venous cannula, a venous reservoir, arterial line filter, and arterial cannula. The heparinized blood of the patient is drained into the venous reservoir by inserting cannula in the venous side of the heart (right atrium, superior vena cava, inferior vena cava, femoral vein, internal jugular vein). This venous blood passes through the oxygenator for gaseous exchange (oxygenation and

removal of CO_2). The mechanical pump returns the oxygenated blood to the arterial side of circulation (the aorta or one of the major arteries). To arrest the electromechanical activity of the heart, cardioplegia solution (especially formulated hyperkalemic solution) is delivered to the coronary circulation by a cardioplegia delivery system. In addition, a cardiotomy suction system aspirates blood from open cardiac chambers and the surgical field. With a modern CPB circuit, it is possible to regulate flow rate, gaseous exchange, temperature of perfusate, hematocrit, water and electrolyte contents, oncotic pressure, and pH.

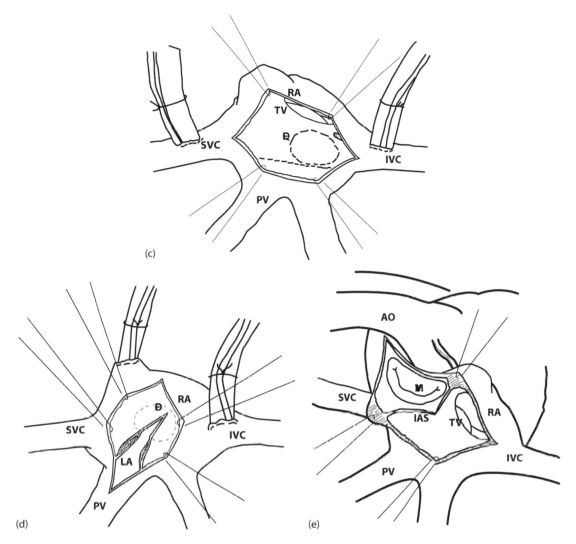

Figure 14.8 (Continued) Various approaches to the mitral valve. **(c)** transseptal approach; **(d)** biatrial approach; **(e)** extended transseptal approach. AO: Aorta; FO: fossa ovalis; IAS: interatrial septum; IVC: inferior vena cava; MV: mitral valve; PV: pulmonary vein; RA: right-atrial free wall; SVC: superior vena caca; TV: tricuspid valve.

SURGICAL TECHNIQUE OF OMC

After initiating cardiopulmonary bypass, the heart is arrested with cardioplegia solution. The left atrium is opened to expose the mitral valve and a search is made for any clot/thrombus. The LAA is invaginated into the atrium and inspected. Any thrombus or clot, if present, is removed. The mitral valve is inspected. The process of commissurotomy is started at one of the commissures. Two blunt-ended, long-handled hooks are placed beneath each leaflet on either side of the commissure and

gentle traction is applied (Figure 14.10a). This displays and spreads out the region of the commissure. The fused commissure is incised with a No. 11 blade (Figure 14.10b and c). Subsequently, the fused chordae are separated with a knife or scissors and, when appropriate, the incision is carried down into the center of the papillary muscle (Figure 14.10d). A similar procedure is repeated on the other commissure. After release of fused commissural and subvalvular components, the fibrous layer on the atrial surface of both the leaflets is peeled off (Figure 14.10e). This restores the

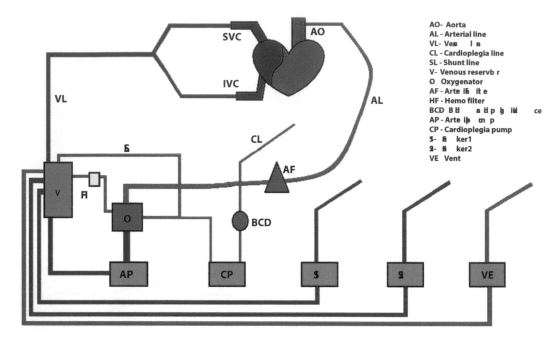

AO- Aorta
AL - Arterial line
VL- Ve‍n‍‍ l‍‍‍‍ a
CL - Cardioplegia line
SL - Shunt line
V- Venous reservb r
O Oxygenator
AF - Arte i‍f‍ it‍ e
HF - Hemo filter
BCD B ‍f‍‍‍‍ a ‍‍‍‍p ‍‍b‍ i‍‍‍ ce
AP - Arte ‍‍i‍p‍ m p
CP - Cardioplegia pump
S- ‍‍f‍ ker1
S- ‍‍f‍ ker2
VE Vent

Figure 14.9 Schematic representation of cardiopulmonary bypass circuit.

pliability of mitral leaflets. Calcification from the leaflets is shaved off. At the completion of the procedure, annuloplasty is performed. Finally, valve opening and competence of the valve are assessed. The competence of the mitral valve is assessed by injecting a saline solution with a bulb syringe into the left ventricle directly through the mitral valve. If the results are satisfactory, the left atrium is closed, the heart is deaired, and the patient is weaned off cardiopulmonary bypass. Mitral valve function is again assessed using intraoperative transesophageal echocardiography.

Complications

Early mitral regurgitation due to technical failure might occur. This may occur if the commissurotomy incision is extended up to the annulus resulting in a flailing anterior mitral leaflet. It can be managed by commissural plication along with posterior annuloplasty. Progression of the rheumatic heart disease process can result in restenosis in the long term.

Results

OMC provides excellent early and long-term results in a selected group of patients. Excellent

hemodynamic improvement is achieved after OMC.[21-23] Operative mortality ranges from 0 to 2%, and is usually limited to patients who present with advanced failure. In our own experience of 187 patients, there was no mortality related to OMC.[21] The early mitral valve failure rate leading to severe mitral regurgitation ranges from 1%–3% and can be attributed to technical lapses. The late mitral valve failure (severe regurgitation or restenosis) rate ranges from 2% to 5%.[21,22] However, later on, the restenosis rate increases steeply. In our experience, the actuarial freedom from mitral valve failure was 87% ± 3.5% at 10 years. Antunes and colleagues reported nine-year actuarial survival in 96%, freedom from reoperation in 98%, and freedom from all valve-related complications in 92% of patients.[22] In contrast to this, some investigators reported higher reoperation rates.[23]

Open mitral commissurotomy versus mitral valve replacement

Though valve replacement (MVR) is a simple, reproducible, and more durable option for mitral stenosis, OMC definitely has some advantages. All patients with mitral stenosis are not the candidates for OMC. In our experience, we could save

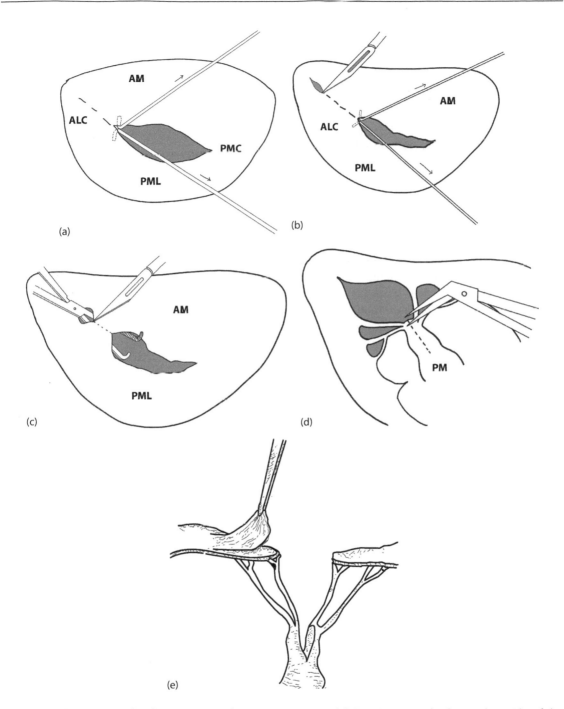

Figure 14.10 Steps involved in open mitral commissurotomy. **(a)** Traction is applied on either side of the commissure; **(b)** a stab incision is made in the fused commissure; **(c)** the commissurotomy is enlarged; **(d)** thickened, fused papillary muscle and chorda are incised longitudinally; **(e)** cusp thinning. ALC: Anterolateral commissure; AML: anterior mitral leaflet; PLC: posterolateral commissure; PM: papillary muscle; PML: posterior mitral leaflet.

only 25% of the valves and the rest of them had to be replaced.[21] Preoperative valve morphology and careful selection of patients is the key for better long-term results. The outcome is dependent on the skills of the operating surgeon. In young patients, OMC may be offered, whenever possible, because of its better long-term survival and freedom from thromboembolism, anticoagulant-related hemorrhage, and other valve-related complications. In addition, the cost-benefit from expensive anticoagulation and its monitoring are some important advantages of OMC, especially for people living in rural and remote areas in developing countries. Glower and colleagues compared the results of OMC with mitral valve replacement with or without chordal preservation.[23] Though survival was better with OMC, the late reoperation rate was much higher with OMC. Anticoagulation-related complications and incidence of thromboembolism were also lower with OMC. Cotrufo and colleagues[24] also reported reduced ten-year survival with MVR, as compared with OMC (98% vs. 93%) due to thromboembolism, anticoagulation-related complications, and other prosthetic valve-related complications that outweigh the durability of MVR.

MITRAL VALVE REPLACEMENT

If the valve is badly damaged and calcified, mitral valve replacement (MVR) is performed with a suitable prosthesis. The presence of severe subvalvular disease that is not amenable to OMC also necessitates valve replacement. MVR is performed using cardiopulmonary bypass and cardioplegic arrest. The mitral valve is excised and replaced with a sewable prosthesis using interrupted or continuous suture technique. Information based on experimental observation and clinical findings indicate that partial or total retention of subvalvular apparatus of the mitral valve results in reduced operative mortality, better ventricular function in the postoperative period, and better early and long-term survival.[25-27]

Technique of operation

Mitral valve replacement is done under cardiopulmonary bypass and cardioplegic arrest. Median sternotomy is the most commonly used approach. However, any other approach, as shown in Figure 14.7, can be used. Standard aortic and bicaval cannulation is used. The interatrial groove is dissected. The ascending aorta is clamped and the cardioplegia solution is delivered to the aortic root to arrest the heart. Left atriotomy is made near and parallel to the interatrial groove. The left-atrial cavity and appendage are inspected for any thrombus/clot. If any thrombus/clot is present, it is removed. A valve hook is engaged into the valve orifice and the anterior leaflet is pulled. With a sharp no. 11 blade, a horizontal nick is made 2 mm away from the anterior annulus at the "12 o'clock" position (Figure 14.11a). The incision is carried onto both the commissures, leaving behind a thin strip of valve tissue approximately 2 mm wide (Figure 14.11b). The separated anterior mitral leaflet is incised in two equal halves (Figure 14.11c). Excessive cusp tissue and thickened chordae are excised, leaving behind small island of cuspal tissue and the healthy long chordae. The two chordal segments thus created are sutured to the respective anterolateral and posteromedial commissures (Figure 14.11d). The posterior mitral leaflet is divided in the center and thickened, and the cuspal tissue is removed. The remaining chordae, especially thickened and fibrosed or calcified, are transected at their attachment with the papillary muscles. The annulus is sized with an appropriate valve sizer. The prosthetic valve is chosen and sutured in the annulus (Figure 14.11e and f). At completion, the prosthetic valve is assessed for satisfactory function. The left atrium is closed and the heart is deaired. The aortic cross clamp is removed and the heart is revived. Once the heart resumes its function satisfactorily, the cardiopulmonary bypass is weaned off.

Intraoperative complications

Faulty surgical technique is responsible for intraoperative complications. Prosthetic valve malfunction can happen if it is not opening or closing properly. It is more common when complete chordal preservation is done. Paravalvular leaks may also occur if the annulus is heavily calcified. Injury to the ventricular wall can result in life-threatening hemorrhage. Deep sutures can cause injury to adjacent structures, namely, the aortic valve, left circumflex coronary artery, coronary sinus, and atrioventricular conduction system.

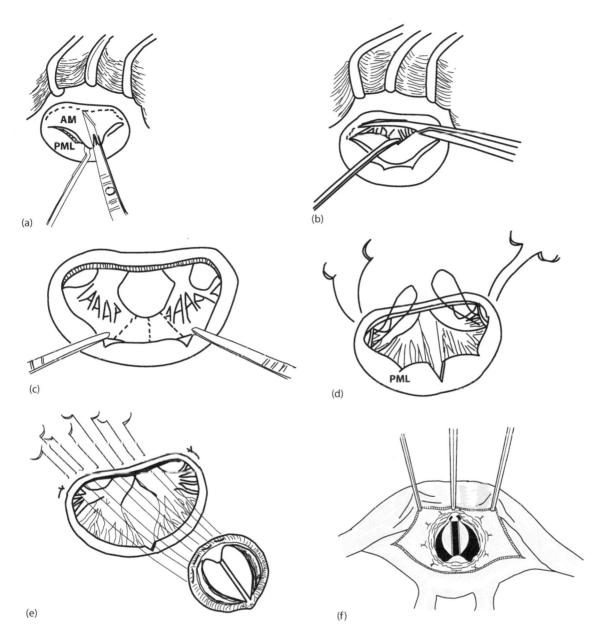

Figure 14.11 Steps involved in mitral valve replacement. **(a)** The AML is incised near the annulus; **(b)** the incision in AML is extended towards commissures; **(c)** the separated AML is divided in two halves. Thickened cusp is removed; **(d)** cusp islands with chordal attachments are sutured to the annulus; **(e)** the mitral prosthesis is being sutured in the annulus using interrupted sutures; **(f)** mitral valve replacement, completed picture. AML: anterior mitral leaflet; PM: papillary muscle; PML: posterior mitral leaflet.

Results

The operative mortality of MVR ranges from 2 to 8%. The Society of Thoracic Surgeons Adult Cardiac Surgery Database reported a mortality of 5.7% for isolated MVR.[28] Advanced age (>65 years), left-ventricular dysfunction, a large left atrium, atrial fibrillation, emergency surgery, renal dysfunction, associated tricuspid valve disease, and higher NYHA class contribute to higher operative mortality and reduced long-term survival. The actuarial survival after MVR ranges between 50% and 60% at 10 years. In a recent study, one-, five-, and ten-year Kaplan-Meier survival estimates for patients undergoing replacement were 82.6%, 64.7%, and 37.2%.[29]

MITRAL VALVE REPLACEMENT: LONG-TERM COMPLICATIONS

Although replacement of the diseased mitral valve with a suitable prosthesis provides the immediate relief of symptoms and improvement in the general condition of the patient, a prosthetic valve brings its own inherent problems to the patient. Some of the important problems of prosthetic valves are mentioned here briefly.

Anticoagulation-related hemorrhage

Mechanical valves, and stented bioprostheses in the early phase, require anticoagulation therapy for proper function. Anticoagulation therapy can occasionally result in internal or external bleeding episodes that can cause death, stroke, reoperation, and hospitalization. The annual risk of a major bleeding episode is approximately 1%–2% per patient-year and is higher in patients with mechanical valves.[30,31] The risk of bleeding is much higher in elderly patients.

Valve thrombosis

Thrombosis of a mechanical valve may occur as a catastrophic event with the acute onset of heart failure, pulmonary edema, or cardiogenic shock. Acute valve thrombosis requires urgent thrombolytic therapy or emergency surgery, but mortality remains high. The incidence of obstructive valve thrombosis varies between 0.3% and 1.3% per patient-year.[30,32]

Thromboembolism

All prosthetic valves are susceptible to the formation of thrombus that can subsequently embolize and can result in stroke or loss of function of other organs. The incidence ranges from 0.6% to 2.3% per patient-year.[30,33,34] The risk factors for thromboembolism include mechanical valve, left-ventricular dysfunction, cardiomegaly, atrial fibrillation, hypertension, and smoking.

Structural valve deterioration

Structural valve deterioration is extremely rare in mechanical prostheses. However, all bioprostheses develop structural valve deterioration and ultimately fail. Various risk factors for structural valve deterioration include younger age at implantation, older generation of bioprosthesis, renal insufficiency, hyperparathyroidism, hypertension, and left-ventricular dysfunction.[30,33,35–37] Structural valve deterioration in bioprosthetic valves starts 7 to 8 years after implantation. With conventional stented bioprostheses, the freedom from structural valve failure is 70%–90% at 10 years and 50%–80% at 15 years. Bioprosthetic structural valve deterioration is strongly influenced by the age of the patient at the time of implantation. The rate of failure of bioprostheses is <10% at 10 years in elderly patients (>70 years of age), but is 20%–30% in patients <40 years of age.[35–37]

Prosthetic valve endocarditis

Prosthetic Valve Endocartitis (PVE) is the worst complication after valve replacement, with a mortality rate of 30%–50%.[30,38] The incidence of PVE is 0.3%–1% per patient-year, with a cumulative incidence of 3% at 5 years and 5% at years.[39] The risk of PVE to the patient is lifelong. However, the risk of infection appears to be greatest during the first three months after valve implantation. Then it falls steadily, and after 12 months attains a constant low level.[40,41] Most large series have found the incidence of PVE to be the same whether a mechanical or a bioprosthetic valve is used.[42,43] However, mechanical valves appear to be at higher risk of infection within the first three months after implantation than bioprosthetic valves.[44]

Paravalvular regurgitation

Moderate or severe paravalvular regurgitation is rare (1%–2%). In the early postoperative period, it is mostly due to technical glitches and suture dehiscence. In the late postoperative period, it may be related to operative technical factors but is most often caused by endocarditis.

Hemolysis

Some degree of intravascular hemolysis occurs in a large proportion (50%–95%) of patients with mechanical valves.[30] However, anemia caused by hemolysis is rare unless prosthetic regurgitation has occurred.

Patient prosthesis mismatch

Patient prosthesis mismatch (PPM) occurs when a normally functioning prosthesis is too small in relation to the patient's cardiac output requirements.[45] It results in abnormally high postoperative gradients. PPM is usually defined and graded on the basis of indexed effective orifice area (EOA).[34,46,47] Severe PPM occurs in 2%–10% of patients and is associated with less improvement in symptoms and functional class, impaired exercise capacity, and higher short-term and long-term mortality.[34,48]

Reoperation

All the bioprostheses develop structural valve deterioration and ultimately fail. Major determinants of structural valve deterioration include age at implantation and type of prosthesis. Earlier bioprostheses without anti-calcification treatment degenerate much faster. Mechanical valves are also not free from reoperations, 0.3%–1.2% per year risk of reoperation for a mechanical valve is reported in the literature.[31,49] In contrast to bioprostheses, there is a constant hazard of reoperation with mechanical valves. Most of the mechanical valves needed emergency reoperations for valve thrombosis and came with a mortality of 20%–24%.[50,51]

HEART VALVE SUBSTITUTES

In the 1950s, Harken defined "Ten Commandments" for the prosthetic valve (Table 14.3).[52] The ideal valve

Table 14.3 Harken's "Ten Commandments" for an ideal valve

SN	Commandment
1	It must not propagate emboli
2	It must be chemically inert and not damage blood elements
3	It must offer no resistance to physiological flows
4	It must close promptly (less than 0.05 seconds)
5	It must remain closed during the appropriate phase of the cardiac cycle
6	It must have lasting physical and geometric features
7	It must be inserted in a physiological site (generally the normal anatomical site)
8	It must be capable of permanent fixation
9	It must not annoy the patient
10	It must be technically practical to insert

should be inert, durable, non-thrombogenic, non-obstructive, competent, noise-free, easily implanted, readily available, should not need anticoagulation, and should not cause trauma to blood elements. In addition, it should have the potential for self-repair and growth. A number of valve substitutes are available, but none fulfills all the criteria. Currently, mechanical prostheses and stented xenografts (bioprosthesis) are most commonly used substitutes for mitral valve replacement. Table 14.4 shows a summary of advantages, disadvantages, and suitability of both types of valve.

Mechanical valves

Mechanical valves are the most commonly used valve substitutes (Figure 14.12). Easy availability and durability are the advantages of mechanical valves. However, mechanical valves require life-long anticoagulation. Thus, there is risk of anticoagulation hazards. Besides this, there is increased risk of thromboembolic episodes and endocarditis. Commonly available mechanical valves are shown in Table 14.5.

Stented bioprostheses

Stented bioprostheses (or xenografts; Figure 14.13) are either porcine aortic valves or prepared from

Table 14.4 Various valve substitutes in the mitral position

Type of valve	Advantages	Disadvantages	Suitable for implantation	Not suitable for implantation
Mechanical	Durable, competent, readily available, easy to implant, requires less reoperation	Needs anticoagulation, thromboembolism, valve thrombosis, catastrophic malfunction, difficult to treat if infected, noisy, smaller sizes not available, makes other surgical procedures more difficult, in some valves PI is low	Young patients with good life expectancy where anticoagulation is not a problem	Where anticoagulation is not possible/desirable, with possibility of bleeding, patients with hazardous professions, cases of potential non-compliance, in remote areas, in patients with short life expectancy, patients planning for pregnancy, patients with active endocarditis
Bioprosthesis	Competent, readily available, easy to implant, no long-term anticoagulation is required, no catastrophic malfunction	Degeneration, reoperation, high profile, less PI in older valves, smaller sizes unavailable	Anticoagulation is contraindicated or not desirable, possibility of bleeding, patients with hazardous professions, in cases of potential non-compliance, in remote areas, in patients planning for pregnancy, in patients with short life expectancy or old age, in comorbid conditions	Children, younger patients with good life expectancy, patients with high calcium metabolism (renal failure, hyperparathyroidism)

Abbreviation: PI: The performance index is the measure of the valve's ability to allow non-obstructed flow.

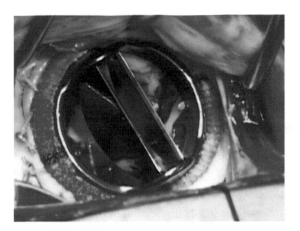

Figure 14.12 Intraoperative view. Bileaflet mechanical valve in mitral position.

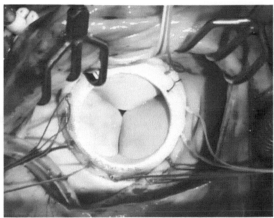

Figure 14.13 Intraoperative view. Bovine pericardial bioprosthesis in mitral position.

bovine pericardium and mounted on a metallic stent. The advantage of bioprostheses is that anticoagulation is not required after a period of 3 to 6 months. However, depending upon the age at implantation, bioprostheses start degenerating after 5 to 7 years and the average lifespan of a valve is 10 to 12 years. Depending upon the age of the patient, reoperation is required. Commonly used bioprostheses are listed in Table 14.6.

CHOICE OF VALVE PROSTHESIS

Mechanical valves impose the mortality and morbidity related to anticoagulation. On the other hand, with bioprostheses, if the patient survives long enough, there is mandatory risk of reoperation. Selection of the prosthesis should be based upon the informed choice of the patient, life expectancy, indication/contraindication for warfarin therapy, and comorbidities, socioeconomic and educational background, occupation of the patient, availability, cost, monitoring of anticoagulation,

monitoring of valve function and other valve-related complications, and possibility of reoperation. The cut-off age, suggested in the various guidelines,[53,54] is based on the average life expectancy of the Western population and may not hold valid in Indian circumstances where average life expectancy is much lower. Life expectancy should not just rely on the age of the patient but should consider all biological and socioeconomic factors. If the life expectancy of a patient is less than the average life of a bioprosthesis, the patient should receive a bioprosthesis. If the life expectancy of the patient is reduced because of cardiac condition (Table 14.7) or other comorbidities, a bioprosthesis is preferred. Similarly, if reliable anticoagulation is not possible (Table 14.8), a bioprosthesis should be considered.

The choice of prosthetic heart valve should be a shared decision-making process that accounts for the patient's values and preferences, with full disclosure of the indications for and risks of anticoagulant therapy and the potential need for and

Table 14.5 Commonly used mechanical valves

Type	Common valves	Comments
Caged ball valve	Starr Edwards	Not available anymore. Large number of patients in follow-up
Tilting disc or mono-leaflet valve	Medtronic-Hall, Omnicarbon, TTK-Chitra	Hemodynamically less efficient than bileaflet valves. Valve thrombosis is more catastrophic
Bileaflet valve	St. Jude Medical, Medtronic ATS, On-X, Carbomedics (Sorin)	Most commonly used valves globally

Table 14.6 Commonly used stented mitral bioprostheses

Type	Common valves	Comments
Bovine pericardial	Edwards Perimount Magna, Carbomedics Mitraflow	Anti-calcification treatment retards degeneration
Porcine aortic valve	St. Jude Epic Medtronic Hancock, Medtronic Mosaic, Carpentier Edward Porcine, St. Jude Biocor	St. Jude Epic and Medtronic Mosaic have anti-calcification treatment

Table 14.7 Cardiac factors predicting reduced survival and, thus, favoring bioprosthesis

SN	Cardiac factor
1	Left-ventricular dysfunction
2	Severe pulmonary arterial hypertension
3	Tricuspid valve involvement
4	Atrial fibrillation
5	Cardiomegaly
6	Advanced functional class
7	Coronary artery disease
8	Mechanical valve in aortic position

Table 14.8 Socioeconomic factors increasing difficulty of anticoagulation and, thus, favoring bioprosthesis

SN	Socioeconomic factor
1	Rural background, underdeveloped region, inadequate medical services, lack of monitoring
2	Female gender
3	Non-earning member of family
4	Poor socioeconomic status
5	Lack of education
6	Non-availability of anticoagulants
7	Mental illness

risk of reoperation.[54] A mechanical valve is favored in circumstances where: (1) the informed patient wants a mechanical valve and has no contraindication for long-term anticoagulation; (2) the patient is already on anticoagulation (mechanical prosthesis in another position or at high risk for thromboembolism); (3) the patient is at risk of accelerated bioprosthesis structural deterioration (young age, hyperparathyroidism, renal insufficiency); and (4) a patient with a longer life expectancy. On the other hand, a bioprosthesis may be preferred in cases where: (1) the informed patient wants a bioprosthesis; (2) good-quality anticoagulation is unavailable (contraindication or high risk, compliance problems, lifestyle); (3) the patient has limited life expectancy; and (4) the patient is a woman of childbearing age who has a history of repeated abortions and who intends to be pregnant.

In addition to the above factors, certain etiological/morphological factors also dictate the choice of valve substitute. An elderly patient with a small left-ventricular cavity will be unlikely to accommodate a bioprosthesis with a high-profile stent. Such a patient may be best served by a mechanical prosthesis.

ACKNOWLEDGMENT

The authors are thankful to Dr. Palleti Rajashekar, Associate Professor, Department of CTVS, AIIMS, New Delhi for preparing several figures in this chapter.

REFERENCES

1. Brunton L, Edin MD. Preliminary note on the possibility of treating mitral stenosis by surgical methods. *Lancet* 1902;159:352.
2. Cutler EC, Levine SA. Cardiotomy and valvulotomy for mitral stenosis: Experimental observations and clinical notes concerning an operated case with recovery. *Boston Med Surg J* 1923;188:1023.
3. Souttar HS. The surgical treatment of mitral stenosis. *Br Med J* 1925;2:603.
4. Bailey CP. The surgical treatment of mitral stenosis (mitral commissurotomy). *Dis Chest* 1949;15:377.
5. Baker C, Brock RC, Campbell M. Valvulotomy for mitral stenosis: Report of six successful cases. *Br Med J* 1950;1:1283.

6. Harken DW, Ellis LB, Ware PF, Norman LR. The surgical treatment of mitral stenosis. I. Valvuloplasty. *N Engl J Med* 1948;239:801.

7. Austen WG, Wooler GH. Surgical treatment of mitral stenosis by the transventricular approach with a mechanical dilator. *N Engl J Med* 1960;263:661.

8. Edmunds Jr LH. Evolution of prosthetic heart valves. *Am Heart J* 2001;141 (5):849–55.

9. Starr A, Edwards ML. Mitral replacement: Clinical experience with a ball valve prosthesis. *Ann Surg* 1961;154:726–40.

10. Bjork VO. The central flow tilting disc valve prosthesis (Björk-Shiley) for mitral valve replacement. *Scand J Thorac Cardiovasc Surg* 1970;4:15–23.

11. Emery RW, Nicoloff DM. St. Jude Medical cardiac valve prosthesis: In vitro studies. *J Thorac Cardiovasc Surg* 1979;78:269–76.

12. Kaiser GA, Hancock WD, Lukban SB, Litwak RS. Clinical use of new design stented xenograft heart valve prosthesis. *Surg Forum* 1969;20:137–8.

13. Carpentier A. Principles of tissue valve transplantation. In Ionescu MI Ross N Wooler GH. *Biological tissue in heart valve replacement.* London: Butterworths; 1971:49–82.

14. John S, Bashi VV, Jairaj PS et al. Closed mitral valvulotomy: Early results and long-term follow-up of 3,723 consecutive patients. *Circulation* 1983;68: 891–6.

15. Tutun U, Ulus AT, Aksöyek AI, Hizarci M, Kaplan S, Erbas S, Köse K, Katircioglu SF, Kutsal A. The place of closed mitral valvotomy in the modern cardiac surgery era. *J Heart Valve Dis* 2003 Sep;12(5):585–9.

16. Turi ZG, Reyes VP, Raju BS, Raju AR, Kumar DN, Rajagopal P, Sathyanarayana PV, Rao DP, Srinath K, Peters P. Percutaneous balloon versus surgical closed commissurotomy for mitral stenosis. A prospective, randomized trial. *Circulation* 1991 Apr 1;83(4):1179–85.

17. Ommen SR, Nishimura RA, Grill DE, Holmes DR, Rihal CS. Comparison of long-term results of percutaneous mitral balloon valvotomy with closed transventricular mitral commissurotomy at a single North American Institution. *Am J Cardiol* 1999 Sep 1;84(5):575–7.

18. Arora R, Nair M, Kalra GS, Nigam M, Khalilullah M. Immediate and long-term results of balloon and surgical closed mitral valvotomy: A randomized comparative study. *Am J Cardiol* 1993 Apr 1;125(4):1091–4.

19. Farhat MB, Ayari M, Maatouk F, Betbout F, Gamra H, Jarrar M, Tiss M, Hammami S, Thaalbi R, Addad F. Percutaneous balloon versus surgical closed and open mitral commissurotomy. *Circulation* 1998 Jan 27;97(3):245–50.

20. Patel JJ, Shama D, Mitha AS, Blyth D, Hassen F, Le Roux BT, Chetty S. Balloon valvuloplasty versus closed commissurotomy for pliable mitral stenosis: A prospective hemodynamic study. *J Am Coll Cardiol* 1991 Nov 1;18(5):1318–22.

21. Choudhary SK, Dhareshwar J, Govil A, Airan B, Kumar AS. Open mitral commissurotomy in the current era: Indications, technique, and results. *Ann Thorac Surg* 2003 Jan 31;75(1):41–6.

22. Antunes MJ, Vieira H, Ferrao de Oliveira J. Open mitral commissurotomy: The "golden standard". *J Heart Valve Dis* 2000 Jul 1;9(4):472–7.

23. Glower DD, Landolfo KP, Davis RD, Cen YY, Harrison JK, Bashore TM, Lowe JE, Wolfe WG. Comparison of open mitral commissurotomy with mitral valve replacement with or without chordal preservation in patients with mitral stenosis. *Circulation* 1998 Nov;98(19 Suppl):II120–3.

24. Cotrufo M, Renzulli A, Vitale N et al. Long-term follow-up of open commissurotomy versus bileaflet valve replacement for rheumatic mitral stenosis. *Eur J Cardiothorac Surg* 1997;12:335–9.

25. Lillehei CW, Levy MJ, Bannabeau RC. Mitral valve replacement with preservation of papillary muscles and chordae tendinae. *J Thorac Cardiovasc Surg* 1964;47:532–43.

26. Moon MR, DeAnda A Jr, Daughters GT 2nd, Ingels NB, Miller DC. Effect of mitral valve replacement on regional left ventricular systolic strain. *An Thorac Surg* 1999;68:894–902.

27. Talwar S, Jayanthkumar HV, Kumar AS. Chordal preservation during mitral valve replacement: Basis, techniques and results. *Indian J Thorac Cardiovasc Surg* 2005 Jan 1;21(1):45–52.

28. O'Brien SM, Shahian DM, Filardo G et al. The Society of Thoracic Surgeons 2008 cardiac surgery risk models: Part 2—Isolated valve surgery. *Ann Thorac Surg* 2009;88:23–42.

29. Vassileva CM, Mishkel G, McNeely C, Boley T, Markwell S, Scaife S, Hazelrigg S. Long-term survival of patients undergoing mitral valve repair and replacement. *Circulation* 2013 May 7;127(18):1870–6.

30. Vesey JM, Otto CM. Complications of prosthetic heart valves. *Curr Cardiol Rep* 2004;6:106–11.

31. Hammermeister K, Sethi GK, Henderson WG, Grover FL, Oprian C, Rahimtoola SH. Outcomes 15 years after valve replacement with a mechanical versus a bioprosthetic valve: Final report of the Veterans Affairs randomized trial. *J Am Coll Cardiol* 2000;36:1152–8.

32. Roudaut R, Serri K, Lafitte S. Thrombosis of prosthetic heart valves: Diagnosis and therapeutic considerations. *Heart* 2007;93:137–42.

33. Bonow RO, Carabello BA, Kanu C et al. ACC/AHA 2006 guidelines for the management of patients with valvular heart disease: A report of the American College of Cardiology/American Heart Association Task Force on Practice Guidelines. *Circulation* 2006;114:e84–e231.

34. Pibarot P, Demesnil JG. Prosthetic heart valves: Selection of the optimal prosthesis and long-term management. *Circulation* 2009;119:1034–48.

35. Jamieson WR, Cartier PC, Allard M et al. Surgical management of valvular heart disease 2004. *Can J Cardiol* 2004;20(suppl E):7E–120E.

36. Schoen FJ, Levy RJ. Calcification of tissue heart valve substitutes: Progress toward understanding and prevention. *Ann Thorac Surg* 2005; 79:1072–80.

37. Ruel M, Kulik A, Rubens FD, Bedard P, Masters RG, Pipe AL, Mesana TG. Late incidence and determinants of reoperation in patients with prosthetic heart valves. *Eur J Cardiothorac Surg* 2004;25:364–70.

38. Butchart EG, Gohlke-Barwolf C, Antunes MJ et al. Recommendations for the management of patients after heart valve surgery. *Eur Heart J* 2005;26:2463–71.

39. Sohail MR, Martin KR, Wilson KWR, Baddour LM, Harmsen WS, Steckelberg JW. Medical versus surgical management of Staphylococcus aureus prosthetic valve endocarditis. *Am J Med* 2006; 119:147–54.

40. Ivert TSA, Dismukes WE, Cobbs CG et al. Prosthetic valve endocarditis. *Circulation* 1984;69:223–32.

41. Calderwood SB, Swinski LA, Waternaux CM et al. Risk factors for the development of prosthetic valve endocarditis. *Circulation* 1985;72:31–7.

42. Grover FL, Cohen DJ, Oprian C et al. Determinants of the occurrence of and survival from prosthetic valve endocarditis: Experience of the Veterans Affairs Cooperative Study on Valvular Heart Disease. *J Thorac Cardiovasc Surg* 1994;108:207–14.

43. Sabik JF, Lytle BW, Blackstone EH et al. Aortic root replacement with cryopreserved allograft for prosthetic valve endocarditis. *Ann Thorac Surg* 2002;74:650–9.

44. Habib G, Thuny F, Avierinos JF. Prosthetic valve endocarditis: Current approach and therapeutic options. *Prog Cardiovasc Dis* 2008;50:274–81.

45. Rahimtoola SH. The problem of valve prosthesis-patient mismatch. *Circulation* 1978;58:20–4.

46. Pibarot P, Dumesnil JG. Hemodynamic and clinical impact of prosthesis-patient mismatch in the aortic valve position and its prevention. *J Am Coll Cardiol* 2000;36:1131–41.

47. Pibarot P, Dumesnil JG. Prosthesis-patient mismatch: Definition, clinical impact, and prevention. *Heart* 2006;92:1022–9.

48. Magne J, Mathieu P, Dumesnil JG, Tanné D, Dagenais F, Doyle D, Pibarot P. Impact of prosthesis-patient mismatch on survival after mitral valve replacement. *Circulation* 2007;115:1417–25.

49. Ruel M, Chan V, Bédard P, Kulik A et al. Very long-term survival implications of heart valve replacement with tissue versus mechanical prostheses in adults <60 years of age. *Circulation* 2007;116(11 Suppl):I294–I300.

50. Roques F, Michel P, Gladstone AR, Nashef SAM. The logistic EuroSCORE. *Eur Heart J* 2003;24:1–2.

51. Oakley RE, Kliene P, Bach DS. Choice of prosthetic heart valve in today's practice. *Circulation* 2008;117:253–6.

52. Harken DE. Heart valves: Ten commandments and still counting. *Ann Thorac Surg* 1989;48(Suppl. 3):S18–S19.

53. Vahanian A, Alfieri O, Andreotti F et al. Guidelines on the management of valvular heart disease (version 2012). Joint Task Force on the Management of Valvular Heart Disease of the European Society of Cardiology (ESC); European Association for Cardio-Thoracic Surgery (EACTS). *Eur Heart J* 2012;33(19):2451–96.

54. Nishimura RA, Otto CM, Bonow RO et al. 2014 AHA/ACC guideline for the management of patients with valvular heart disease. *J Am Coll Cardiol* 2014;63(22):2438–88.

Special situations

15

Juvenile mitral stenosis

ARIMA NIGAM AND RAVI S. MATH

INTRODUCTION

Sujoy B Roy from India coined the term "juvenile mitral stenosis" for patients presenting with severe MS at <20 years of age.[1] A landmark publication by Roy et al. identified that:

1. Rheumatic mitral stenosis (MS) does not require two decades to become symptomatic in India
2. Symptomatic critical MS is often seen below the age of 20 years

3. Mitral stenosis can be severe enough to cause congestive heart failure (CHF) without active carditis. Thus, the presence of CHF should not be considered synonymous with active rheumatic fever and carditis in children and adolescents in India by default.[1]

In several developing countries in Africa and South Asia, severe MS develops at a very young age.[1-5] It is generally believed that, in developing countries, 25% of patients with MS are <20 years of age, and 10% of patients are <12 years of age.[1,2]

The data available in the literature for juvenile MS, regarding its epidemiology, clinical features, hemodynamics, and pathology, is mostly from the pre-echocardiography era. Nothing much has been added in the literature regarding preventive aspects of the disease in recent years.

CAUSES OF MITRAL STENOSIS IN THE YOUNG

The term "juvenile MS" should be reserved for rheumatic mitral stenosis, because when Roy et al.[1] coined the term he ascribed rheumatic etiology to all the cases of mitral stenosis encountered. In this era of modern diagnostic techniques, especially echocardiography, some cases of MS in the young may rarely be attributed to other etiologies, such as congenital MS, malignant carcinoid disease, systemic lupus erythematosus, rheumatoid arthritis, mucopolysaccharidoses of the Hunter-Hurler phenotype, Fabry disease, Whipple disease, and methysergide therapy. We can conclusively attribute rheumatic etiology to MS if :

1. Clinically, prior history of rheumatic fever is present, and/or
2. There is pathological evidence of rheumatic etiology (Aschoff nodules), and/or
3. A good echocardiographic examination has ruled out typical congenital morphologies (i.e., parachute or double-orifice mitral valve)

Since all other causes of mitral stenosis are extremely rare in this age group, almost all the cases of MS can be attributed to rheumatic etiology even in the absence of clinical history of rheumatic fever or pathological evidence if echocardiography otherwise rules out congenital etiology.

There are certain echocardiographic features which are suggestive of rheumatic etiology. The mitral leaflets are typically pliable, with restricted mobility of the leaflet tips, which results in doming and a "hockey-stick" appearance of the anterior mitral leaflet in diastole in parasternal long-axis view. On parasternal short-axis examination, there is a typical fish-mouth appearance because of commissural fusion. Subvalvular thickening and fusion may or may not be present. Two papillary muscles are well identified.

EVIDENCE OF RHEUMATIC PROCESS IN JUVENILE MITRAL STENOSIS

In the 108-patient series by Roy et al.,[1] a history of rheumatic fever was present in only 71 (66%) cases. In the Cherian series,[6] such history was present in only 53% of cases. In the Huntarian lecture by ATS Paul[7] only 55% of patients gave a history of rheumatic fever; however, 59% of those MS patients who had no history of acute rheumatic fever had typical Aschoff nodules on auricular biopsy. Fifty percent of those with positive rheumatic history had negative auricular biopsy. So, there are cases where there is neither clinical nor biopsy evidence of rheumatic process. In Paul's series, 16% of patients were said to be such silent cases of unknown etiology. Importantly, in this series, the number of rheumatic attacks did not appear to increase the incidence of mitral stenosis.

SUBCLINICAL CARDITIS

Rheumatic fever is a clinical diagnosis, made with the help of modified Jones criteria. Carditis is one component of it and rheumatic fever can be diagnosed even in the absence of clinical carditis if other major/minor criteria are present. Rheumatic fever may occur without clinical carditis (heart failure, new-onset murmur, pericardial friction rub, etc.). Subclinical carditis is the term given to those cases of rheumatic fever where carditis is diagnosed by echocardiography and there is no clinical evidence of carditis. Patients with subclinical carditis suffer the same fate as that of manifest carditis. Since all cases of rheumatic fever (with or without carditis) need to get penicillin prophylaxis, the therapeutic significance of subclinical carditis lies in the duration of penicillin prophylaxis.[8–10]

DIFFERENCES BETWEEN ADULT AND JUVENILE MITRAL STENOSIS

Time interval between the onset of rheumatic fever and mitral stenosis

In the Western literature it is generally agreed that a time interval of several years has to elapse between the initial attack of carditis and the time when definite clinical evidence of MS becomes apparent. Paul Wood[11] states that the average duration between rheumatic fever and critical mitral stenosis is 19 years. Bland and Jones[12] in their 20-year follow-up study of children with acute rheumatic fever showed that nearly 66% of those who had MS at the end of the study did not show it at the 10-year halfway point. Thus, both these Western series practically rule out the possibility of severe MS in the young. But one of the most puzzling features of juvenile MS is the short time interval between the appearance of the rheumatic symptoms and development of tight MS. In the Roy et al.[1] series from Delhi, 70% of the patients with a history of rheumatic fever had symptoms within 5 years of the first attack. In the Shah[13] series from Mumbai, the time interval between the first episode of rheumatic fever and MS in a vast majority of cases was less than 3 years.

The inference from the West is supported by echocardiography-based longitudinal studies that have estimated the average decline in valve area to be as low as 0.09 cm^2/year.[14,15] In contrast, studies from developing countries document the rapid progression of MS leading to serious disability early in life that requires treatment.[2,16-17] In the developing regions of the world this rapid progression can be attributed to recurrent attacks of rheumatic fever in the absence of adequate penicillin prophylaxis and poor socioeconomic conditions of the population.

Juvenile mitral stenosis as isolated lesion or pure mitral stenosis

Roy et al.[1] who coined the term juvenile MS, confined their description to those patients under 20 years who had pure or predominant MS. Mitral stenosis patients who had significant mitral regurgitation (MR) or associated aortic valve disease were not included in the study. Vaishnava et al.,[18] in their series of 133 patients, reported the prevalence of juvenile MS (without MR) to be 26%. However, a series from the West by Bland and colleagues[19] found only 1.7% patients with pure MS and 49% with MS and MR.

Sex ratio

Boys are affected more often than females, with a ratio of 1.6:1.[18] ATS Paul[7] in his Hunterian lecture makes note of a 1:1 male:female ratio in juvenile MS patients. This is quite unlike the 3:1 or 4:1 female preponderance noted in all adult series.[11] The reason for this difference in sex ratio between the adult and juvenile series is unclear. Paul theorized the influence of sex hormones on the female preponderance after puberty as both the sexes are equally exposed to rheumatic infection.

PATHOLOGICAL FINDINGS IN JUVENILE MITRAL STENOSIS

Lung biopsy

Prominent features in lung biopsy are: 1) pronounced medial hypertrophy and intimal thickening of small muscular pulmonary arteries, arterioles, and venules; 2) alveolar capillary sclerosis and; 3) hypertrophic smooth muscle bands in distal respiratory passages. This picture was described as "musculare lungencirhose" of mitral stenosis by Davidson in 1905.[1] Paul Wood[11] noted that pulmonary hypertension in mitral stenosis is predominantly because of spasm. ATS Paul[7] concluded that since biopsy evidence of hypertension is present in only 10% of cases (though incidence in clinical and intra-operative pressure studies is about 70%), successful surgery should give excellent results since pulmonary arteriolar changes are still reversible. A high percentage of minute orifices are encountered at surgery in this age group.

Size of left atrium

Chadha and colleagues[20] noted that at the time of surgery the LA and LAA size were less than ideal in more than 50% of patients, out of which 8% of the cases had a very small appendage. This group was more vulnerable for appendage tear during surgery. The small left atrium in this age group is attributed to rapid progression of the disease. There is no time for left-atrial distension and the brunt of back pressure falls on the pulmonary vasculatures.

Valve morphology

Six types of valve morphologies encountered during surgery were described by Paul.[7] Four of these were met with in adult series as well but two types were especially unique to children, i.e., elastic valves and sclerotic valves.

Elastic valves that stretched like India rubber. According to Paul these valves are occasionally seen in early adult cases and are possibly due to early disease.

Dense cartilaginous sclerotic type is peculiar to childhood cases. These are present in 25% of cases and the valve is button hole, densely sclerotic with fibrous tissue that resembles cartilage in consistency. This was impossible to fracture with fingers and controlled fracture even with ventricular dilators was difficult. When it fractured it occurred with explosive force. This dense sclerotic cartilaginous valve had no counterpart in the adult series of 700 patients of the same author.

SYMPTOMS

Common presenting features are significant dyspnea, CHF, angina, and hemoptysis. Angina in juvenile MS is unlikely to be due to coronary atherosclerotic disease. Since juvenile patients have higher incidence of pulmonary hypertension, Wood's view about angina makes sense.[11] According to him, MS patients with severe pulmonary vascular obstruction have severe impairment of coronary flow caused by limitation of cardiac output, leading to angina. Thromboembolism is rare (1%). The incidence of hemopytsis is roughly 10%. Atrial fibrillation is very uncommon. This may be because the left atrium (LA) is relatively small in such patients, having not attained the critical mass needed for persistent atrial fibrillation to develop.

We should also recognize that symptoms in young children may be predominantly respiratory limited to tachypnea, dyspnea, or failure to thrive (Table 15.1).

GENERAL APPEARANCE

These patients can be said to have a fragile look. The patients with severe pulmonary vascular obstruction have a dusky look owing to a combination of extreme pallor and slight cyanosis.

Paul Wood[11] conferred the term mitral facies for a group of patients who had extreme pulmonary vascular resistance (>10 wood units), decreased cardiac output, and reduced arterial oxygen saturation of less than 90%.

CHF IN JUVENILE MITRAL STENOSIS

Until Roy et al. recognized juvenile MS, acute rheumatic activity was considered to be the most important cause of CHF. Dr. Roy concluded that CHF in patients with juvenile MS below the age of 20 may be due to mitral stenosis per se and not due to acute rheumatic activity. This conclusion was extremely relevant in the pre-echocardiography era as the patients were sent for surgery on the basis of clinical findings alone. Left-ventricular (LV) dysfunction as evaluated by LV end diastolic pressure (EDP) and LV angiogram has been reported by Srivastava et al.[2] They mentioned the presence of global LV

Table 15.1 Incidence of various symptoms in different series

Symptoms	Roy,[1] N = 108	Shrivastava et al.,[2] N = 125 (<12 years)	Wood,[11] N = 300 (adults)	Paul,[7] N = 100 (<16 years)	Cherian,[6] N = 126	Bhayana,[21] N = 140
Dyspnea (Mod-severe)	78%	73.6%	80%	67%	75%	100%
PND	16%	24%	35%	8%	NA	20.7%
Hemoptysis	27%	16%	44–50%	10%	18%	25%
Chest pain/angina	12%	9%	12%	16%	22% (1% with angina)	19.3%
Embolism	2%	1%	13%	1%	1%	2.1%
Rheumatic activity	22%	NA	NA	56% (biopsy)	NA	NA
Asymptomatic	9%	1%	NA	NA	NA	0%
Male:Female	1.6:1	1.4:1	1:3	1:2	1.3:1	1:1
CHF	45%	23%	NA	NA	33%	17.1%
H/o rheumatic fever	66%	51%	68%	55%	53%	NA

Abbreviations: CHF, congestive heart failure; PND, Paroxysmal nocturnal dysprea; NA, not available.

hypokinesia as well as regional wall motion abnormalities. They attributed it to rheumatic myocardial damage, subvalvular fibrosis, or secondary to right-ventricular volume overload.

CAUSES FOR SEVERE PULMONARY HYPERTENSION IN JUVENILE MITRAL STENOSIS

Despite the short duration of the disease process, a significant proportion of patients with juvenile MS develop severe pulmonary hypertension and elevated pulmonary vascular resistance. A number of theories have been proposed to explain this rapid progression of pulmonary vascular disease. These include:

1. Hypersensitive reaction of pulmonary vasculature to a fulminating rheumatic process[1]
2. Tissue response to multiple attacks of rheumatic fever[1]
3. Continued smoldering rheumatic activity[1]
4. Right-atrial clots leading to recurrent pulmonary emboli[20]

ECHOCARDIOGRAPHY IN JUVENILE MITRAL STENOSIS

The mitral valve of juvenile MS patients shows almost the same features as an adult MS patient, with the following exceptions. Mitral valve calcification is usually absent. Minute orifices as small as 0.5 cm² are more commonly seen (Figure 15.1,

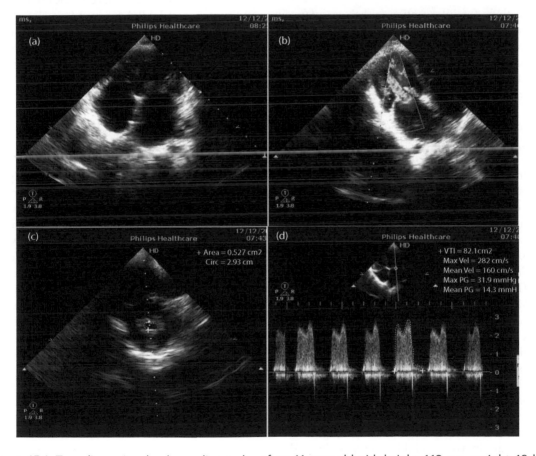

Figure 15.1 Two-dimensional echocardiography of an 11-year-old girl, height 119 cm, weight 12 kg, BSA-0.66 m², **(a)** Apical four-chamber view with dilatation of LA and RA and thickened AML and PML. **(b)** Parasternal long axis view showing severe subvalvular disease. **(c)** Short axis view shows bilateral commissural fusion with diffuse thickening of MV. MVA-0.5 cm², MVAI- 0.75 cm²/m², **(d)** continous wave doppler across mitral valve. Mean gradient 14 mmHg. BSA: Body surface area; LA-left atrium; RA-right atrium; AML-anterior mitral leaflet; PML-posterior mitral leaflet; MVA (I): mitral valve area (indexed) (See Videos 15.1 through 15.3).

Videos 15.1 through 15.3). More severe subvalvular disease and thickened leaflets are seen. The left atrium is unlikely to be enlarged too much. This may be the reason for decreased incidence of atrial fibrillation and absence of left-atrial thrombus in this patient population. Right-atrial and right-ventricular dilatation may be present because of significant pulmonary hypertension. Right-ventricular systolic pressures as measured by tricuspid regurgitation jet velocity may be suprasystemic.

TREATMENT

Indications for percutaneous or surgical intervention

Indications for intervention (either percutaneous or surgical) are well documented in adults.[22,23] According to these guidelines PTMC should be performed in all patients with symptomatic severe MS (valve area less than <1.5 cm²) and even in asymptomatic patients with very severe MS (valve area <1 cm²) if valve morphology is favorable and there are no contraindications (LA thrombus, significant mitral regurgitation). It should be noted that whereas in the 2006 ACC/AHA guidelines pulmonary hypertension (defined as pulmonary artery systolic pressure greater than 50 mmHg at rest or greater than 60 mmHg on exercise) in an asymptomatic patient with MVA <1.5 cm² was considered a class-I indication (level of evidence C) for PTMC, the current guideline update of 2014 is silent on this issue.

These criteria for selection of patients for PTMC, based on cut-off values of mitral valve area, can be applied to a relatively older subgroup (>14 years) of juvenile MS patients but the applicability of these criteria in younger children (<12 years) is questionable. Unfortunately, there are no validated thresholds for interventions in this group of patients on the basis of large series. Children often have a much smaller body surface area and mitral valve area. We should also recognize that symptoms in young children may be limited to tachypnea, dyspnea, or failure to thrive. Taking these facts into cognizance, the AHA guidelines on pediatric interventions[24] have suggested the following indications for intervention in mitral stenosis in children: (1) peak transmitral gradient ≥20 mmHg; (2) mean transmitral gradient ≥15 mmHg;

(3) near-systemic pulmonary artery pressure; and (4) calculated mitral valve area <1 cm²/m² with respiratory symptoms and failure to thrive.

Percutaneous transvenous mitral commissurotomy

Percutaneous transvenous mitral commissurotomy (PTMC) with the Inoue technique (Inoue balloon, Accura balloon) is the first-line therapy in juvenile MS patients at experienced centers, with mitral valve replacement (MVR) and repair being reserved for cases with extremely bad valve morphology. The only absolute contraindication for PTMC in children is probably bicommisural calcification (which itself is rare in children). Other contraindications include severe MR (>Grade 2/4) and presence of LA/LAA appendage clot. PTMC may be performed in the later after anticoagulation for two to six months if the patient is hemodynamically stable. No specific echocardiography score constitutes a contraindication for PTMC, especially in children.

TECHNICAL ASPECTS OF PTMC IN CHILDREN

In our experience, if the patient of juvenile MS is beyond 14 years of age and has attained a height of 140 cm, all the steps of PTMC, including transseptal puncture, can be done in a routine way (as in an adult). Prior correction of anemia, infection, and heart failure stabilization is advisable. However, a critically ill child may need intervention on an urgent/emergent basis. PTMC may also be performed even in the presence of rheumatic activity if needed as the success rate in this subgroup is almost the same, albeit with higher rates of restenosis.[25]

For children younger than 14 years, certain modifications to the routine ("adult") PTMC procedure needs to be made. Rarely, if the child is extremely uncooperative, the procedure may require general anesthesia. Most often, the procedure is performed under local anesthesia with conscious sedation. Meticulous attention should be paid to vascular access. The smallest possible arterial sheath (4–5F) should be used to avoid loss of femoral pulse. Transseptal puncture should ideally be performed with a pediatric transseptal set in the usual manner under fluoroscopic guidance. The differences between the adult and pediatric transseptal set are summarized in Table 15.2. If the

Table 15.2 Difference between adult and pediatric transseptal puncture equipment

	Adult	Pediatric
Brockenbrough needle	71 cm length, 18 G shaft, and 21 G tip	56 cm length, 19 G shaft, and 22 G tip
Mullins sheath/dilator length	63/67 cm	44/52 cm
Size (French)	7/8F	6F
Maximum wire diameter	0.032″	0.025″

patient has suprasystemic pulmonary artery pressure, it will be difficult to appreciate septal pulsations. Probing for the fossa ovalis is safer, with a reported success rate of 80%–90%.

BALLOON SIZE

As in adults, the selection of balloon size is done by Hung's formula (height in cm rounded to nearest zero/10) + 10. However, the relationship of the patients' height with mitral valve orifice diameter is not linear and this formula is not validated in children. When this formula is used in children, it is better to start with an undersized balloon that is 2–4 mm less than the calculated balloon size, in order to avoid severe mitral regurgitation.[26] The smallest available Inoue balloon is 20 mm (effective

range 18–20 mm), whereas, for the Accura balloon, the smallest available size is 22 mm (effective range 19–22 mm). The length and shaft diameter of the Inoue and Accura balloon are 70 and 80 cm, and 12F and 11F, respectively. A stepwise inflation technique is recommended, beginning with the smallest volume and progressively increasing by 0.5–1 mm. Following each inflation, an echocardiogram is performed to assess for MR and commissural splitting. A successful PTMC in the pediatric population has been defined as a MVA >1 cm^2/m^2 and/or an increase in MVA >50% from the baseline in the absence of any major complications.

Overall, the technical steps of PTMC in children are similar to those for an adult patient (Figure 15.2, Videos 15.4 through 15.7). A few challenges

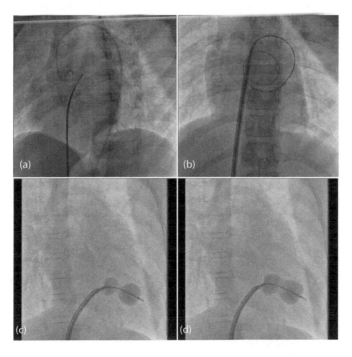

Figure 15.2 PTMC in an 11-year-old girl, weight 20 kg, height 133 cm. **(a)** Transseptal puncture using a pediatric transseptal needle; **(b)** septal dilatation using 14F dilator; **(c)** 22-mm Accura balloon inflated at 20 mm; **(d)** lateral commissure split (left-atrial mean pressure decreased from 29 mmHg to 17 mmHg, MVA increased from 0.5 cm^2 to 1 cm^2) (see Videos 15.4 through 15.7).

may be encountered due to the small LA; the smaller LA in children may not accommodate the slenderized Inoue balloon (which has a length of 4 cm). On the other hand, the deslenderized Inoue balloon (length 2.5 cm) has a larger profile and gets entrapped in the IAS. Partial deslenderizing of the balloon may be helpful.[27] In addition, LV entry may be hampered as the small LA may prevent the balloon from pointing downwards. Attempts to further withdraw the balloon may lead to entrapment in the IAS. To overcome this, the double-loop technique[27] or over-the-wire technique[28] can be tried.

OUTCOMES OF PTMC IN JUVENILE MITRAL STENOSIS

A number of moderate to large series pertaining to PTMC in juvenile MS are now available in the literature.[28–37] These studies can be divided into those enrolling patients younger than 20 years old and those enrolling very young patients (<12 years). Studies enrolling patients <20 years have noted PTMC results that are at least as good or better than the adult population. Success rates have ranged from 93%–100%, with almost nil mortality (Table 15.3). In the series by Karur and colleagues,[31] the immediate results in juvenile MS patients were better than in adults with significantly larger mitral valve area index and no significant complications. In the Gamra series[32] the better results in juvenile patients were attributed to small left-atrial dimensions and more pliable valves. Rates of severe MR ranged from 3.8 to 6%.

PTMC success rates in very young children (<12 years) are good (93%–94%), although a little lower than the former group (Table 15.3). This probably results from the aggressive nature of the disease in this group leading to severe subvalular deformity. Reported mortality was nil.

There is an apprehension that restenosis rates after PTMC may be higher among patients with juvenile MS. This may be due to smoldering rheumatic activity or the recurrence of rheumatic fever in this age group. The rates of restenosis ranged from 16% at intermediate follow-up (mean follow-up: 34 months) to 26% on long-term follow-up (mean follow-up: 8.5 ± 4.8 years). Thus, these results are comparable to the adult population. Echo score rather than age was a predictor of restenosis.

Optimal immediate and long-term results are seen in children and young adults with favorable valve morphology. Among 100 children younger than 12 years of age from India, event-free survival

at 1, 3, and 5 years was 97.1%, 91.4%, and 88.5%, respectively.[26] In the study from Saudi Arabia of 57 patients aged <18 years, event-free survival rates at 10, 15, and 18 years were 87% ± 6%, 62% ± 1%, and 20% ± 2%, respectively.[33] Repeat PTMC has been successfully performed in patients with restenosis with suitable anatomy with good success rates (85%–100%). However, the need for MVR rises with restenosis due to a higher incidence of unfavorable valve anatomy.

MITRAL VALVE REPLACEMENT IN CHILDREN AND YOUNG PATIENTS

Advanced mitral valve disease with severe fibrosis and distortion makes mitral valve replacement (MVR) often necessary in children and young patients. Replacement of the diseased mitral valve with the prosthesis is associated with the risks of anticoagulation, suboptimal preservation of ventricular function, and reduced survival.[38] Bioprosthetic valves have high rates of degeneration and are not usually preferred over mechanical valves. Children who have small prostheses implanted are at an increased risk of restrictive hemodynamics and the certainty that the child will outgrow the prosthesis.[39]

The long-term prognosis is not good for young MVR patients. Actuarial freedom from late reoperation at 10 and 14 years for patients with MVR is 88% and 73%, respectively. Actuarial freedom from thrombotic, embolic, and hemorrhagic events at 10 and 14 years is 63% and 45%, respectively.[40] MVR in children continues to be a high-risk procedure, and efforts to preserve native valve function should be attempted whenever technically feasible.

IS ACUTE RHEUMATIC FEVER MORE SEVERE IN SOUTH ASIA?

It is generally believed that acute rheumatic fever (RF) is more severe in the Indian subcontinent, leading to devastating sequelae, but this issue is controversial. Desilva[41] and Padmavati[42] emphasized the paucity of severe manifestation of RF in children from Sri Lanka and New Delhi, respectively. On the other hand, Roy et al. reported a much higher incidence of carditis and congestive heart failure. However, these were retrospective series. A prospective series from North India[43] reported that with continuous prophylaxis, the prevalence, rate, evolution, and clinical spectrum

Table 15.3 PTMC results in patients

Author, year	No.	Country	Age (range)	Success (%)	Death (%)	Tamponade (%)	Severe MR (%)	Stroke/ embolism (%)
(a) <20 years of age								
Karur et al., 2014[31]	40	India	10–20 (16.98 ± 3.22)	95	0	0	5%	0
Fawzy et al., 2008[33]	57	Saudi Arabia	10–18 (15.3 ± 2.4)	98.3	0	1.7	0	0
Harikrishan et al., 2006[30]	66	India	18.1 + 2.1	93	0	1.5	6%	0
Fawzy et al., 2005[34]	84	Saudi Arabia	10–20 (16.7 + 3.3)	98	0	1.2	0	0
Gamra et al., 2003[32]	110	Tunisia	<20 (16 ±2.8)	100	0	0	0	0
Yonga et al., 2003[35]	45	Kenya	9–20 (14 ± 2.6)	100	0	0	0	0
Joseph and Bonhoeffer, 1997[29]	107	India	10–18 (14.5 + 2.3)	98%	0	0.9	0.9	0
(b) <12 years of age								
Shrestha et al., 2015[36]	100	Nepal	7–15 (13 + 1.6)	94%	0	0	0	0
Kothari et al., 2005[26]	100	India	7–12 (11 + 1.2)	94%	0	0	4%	0
Krishnamoorthy et al., 2003[37]	13	India	<12	93%	0	0		0

of sequelae of RF in children from India do not differ significantly from Western series. This series emphasized the importance of adequate health-care delivery, which, in the long-term, can help curtail the prevalence of juvenile mitral stenosis.

To summarize, juvenile MS is widely prevalent in developing regions of the world, with prevalence as high as 25% of all MS patients. After an initial attack of rheumatic fever, the disease progresses rapidly and patients may develop severe stenosis within 3 to 5 years. These patients present in advanced functional class and have evidence of severe pulmonary hypertension. The majority of juvenile MS patients continue to maintain sinus rhythm and thromboembolic episodes are uncommon. If valve morphology is suitable, PTMC should be the first treatment offered. It provides good short-term and long-term outcomes. Finally, with improvement of socioeconomic conditions and appropriate health-care delivery, the prevalence of juvenile MS can be decreased.

VIDEOS

Two-dimensional echocardiography of 11-year-old girl with severe MS (MVA 0.5 cm², corresponding to Figure 15.1)

Video 15.1. Parasternal long axis view shows severe subvalvular disease. https://youtu.be/DaRSwP8nveY

Video 15.2. Apical four-chamber view with dilatation of LA and RA and thickened AML and PML. https://youtu.be/3doVhkoCSeU

Video 15.3. Short axis view shows bilateral commissural fusion with diffuse thickening of MV. https://youtu.be/8eE4-BxS2Vs

PTMC in 11-year-old girl, weight 20 kg, height 133 cm (corresponding to Figure 15.2, Courtesy of Prof. Jayaranganath M and Prof. K. H. Srinivasa)

Video 15.4. TSP using a pediatric Brockenbrough transseptal needle. https://youtu.be/0ygI9hlfOkw

Video 15.5. Septal dilatation using 14 Fr dilator. https://youtu.be/ICbePAGZ7sE

Video 15.6. LV entry. https://youtu.be/r2tc_fvWiEc

Video 15.7. PTMC with Accura 22 balloon inflated to 20 mm with splitting of lateral commissure. https://youtu.be/pBpYbh645nM

REFERENCES

1. Roy SB, Bhatia ML, Lazaro EJ, Ramalingaswami V. Juvenile mitral stenosis in India. *Lancet* 1963:2;1193–5.
2. Shrivastava S, Tandon R. Severity of mitral stenosis in children. *Int J Cardiol* 1991;30:163–7.
3. Oli K, Tekle-Haimanot R, Forsgren L, Ekstedt J. Rheumatic heart disease prevalence among school children of an Ethiopian rural town. *Cardiology* 1992;80:152–5.
4. Oli K, Porteous J. Prevalence of rheumatic heart disease among school children in Addis Ababa. *East Afr Med J* 1999;76:601–5.
5. Yuko-Jowi C, Bakari M. Echocardiographic patterns of juvenile rheumatic heart disease at the Kenyatta National Hospital. Nairobi. *East Afr Med J* 2005;82:514–9.
6. Cherian G, Vytilingam KI, Sukumar IP, Gopinath M. Mitral valvotomy in young patients. *Brit Heart J* 1964;26:157.
7. Paul ATS. The problem of mitral stenosis in childhood. *Ann R Coll Surg Engl* 1967;41:387–401.
8. Minich LL, Tani LY, Pagotto LT, Shaddy RE, Veasy LG. Doppler echocardiography distinguishes between physiologic and pathologic "silent" mitral regurgitation in patients with rheumatic fever. *Clin Cardiol* 1997;20:924–6.
9. Figueroa FE, Fernandez MS, Valdes P et al. Prospective comparison of clinical and echocardiographic diagnosis of rheumatic carditis: Long term follow-up of patients with subclinical disease. *Heart* 2001;85:407–10.
10. Caldas AM, Terreri MT, Moises VA et al. What is the true frequency of carditis in acute rheumatic fever? A prospective clinical and Doppler blind study of 56 children with up to 60 months of follow-up evaluation. *Pediatr Cardiol* 2008;29:1048–53.
11. Paul Wood. An appreciation of mitral stenosis. *Br Med J* 1954 May 15;1(4871):1113–24.

12. Bland EF, Jones TD: Rheumatic fever and rheumatic heart disease. A 20-year report on 1000 patients followed since childhood. *Circulation* 1961:24;836.

13. Shah SJ, Goyal BK, Sheth A et al. Juvenile MS in India. *Indian Heart Journal* 1974;27:6–12.

14. Gordon SPF, Douglas PS, Come PC, Manning WJ. Two-dimensional and doppler echocardiographic determinants of the natural history of mitral valve narrowing in patients with rheumatic mitral stenosis: Implications for follow-up. *J Am Coll Cardiol* 1992;19:968–73.

15. Sagie A, Freitas N, Padial LR et al. Doppler echocardiographic assessment of long-term progression of mitral stenosis in 103 patients: Valve area and right heart disease. *J Am Coll Cardiol* 1996;28:472–9.

16. Borman JB, Stern S, Shapira T, Milvidsky H, Braun K. Mitral valvotomy in children. *Amer Heart J* 1961;61:763.

17. Al-Bahrani IR, Thamer MA, Al-Omeri MM, Al-Namaan YD. Rheumatic heart disease in the young in Iraq. *Brit Heart J* 1966;28:824.

18. Vaishnava S, Webb JK, Cherian J. Juvenile rheumatism in south India. A clinical study of 166 cases. *Indian J Child Health* 1960;9:290–9.

19. Bland EF, White PD, Jones TD. The development of mitral stenosis in the young people. *Am Heart J* 1935;10(8):995–1004.

20. Chadha SK, Thareja RN, Durairaj M et al. Mitral valve disease in young; review of surgical treatment. *Indian J Thorac Cardiovasc Surg* 1983;2:29–35.

21. Bhayana JN, Khanna SK, Gupta BK et al. Mitral stenosis in the young in developing countries. *J Thorac Cardiovasc Surg* 1974;68:126–30.

22. Nishimura RA, Otto CM, Bonow RO et al. American College of Cardiology/American Heart Association Task Force on Practice Guidelines. 2014 AHA/ACC guideline for the management of patients with valvular heart disease. *J Am Coll Cardiol* 2014;63:e57–185.

23. Bonow RO, Carabello BA, Chatterjee K et al. ACC/AHA 2006 Guidelines for the Management of Patients with Valvular Heart Disease. *JACC* 2006;48:e1–148.

24. Feltes TF, Bacha E, Beekman RH. Indications for cardiac catheterization and intervention in pediatric cardiac disease: A scientific statement from the American Heart Association. *Circulation* 2011;123:2607–52.

25. Kothari SS, Ramakrishnan S, Juneja R, Yadav R. Percutaaneous transvenous mitral commissurotomy in patients with severe mitral stenosis and acute rheumatic fever. *Pediatr Cardiol* 2006:27;347–50.

26. Kothari SS, Ramakrishnan, Kumar CK, Juneja R, Yadav R. Intermediate-term results of percutaneous transvenous mitral commissurotomy in children less than 12 years of age. *Catheter Cardiovasc Interv* 2005;64:487–90.

27. Trehan V, Metha V, Mukhopadhyay S et al. Difficult percutaneous transvenous mitral commissurotomy: A new technique for left atrium to left ventricular entry. *Indian Heart J* 2004;56:158–62.

28. Manjunath CN, Srinivasa KH, Patil CB et al. Balloon mitral valvuloplasty: Our experience with a modified technique of crossing the mitral valve in difficult cases. *Catheter Cardiovasc Interv* 1999;46:117–8.

29. Joseph PK, Bhat A, Sivasankaran S et al. Percutaneous transvenous mitral commissurotomy using an Inoue balloon in children with rheumatic mitral stenosis. *Int J Cardiol* 1997;62:19–22.

30. Harikrishnan S, Nair K, Tharakan JM, Titus T, Kumar VK, Sivasankaran S. Percutaneous transmitral commissurotomy in juvenile mitral stenosis—Comparison of long term results of Inoue balloon technique and metallic commissurotomy. *Cathet Cardiovasc Interv* 2006;67:453–9.

31. Karur S, Veerappa V, Manjunath CN. Balloon mitral valvotomy in juvenile rheumatic mitral stenosis: Comparison of immediate results with adults. *Heart Lung Circ* 2014;12: 1165–8.

32. Gamra H, Betbout F, Ben Hamda K et al. Balloon mitral commissurotomy in juvenile rheumatic mitral stenosis: A ten year clinical and echocardiographic actuarial results. *Eur Heart J* 2003;24:1349–56.

33. Fawzy ME, Stefadouros MA, El Amraoui S et al. Long-term (up to 18 years) clinical and echocardiographic results of mitral balloon

valvuloplasty in children in comparison with adult population. *J Interven Cardiol* 2008;21:252–9.

34. Fawzy ME, Stefadouros MA, Hegazy H, El Shaer F, Chaudhary MA, Al Fadley F. Long term clinical and echocardiographic results of mitral balloon valvotomy in children and adolescents. *Heart* 2005;91(6):743–8.

35. Yonga GO, Bonhoeffer P. Percutaneous transvenous mitral commissurotomy in juvenile mitral stenosis. *East Afr Med J* 2003;80(4):172–4.

36. Shrestha M, Adhikari CM, Shakya U, Khanal A, Shrestha S, Rajbhandari R. Percutaneous transluminal mitral commissurotomy in Nepalese children with rheumatic mitral stenosis. *Nepalese Heart J* 2013;10:23–6.

37. Krishnamoorthy KM, Tharakan JA. Balloon mitral valvotomy in children < or = 12 years. *J Heart Valve Dis* 2003;12:461–8.

38. Antunes MJ, Wessels A, Sadowski RG et al. Medtronic Hall valve replacement in a third-world population group. *J Thorac Cardiovasc Surg* 1988;95:980–93.

39. Raffa H, Khateeb H, Tunisi T. Mitral valve replacement in children. *Aust. N.Z.J Surg* 1988;58:647–9.

40. Remenyi B, Webb R, Gentles T et al. Improved long term survival for rheumatic mitral valve repair compared to replacement in the young. *World J Pediatr Congenit Heart Surg* 2013 Apr;4(2):155–64.

41. Desilva S. Incidence of rheumatic fever in Ceylon. *Arch Dis Child* 1959;34:347.

42. Padmavati S. Epidemiology of cardiovascular disease in India. Rheumatic heart disease. *Circulation* 1962;25:703.

43. Sanyal SK, Berry AM, Duggal S et al. Sequelae of initial attack of rheumatic fever in children from north India. A prospective 5 year follow-up study. *Circulation* 1982;65:375–9.

16

Pregnancy and mitral stenosis

RAGHAV BANSAL, PREETI YADAV, AND SIVASUBRAMANIAN RAMAKRISHNAN

INTRODUCTION

Pregnancy is associated with a significant hemodynamic burden on the heart leading to the worsening of maternal cardiac disease and adverse maternal and fetal outcomes.[1] Though on decline in the Western world, rheumatic heart disease (RHD) still remains a common cardiovascular problem encountered in clinical practice in the developing world. Mitral stenosis (MS) in isolation or in combination with other valvular lesions remains the most common valvular problem encountered during pregnancy. Severe MS during pregnancy is poorly tolerated and is reported to be associated with mortality rates as high as 5%. Careful selection and timing of a specific management strategy remains the cornerstone for achieving the best possible maternal and fetal outcomes. This chapter discusses the pathophysiology, evaluation, management options, and outcomes of MS during pregnancy, with a special emphasis on the optimal use of percutaneous intervention.

EPIDEMIOLOGY

Developed countries have witnessed a significant decline in the prevalence of RHD over the past few decades, attributed to improved socioeconomic conditions. This has also been reflected in the pattern of heart disease during pregnancy. In a prospective multicenter study of 562 pregnant patients with heart disease, only 14% had valvular heart disease.[2] However, many parts of the world, including Asia, Africa, and South America, continue to face RHD as a major public health problem.[3] Due to greater prevalence in females of reproductive age, MS remains the most commonly encountered rheumatic valvular lesion during pregnancy.[4] In a study of 486 pregnant patients with RHD in India, only a single valve was affected in 63% of cases. MS was the abnormality in 90% of these patients.[5] In another series from India, MS constituted 88% of the pregnant patients complicated by heart disease being referred to a tertiary care hospital.[6]

CARDIOVASCULAR PHYSIOLOGY OF NORMAL PREGNANCY

The blood volume begins to expand from the sixth week of gestation. There is an initial rapid increase in volume up to 20 weeks, after which further increase is slower.[7] The maximum blood volume is reached at around 32 weeks of gestation, when the blood volume is around 50% more than the pre-pregnancy level.[7-9] The change in blood volume is also accompanied by redistribution of fluid, with a disproportionate rise in interstitial fluid and extra-cellular intravascular volume.[10] The red cell mass also increases (by 17%–40%) but fails to parallel the rise in blood volume, leading to a state of physiologic anemia of pregnancy associated with an increased demand for iron by 500 mg.[11]

Cardiac output (the product of heart rate and stroke volume) also increases by as much as 50%, peaking at 25 to 35 weeks of gestation.[12] Initially this rise is mainly driven by increase in stroke volume, which increases to a maximum at around 20 weeks of gestation and then plateaus. Later, heart rate becomes the dominant factor, contributing to an increase in cardiac output during the third trimester.[12] Cardiac output falls with supine position during pregnancy due to the compression of the inferior cava by the gravid uterus leading to decreased preload.[13] The changes in blood pressure during pregnancy are mainly driven by changes in the systemic vascular resistance (SVR). The SVR starts decreasing from the fifth week of gestation, reaches a trough level at 20 weeks (35% below the baseline), remains constant up till 32 weeks followed by a small increase up to term.[13] Oxygen consumption progressively increases with the course of pregnancy, peaking at term, with a peak increase of 20%–30% over the baseline.[14]

Labor and delivery are accompanied by abrupt fluid shifts and hemodynamic changes posing a greater stress on the cardiovascular system. With each uterine contraction around 500 mL blood is squeezed into maternal circulation, further increasing the cardiac output (up to 30% in the first stage and 50% in the second stage of labor, peaking at the time of delivery).[15,16] Immediately after the delivery, venous return increases rapidly mainly due to autotransfusion from the uterus and also due to the release of compression of the inferior vena cava by the gravid uterus. The increment in cardiac output is up to 60%–80% immediately after

delivery and begins to settle after 10 minutes.[15,16] However, autotransfusion continues to occur over a period of 24–72 hours post-delivery, marking the time frame when a patient might go into pulmonary edema secondary to mitral stenosis.[15,16] The hemodynamic changes of pregnancy revert to baseline gradually over a period of 6 to 12 weeks.

PATHOPHYSIOLOGY OF MITRAL STENOSIS DURING PREGNANCY

MS is characterized by obstruction to the blood flow from the left atrium (LA) to the left ventricle (LV) during diastole, limiting the preload and thus the cardiac output. To overcome the resistance, the left-atrial pressure rises, resulting in pulmonary venous congestion. The increase in heart rate shortens the diastole, further compromising the cardiac output by decreasing left-ventricular filling. Thus, pregnant females with MS often develop worsening symptoms during the second trimester due to pulmonary congestion and tachycardia. This is marked by the appearance of symptoms in previously asymptomatic patients or the worsening of functional class of symptomatic patients. Not uncommonly, the patients decompensate and develop pulmonary edema, which might be the first presentation of disease.

There is a progressive increase in left-atrial pressure and volume during pregnancy. This is accompanied by risk of atrial fibrillation (AF), especially during the third trimester. With the onset of AF, loss of atrial kick may lead to rapid decompensation to pulmonary edema. Also, the increased LA pressure is transmitted to the pulmonary circulation leading to pulmonary arterial hypertension (PAH). With longstanding PAH reactive changes develop in the pulmonary circulation leading to a pathologic rise in pulmonary vascular resistance (PVR). PAH due to high PVR is life-threatening in pregnancy and may also precipitate right-ventricular failure in the postpartum period. Atrial fibrillation and left-atrial stasis in the milieu of hypercoagulable state during pregnancy also increase the risk of systemic thromboembolism.

Labor and delivery frequently precipitate decompensation and pulmonary edema in patients with critical MS. Uterine contractions cause pain leading to tachycardia, and auto-transfusion leading to pulmonary congestion. Cardiac workload is also increased due to the active phases of labor. All these factors contribute to the development of pulmonary edema. It is pertinent to remember that the risk of pulmonary edema continues in the early postpartum period due to the continued autotransfusion as mentioned above.

MATERNAL AND FETAL OUTCOMES OF MITRAL STENOSIS

Although pregnancy with MS may lead to precipitation of complications (including pulmonary edema, right-sided heart failure, atrial arrhythmia, and systemic embolization), pregnancy, once completed, does not alter the natural history of MS. Chesley reviewed case histories of 134 women with functionally severe MS who became pregnant between 1931 and 1943.[17] This study represented the natural history of disease, since these cases were studied before the advent of modern management of MS. Women with subsequent pregnancies had similar survival as compared to those who did not become pregnant again. Thus, pregnancy does not affect the long-term outcome of MS.

Pulmonary edema and AF remain the most common complications of MS in pregnancy. In a case series of 80 pregnant patients with MS, pulmonary edema and arrhythmias were seen in 31% and 11%, respectively.[18] In the same series, the incidence of pulmonary edema and arrhythmias increased to 56% and 33%, respectively, in patients with critical MS (valve area of less than 1 cm^2).[18] The incidence of maternal complications was 67% in severe MS, 38% in moderate MS, and 26% in mild MS.[18] Thus, the severity of MS remains an important predictor of maternal outcomes during pregnancy. The other important predictor is abnormal functional class.[19] The mortality rate amongst pregnant females with MS with minimal symptoms is <1%. This rises to around 5% in patients with severe MS with significant symptoms.[20] It is important for the cardiologist to keep in mind the fetal outcomes while planning the management. The rate of fetal or neonatal mortality is more than 4% with severe left-heart obstruction.[2] However, it rises to as high as 30% in patients with NYHA (New York Heart Association) class IV symptoms.[21] Still, a good fetal outcome can be expected if maternal decompensation can be avoided with current management practices.

PRE-PREGNANCY COUNSELLING AND ASSESSMENT OF RISK

All females of reproductive age with heart disease, including valvular heart disease, should be offered the benefit of pre-conceptional counselling. This should include making an informed decision after detailed discussion regarding the risks and outcomes of pregnancy. Also, this gives a chance for optimization of cardiac status. The importance of safe contraception for those who decide against pregnancy cannot be overemphasized.

Various risk prediction tools are available for ascertaining risk of heart disease in pregnancy. According to the CARPREG (Cardiac Disease in Pregnancy) study, four risk markers have been identified for adverse events[2]: (1) poor functional class (NYHA class III or IV) or cyanosis; (2) systemic ventricular ejection fraction of <40%; (3) left-heart obstruction; (4) cardiac event prior to pregnancy. The modified WHO (World Health Organization) risk classification system is the most widely used tool for risk prediction as it appears reliable in many studies.[22] It classifies cardiac lesions from class I to IV. Class I lesions are at mild or no risk of maternal morbidity. Class II lesions are associated with moderate increase in maternal morbidity or small risk of mortality. Class III lesions are associated with significantly increased risk of maternal mortality and morbidity. And class IV lesions are extremely high-risk lesions where pregnancy is contraindicated.[23] Severe MS, even when asymptomatic, is a WHO class IV lesion with high risk of adverse outcomes. Thus, all females with severe MS should be advised an intervention to relieve the obstruction before becoming pregnant. It remains important to assess the functional capacity; obtain a 12-lead ECG to rule out AF and a transthoracic echocardiogram to ascertain the severity of the valvular lesion. Asymptomatic patients with MS with valve area around 1.5 cm^2 may undergo risk assessment with exercise testing. Exercise testing helps in assessing hemodynamic tolerance to stress in terms of effort tolerance, mitral gradients, and presence or absence of PAH. Patients who have limited functional capacity or who develop PAH on exercise should undergo an intervention for relief of obstruction prior to pregnancy. Another important aspect of pre-conception counselling is planning for safe anticoagulation in patients with an indication to receive warfarin, as warfarin is teratogenic.

DIAGNOSIS AND ASSESSMENT OF SEVERITY

Clinical diagnosis of MS during pregnancy poses special challenges due to the hemodynamic changes of pregnancy. Many pregnant females suffer from symptoms of dyspnea, fatigue, palpitations, increased venous pressure, and pedal edema — similar to symptoms caused by MS. Pregnancy is also associated with increase in heart rate and hyperkinetic circulation. Assessment should be done keeping these facts in mind and echocardiography remains an important tool to confirm the diagnosis in cases of diagnostic dilemmas. Approximately 25% of female patients with MS become symptomatic for the first time due to pregnancy.[24] It is important to make an early diagnosis in these patients for timely management and prevention of complications.

The commonly used Doppler techniques for the assessment of valve severity are also flawed during pregnancy. The gradients are often overestimated due to the increased cardiac output and thus increased flow across the valves. Estimation of valve area remains more accurate, although it is also associated with inaccuracies during pregnancy. Rokey and colleagues compared mitral valve areas during pregnancy using the pressure half-time method and the continuity equation method.[25] They found the continuity equation method to be more reliable, with the pressure half-time method underestimating the degree of stenosis.[25] Determination of valve area is essential during pregnancy due to the non-reliability of valve gradients. Valve area is also commonly determined by the 2D planimetric method, though it remains operator-dependent.

MEDICAL MANAGEMENT

The importance of medical management cannot be overemphasized and remains the first line in all symptomatic patients. Surgical or percutaneous intervention are reserved for refractory cases only. All patients should continue to receive secondary penicillin prophylaxis as recurrent rheumatic fever episodes may translate into significant deterioration. Sulfadiazine is contraindicated due to its teratogenicity. Adequate iron supplementation is a must to avoid anemia. The goal of the medical management in MS during pregnancy is to balance the increase in cardiac output due to pregnancy with the flow limitation across the mitral valve. Patients with severe MS often require restriction of maternal physical activity. This helps in maintaining a balanced state by reducing cardiac work load and maternal tachycardia, thus prolonging diastolic filling and maintenance of cardiac output. Diuretics remains the mainstay of medical management in symptomatic pregnant patients with significant MS. In pregnancy, torsemide may be relatively safer (FDA category B) as compared to fruosemide (FDA category C). Loop diuretics must be used with oral potassium supplementation and aldosterone antagonists are contraindicated in pregnancy. Diuretics, although not having been shown to be teratogenic, carry a risk of volume depletion and utero-placental hypoperfusion leading to intrauterine growth retardation (IUGR). They may also have harmful neurodevelopmental effects in the fetus secondary to electrolyte imbalances. Thus, cautious administration and careful monitoring of volume status and serum electrolytes is required. Daily weight monitoring may be the best method for the assessment of diuretic response.

β-adrenergic blockers are the cornerstone of medical management in patients with symptomatic severe MS.[26] β-blockers improve cardiac output by enhancing diastolic filling by virtue of decreasing the heart rate. In a study of 25 pregnant patients with severe MS receiving β-blockers, Al Kasab and colleagues demonstrated a reduction in the incidence of maternal pulmonary edema without significant adverse effects on the fetus.[27] The same study also demonstrated significant initial deterioration of functional class with pregnancy and subsequent improvement in functional class with β-blocker therapy. According to the European Society of Cardiology guidelines (2011) on the management of cardiovascular diseases during pregnancy, all severe MS patients who are symptomatic or have pulmonary arterial pressure greater than 50 mmHg should receive therapy with β-blockers.[23] Although β-blockers do carry some risk of IUGR, fetal bradycardia, and neonatal hypoglycemia, they are generally safe and their benefits far outweigh the risks in patients with severe MS. It is preferable to use β-1 selective agents to avoid uterine side effects of non-selective agents. Metoprolol has been shown to have a lower incidence of IUGR as compared to atenolol, and remains the β-blocker of choice in pregnancy.[28]

In patients with chronic AF, digoxin and β-blockers are indicated for rate control. Anticoagulation is indicated due to increased risk of systemic embolism. No anticoagulation regimen is perfect. Fetal exposure to warfarin in the first trimester can lead to embryopathy ranging from bone stippling (chondrodysplasia punctata) to nasal hypoplasia, optic atrophy, and mental retardation. However, the effects are dose-related and negligible when daily dose is less than 5 mg.[29] It is suggested that warfarin may be continued even through the first trimester when the daily dose is less than 5 mg. Otherwise, consideration should be given to a switch to low-molecular-weight heparin (LMWH) as early as 6 weeks of gestation and continued up till 13 to 14 weeks of gestation when embryogenesis is complete. Patients can safely receive warfarin during the second and third trimesters with a switch to LMWH at 36 weeks to prevent both maternal and fetal bleeding complications during labor and parturition.[23] A complete discussion over anticoagulation during pregnancy is out of scope of the current discussion. Consideration should be given to cardioversion in patients with acute-onset AF and subsequent decompensation. Amiodarone should be avoided due to risk of IUGR and fetal thyropathy.

A NOTE ON OBSTETRIC MANAGEMENT

Pregnant females with severe MS should be delivered in a unit with 24-hour availability of an expert obstetrician, cardiologist, and anesthetist. The importance of continuous ECG monitoring and careful monitoring of fluid balance cannot be overemphasized. Although it is not routinely required, invasive hemodynamic monitoring may be considered in patients with very high risk of developing pulmonary edema to monitor fluid therapy and diuresis.[30] Intravenous β-blocker administration in the form of bolus doses may also be required for controlling the heart rate and maintenance of cardiac output in the emergency setting.[30] At term, the induction of labor is often electively chosen so that labor can proceed in a planned way. It is best to start with a lower dose of prostaglandin for

the induction of labor due to the risk of uterine hyperstimulation and cardiac decompensation. As compared to an uncomplicated labor delivery, Caesarean section subjects the mother to more stress and should not be the method of delivery just for the sake of presence of cardiovascular disease. Caesarean section should be reserved for obstetric indications only.[30] However, Caesarean section may be considered in cases where complicated labor is expected.

The key to success in managing patients with MS lies in minimizing the cardiovascular stress.[30] This can be achieved effectively by minimizing the pain with the use of regional anesthesia (epidural analgesia) and shortening of the second stage of labor. This may be achieved by assisting the delivery with application of forceps or vacuum. Operative vaginal delivery also minimizes abrupt hemodynamic and blood-pressure changes associated with pushing. Fluid shifts in the immediate postpartum period causes an abrupt rise in pulmonary artery pressure and poses a significant risk of pulmonary edema.[30] Hence, aggressive diuresis should be given in the immediate postpartum period and close monitoring should be continued at least up to 72 hours after delivery.

SURGICAL VERSUS PERCUTANEOUS INTERVENTION: OUTCOMES

Only patients who continue to have NYHA class III or IV symptoms or have a pulmonary artery pressure of greater than 50 mmHg despite medical management require some form of intervention. The options available include closed mitral valvotomy (CMV), open mitral commissurotomy (OMC), mitral valve replacement (MVR), and percutaneous transvenous mitral commissurotomy (PTMC).

CMV during pregnancy was first reported in 1952 followed by several reports being published.[31] CMV carries an average maternal mortality rate of 1.7% and a fetal mortality rate of 5%–15%.[31] However, in a more recent series of eight pregnant patients with severe MS undergoing CMV, all patients improved clinically without any major morbidity or mortality.[32] OMC and MVR are reserved for patients having severe refractory disease with left-atrial thrombus or calcified mitral valve rendering the patient non-amenable to PTMC. Due to the need for cardiopulmonary

Table 16.1 Summary of various studies regarding outcomes of PTMC during pregnancy

Study	Number of patients	Mean age (years)	Mean gestational age (weeks)	Procedural success	Post-procedure severe MR	Maternal mortality	Fetal loss
Mishra et al.[34]	85	23 ± 4	25 ± 5	94%	1.2%	0	0
Esteves et al.[35]	71	27 ± 6	24 ± 7	100%	4.6%	0	4.2%
Nercolini et al.[36]	44	28 ± 6	23 ± 6	95%	0	0	8.1%
Farhat et al.[37]	44	29 ± 6	26 ± 6	97.7%	2.3%	0	0
Routray et al.[38]	40	23 ± 5	24 ± 5	95%	0	0	2.5%
Gupta et al.[39]	40	24 ± 5	21 ± 11	97.5%	2.5%	2.5%	3.4%
Kalra et al.[40]	27	25 ± 3	22 ± 4	96.3%	3.7%	0	3.7%
Esteves et al.[41]	13	26 ± 7	25 ± 6	100%	0	0	0

bypass they carry a high risk of maternal mortality (1.5%–5%) and a high rate of fetal loss (16%–33%).[33]

PTMC has been shown to achieve success with a low rate of complications in multiple case series.[34–41] Data from recently published case series are presented in Table 16.1. To summarize, the procedural success of PTMC during pregnancy is as high as 89%–100%, with a low risk of postprocedural mitral regurgitation (0%–5%) and maternal mortality (0.2%). The rate of fetal loss is low and ranges between 0% and 8% in various studies. Esteves and colleagues also reported long-term follow-up after PTMC done during pregnancy in 71 patients. They reported preterm deliveries in 13%. Of those delivering at term, 88% had normal birth weight babies. At a mean follow-up of 44 months, a 54% event-free maternal survival was reported with all the children exhibiting normal growth and development.[35] In a direct comparison of PTMC to OMC during pregnancy, a similar 95% success rate was achieved with both procedures. PTMC was better in terms of fetal outcome, with a rate of fetal loss of 5% as compared to 33% with OMC.[42] Thus PTMC is the procedure of choice for severe symptomatic MS during pregnancy due to its low rate of fetal complications as compared to surgical options. However, at the same time it remains important to remember that medical management should be exhausted before offering any intervention due to inherent risks of all interventions.

PTMC: OPTIMAL TIMING AND TECHNICAL ASPECT

Ideally, the best time to perform the procedure is before conception. In patients who present with symptomatic severe MS in early pregnancy, PTMC may be delayed until organogenesis of the fetus is complete (i.e., 12–14 weeks), to avoid radiation exposure to the fetus in the first trimester. The best time frame for performing a PTMC is 14–22 weeks in these circumstances.[43] In the early second trimester the fetus is small and thus causes minimal interference with catheter manipulation. Also, it may be easier to keep the fetus out of the radiation field due to the smaller size of the fetus. However, many patients become symptomatic only after 20 weeks of gestation when the expansion of blood volume peaks. In such cases the procedure should be deferred to 26–30 weeks of gestation, so that fetal viability is achieved in case of inadvertent preterm delivery.[43] The procedure becomes more challenging in the third trimester (due to the size of gravid uterus causing venacaval compression and interfering with catheter manipulation). The risk of maternal complications is also increased in the late third trimester. However, even if a patient becomes symptomatic in the late third trimester, PTMC should not be denied.

PTMC during pregnancy is a technically demanding procedure and has to be done quickly to minimize radiation exposure. Hence, it should be done at a center with adequate expertise and experience, and also with availability of surgical backup in case of severe postprocedural mitral regurgitation. Inoue's single balloon catheter is the preferred technique due to its considerably shorter procedural time.[43] To shorten the fluoroscopy time, right-heart catheterization and left-ventricular angiogram are best avoided. Two-dimensional echocardiography is used to guide PTMC and assess for the success/complications. It is important to remember that the interatrial septum may be more horizontal during pregnancy due to the elevation of the diaphragm secondary to push by the gravid uterus. Thus, adequate evaluation of the lie of the interatrial septum is essential before performing a septal puncture. Further, the gravid uterus compresses the inferior vena cava, making the movement of the balloon catheter and septal dilator painful. As such, catheter exchanges should be performed slowly and gently. Finally, there is the risk of maternal hypotension. This is because of two reasons. First, venous return is hindered due to the venacaval compression by the gravid uterus in the supine position, leading to decreased cardiac output. This is mitigated by giving intravenous fluids during the procedure. Second, hypotension also occurs during balloon inflation across the mitral valve so the inflation times should be kept as short as possible. Maternal hypotension poses a risk for fetal distress that might translate into a Caesarean section, and should be avoided as far as possible. It is also important to realize that the goal of the procedure is not to achieve a complete success with valve dilatation but to achieve a successful pregnancy outcome. One should not be aggressive with balloon sizing, as complication in the form of severe mitral regurgitation may require urgent surgery and its antecedent complications. A stepwise balloon dilatation technique is used starting at low volumes.

RISKS OF FETAL RADIATION EXPOSURE

The safe permissible dose of radiation during pregnancy is considered to be around 5 rad. Termination of pregnancy should be considered if the radiation dose exceeds 10 rad, due to the high risk of adverse outcomes. The effects of radiation on the foetus can be divided into three parts of pregnancy.[44] In the pre-implantation phase (0 to 9 days of gestation), radiation may lead to spontaneous abortion rather than anomalies, with an "all or none" effect. The phase of embryogenesis (9 days to 12 weeks of gestation) is the most vulnerable period, when radiation may lead to severe structural anomalies. A dose of 200 rad will produce congenital anomalies in all babies, whereas a dose of 10 rad increases the incidence by 1% over the baseline risk of 5%–10%. Although the risk of congenital structural anomalies is negligible in

the second and third trimester, the risk of childhood leukemia and other malignancies become a concern. Current estimates suggest a risk of 2–6 per 100,000 live births with 1 rad of radiation.[45] The brain also remains sensitive to radiation with reports of mental retardation and microcephaly occurring with radiation exposure in the second to third trimester.[46]

All patients during the PTMC procedure should receive an abdominal shield (from diaphragm to pubic symphysis) both on the anterior and the posterior walls of the abdomen. Also, fluoroscopy should be used with a lower frame rate and an adequately collimated X-ray beam (with maximal use of shutters) to minimize the radiation exposure. The mean fluoroscopy times reported in various studies are mostly less than 10 minutes, including 3.6 minutes by Mishra and colleagues,[34] 16 minutes by Farhat and colleagues,[37] 5.5 minutes by Routray and colleagues,[38] 7.8 minutes by Gupta and colleagues,[39] and 5.6 minutes by Kalra and colleagues.[40] With adequate shielding the dose of radiation during PTMC is estimated to be less than 0.2 rad. This dose is usually considered to be safe. The same has also been shown in long-term follow-up studies after PTMC during pregnancy with no significant adverse effects noted up to early childhood.[35]

There is a small risk of fetal hypothyroidism with iodine contrast agent exposure after 25 weeks of gestation when the fetal thyroid glands become active. However, with the omission of a left-ventricular angiogram in the current PTMC practice, the contrast dose used during PTMC is negligible and is not expected to cause any adverse effects.

CONCLUSION

Severe symptomatic MS is associated with significant adverse maternal and fetal outcomes. Thus, it is considered as a contraindication for pregnancy before relief of obstruction by an appropriate intervention. When pregnant patients present with MS, the care should be provided at a center with adequate experience and availability of cardiologist, expert obstetrician, and anesthetist. Medical management with diuretics and β-blockers remains first-line, with intervention reserved for patients with severe symptoms (NYHA class III or IV) despite adequate medical management. Risk of fetal adverse outcomes remains high with surgical interventions and PTMC has been shown to be safe and effective in multiple case series with the best time to perform PTMC being early in the second trimester. Caesarean section should be reserved for obstetric indications and regional anesthesia and assisted delivery should be considered during the progress of labor.

REFERENCES

1. Douglas PS. Cardiovascular health and disease in women. Philadelphia: W.B. Saunders Company;1993:305–28.
2. Siu SC, Sermer M, Colman JM et al. Prospective multicenter study of pregnancy outcomes in women with heart disease. *Circulation* 2001;104:515–21.
3. Eisenberg M. Rheumatic heart disease in the developing world. Prevalence, prevention, and control. *Eur Heart J* 1993;14:122–8.
4. Reimold SC, Rutherford JD. Clinical practice. Valvular heart disease in pregnancy. *N Engl J Med* 2003;349:52–9.
5. Sawhney H, Aggarwal N, Srui V et al. Maternal and perinatal outcome in rheumatic disease. *Int J Gynecol Obstet* 2003;80:9–14.
6. Bhatla N, Lal S, Behera G et al. Cardiac disease in pregnancy. *Int J Gynaecol Obstet* 2003;82:153–9.
7. Lund CJ, Donovan JC. Blood volume during pregnancy. *Am J Obstet Gynecol* 1967;98:393–403.
8. Dieckmann WJ, Wegner CR. The blood in normal pregnancy. I. Blood and plasma. *Arch Intern Med* 1934;53:71–86.
9. Berlin NI, Goetsch C, Hyde GM et al. The blood volume in pregnancy as determined by P-32 labelled red blood cells. *Surg Gynecol Obstet* 1953;97:173–6.
10. Brown MA, Gallery ED. Volume homeostasis in normal pregnancy and preeclampsia: Physiology and clinical implications. *Baillieres Clin Obstet Gynaecol* 1994;8:287–310.
11. Chesley LC. Plasma and red cell volumes during pregnancy. *Am J Obstet Gynecol* 1972;112:440–50.
12. Robson SC, Hunter S, Boys RJ et al. Serial study of factors influencing changes in cardiac output during human pregnancy. *Am J Physiol* 1989;256:H1060–5.
13. Lees HM, Taylor SH, Scott BD et al. The circulatory effect of recumbent postural change in late pregnancy. *Clin Sci* 1967;32:453–65.
14. Elkus R, Popovich J. Respiratory physiology in pregnancy. *Clin Chest Med* 1992;13:555–65.
15. Adams JG, Alexander AM. Alterations in cardiovascular physiology during labor. *Obstet Gynecol* 1958;12:542–9.
16. Robson C, Dunlop W, Boys RJ et al. Cardiac output during labour. *Br Med J (Clin Res Ed)* 1987;295:1169–72.
17. Chesley L. Severe rheumatic cardiac disease and pregnancy: The ultimate prognosis. *Am J Obstet Gynecol* 1980;136:552–8.
18. Silversides CK, Colman JM, Sermer M et al. Cardiac risk in pregnant women with rheumatic mitral stenosis. *Am J Cardiol* 2003;91:1382–5.
19. Barbosa PJ, Lopes AA, Feitosa GS et al. Prognostic factors of rheumatic mitral stenosis during pregnancyand puerperium. *Arq Bras Cardiol* 2000;75:220–4.
20. Clark S. Cardiac disease in pregnancy. *Crit Care Clin* 1991;7:777–97.
21. Brady K, Duff P. Rheumatic heart disease in pregnancy. *Clin Obstet Gynecol* 1989;32:21–40.
22. Balci A, Sollie-Szarynska KM, van der Bijl AG et al. for the ZAHARA-II Investigators. Prospective validation and assessment of cardiovascular and offspring risk models for pregnant women with congenital heart disease. *Heart* 2014;100:1373–81.
23. Regitz-Zagrosek V, Lundqvist CB, Borghi C et al. (The Task Force on the Management of Cardiovascular Diseasesduring Pregnancy of the European Society of Cardiology). ESC Guidelines on the management of cardiovascular diseases during pregnancy. *Eur Heart J* 2011;32:3147–97.
24. Szekely P, Julian DG. Heart disease and pregnancy. *Curr Prob Cardiol* 1979;4:1–74.
25. Rokey R, Hsu HW, Moise KJ Jr, Adam K, Wasserstrum N. Inaccurate noninvasive mitral valve area calculation during pregnancy. *Obstet Gynecol* 1994;84:950–5.
26. Norrad RS, Salehian O. Management of severe mitral stenosis during pregnancy. *Circulation* 2011;124:2756–60.

27. Al Kasab S, Sabag T, Al Zaibag M et al. Beta-adrenergic receptor blockade in the management of pregnant women with mitral stenosis. *Am J Obstet Gynecol* 1990;163:37–40.

28. Nishimura RA, Otto CM, Bonow RO et al. 2014 AHA/ACC Guidelines for the Management of Patients With Valvular Heart Disease. *J Am Coll Cardiol* 2014;63(22):e57–e185.

29. Vitale N, De Feo M, De Santo LS et al. Dose-dependent fetal complications of warfarin inpregnant women with mechanical heart valves. *J Am Coll Cardiol* 1999;33:1637–41.

30. Clark S, Phelan J, Greenspoon J et al. Labor and delivery in the presence of mitral stenosis: Central hemodynamic observations. *Am J Obstet Gynecol* 1985;152:984–8.

31. Presbitero P, Prever SB, Brusca A. Interventional cardiology in pregnancy. *Eur Heart J* 1996;17:182–8.

32. Aggarwal N, Suri V, Goyal S, Malhotra S, Manoj R, Dhaliwal RS. Closed mitral valvotomy in pregnancy and labor. *Int J Gynecol Obstet* 2005;88:118–21.

33. Sutton SW, Duncan MA, Chase VA, Marce RJ, Meyers TP, Wood RE. Cardiopulmonary bypass and mitral valve replacement during pregnancy. *Perfusion* 2005;20:359–68.

34. Mishra S, Narang R, Sharma M et al. Percutaneous transseptal miral commissurotomy in pregnant women with critical mitral stenosis. *Indian Heart J* 2001;53:192–6.

35. Esteves CA, Munoz JS, Braga S et al. Immediate and long-term follow up of percutaneous balloon mitral valvuloplasty in pregnant patients with rheumatic mitral stenosis. *Am J Cardiol* 2006;98:812–16.

36. Nercolini DC, Bueno R, Guérios E et al. Percutaneous mitral balloon valvuloplasty in pregnant women with mitral stenosis. *Cathet Cardiovasc Intervent* 2002;57:318–32.

37. Farhat M, Gamra H, Betbout F et al. Percutaneous balloon mitral commissurotomy during pregnancy. *Heart* 1997;77:564–7.

38. Routray SN, Mishra TK, Swain S, Patnaik UK, Behera M. Balloon mitral valvuloplasty during pregnancy. *Int J Gynecol Obstet* 2004;85:18–23.

39. Gupta A, Lokhandwala Y, Satoskar P, Salvi V. Balloon mitral valvotomy in pregnancy: Maternal and fetal outcomes. *J Am Coll Surg* 1998;187:409–15.

40. Kalra GS, Arora R, Khan JA, Nigam M, Khalillulah M. Percutaneous mitral commissurotomy for severe mitral stenosis during pregnancy. *Cathet Cardiovasc Diagn* 1994;33:28–30.

41. Esteves CA, Ramos A, Braga S, Harrison JK, Souza JE. Effectiveness of balloon mitral valvotomy during pregnancy. *Am J Cardiol* 1991;68:930–4.

42. deSouza J, Martinez E Jr, Ambrose J et al. Percutaneous balloon mitral valvuloplasty in comparison with open mitral valve commissurotomy for mitral stenosis during pregnancy. *Am Coll Cardiol* 2001;37:900–3.

43. Hameed A, Mehra A, Rahimtoola S. The role of catheter balloon commissurotomy for severe mitral stenosis in pregnancy. *Obstet Gynecol* 2009;114:1336–40.

44. Jankowki C. Radiation and pregnancy: Putting the risks inproportion. *Am J Nursing* 1986;86:260–5.

45. Stewart A, Webb J, Giles D. Malignant disease in childhoodand diagnostic irradiation in utero. *Lancet* 1956;271:447.

46. Miller R. Intrauterine radiation exposure and mental retardation. *Health Physics* 1988;55:295–8.

17

Lutembacher syndrome

KIKKERI HEMANNASETTY SRINIVAS AND ANAND SUBRAMANIAM

INTRODUCTION

Lutembacher syndrome, better understood by its eponym, is generally defined as a combination of mitral stenosis (MS) and left-to-right shunt at the atrial level. René Lutembacher, a French cardiologist, initially published his findings of a large fossa ovalis defect and coexistent mitral stenosis in a 61-year-old lady in 1916.[1] However, it was Corvisart who described the lesion as early as 1811. Over the last century, the definition has undergone many changes. The syndrome has been defined by some as a combination of atrial septal defect (ASD) and any mitral valve lesion[2] (mitral stenosis, mitral insufficiency, or combined lesion). On the same note, in the present era of percutaneous transmitral commissurotomy (PTMC), iatrogenic ASD secondary to transseptal puncture has also been loosely included in the bracket of "Lutembacher syndrome." By and large, any combination of ASD (congenital or iatrogenic) and mitral stenosis (congenital or acquired) may be referred to as Lutembacher syndrome, though this definition may not be accepted by all. However, a stretched patent foramen ovale or isolated mitral regurgitation is not included, nor does such a combination produce the unique hemodynamic effects which characterize this condition.

PREVALENCE AND PATHOLOGY

The exact prevalence of Lutembacher syndrome is not known. Prevalence is higher in developing countries where rheumatic heart disease is more common. It is more common in females, as both secundum atrial septal defects and rheumatic MS are more common in females. Although age at presentation can vary, maximum prevalence is during the second and third decades. The incidence of mitral stenosis in patients with an ostium secundum atrial septal defect has been estimated to be around 4%.[3-5] Atrial septal defects are seen in 0.6% of patients with mitral stenosis.[3-5] Repeated transseptal punctures for balloon mitral valvotomy generally produce a small defect, which is usually hemodynamically insignificant.[6] The syndrome is likely to be seen with even lesser frequency in the future, not only due to a decrease in the incidence of rheumatic heart disease, but also due to better school health screening programs, with most children undergoing closure of atrial septal defects in early childhood. Interestingly, despite our center having large volumes of patients who have been treated with PTMC and surgical or device closure of ASD, we have seen very few cases of mitral stenosis developing later in life, after closure of ASD. We have had only three patients needing PTMC after previous surgical closure of ASD. Septal puncture can be challenging in this subset.

There have been few studies on the actual pathology of the mitral valve and it has been thought to be of exclusive rheumatic etiology. Vaideeswar et al. have recently published the pathologic findings seen in 44 patients with a diagnosis of Lutembacher syndrome in autopsies carried out over a period of 16 years.[7] 54.4% of their patients had a nonrheumatic etiology for mitral valve disease, based on the lack of features to suggest postinflammatory change or chronic rheumatic involvement. A history of rheumatic fever was obtained in only two of these patients, suggesting that not all acquired mitral valve disease is rheumatic in nature. A clinical diagnosis of atrial septal defect was made in only 18 of these 44 patients. Some of these turned out to be sinus venosus defects, since they may not have been clinically differentiable. They observed involvement of the posteromedial commissure in patients with rheumatic and non-rheumatic etiology. This has been postulated to be a consequence of friction at this region, arising from altered left-ventricular geometry due to right-ventricular volume overload.

HEMODYNAMICS

The hemodynamic consequences and clinical findings of Lutembacher's syndrome are largely determined by the size of ASD, pulmonary vascular resistance, and the severity of MS. In the initial descriptions of Lutembacher's syndrome, ASD was generally considered as large and non-restrictive, providing another route for the exit of blood from the left atrium. The degree of pre-tricuspid shunt is determined by the severity of MS on one side and pulmonary artery pressure, tricuspid valve disease, and right-ventricular compliance on the other side. As more blood is diverted into the right atrium through the ASD, less backward pressure is exerted on pulmonary veins, avoiding pulmonary venous congestion. This causes progressive right-ventricular dilatation and may eventually lead to right-ventricular failure. Patients complain of easy fatigability rather than dyspnea as there is lesser pulmonary venous congestion and reduced

forward flow into the left ventricle. There could be various combinations, such as:

- Small ASD with severe MS
- Large ASD with mild to moderate MS
- Large ASD with severe MS

A patient with a small fossa ovalis defect and severe mitral stenosis would behave no different from a patient with isolated rheumatic mitral stenosis. Similarly, a patient with a large secundum defect and mild mitral stenosis will present as if they have an isolated atrial septal defect.

The presence of a large secundum defect and severe mitral stenosis leads to an interesting interplay of hemodynamics, with a distinct bearing on each condition. The ASD acts as a vent for the hypertensive left atrium of mitral stenosis. Hence, features of pulmonary venous congestion like dyspnea, orthopnea, or paroxysmal nocturnal dyspnea are not seen. The shunt across the ASD is increased and this leads to further enlargement of the right heart and pulmonary artery. An underfilled left ventricle and increase in the shunt fraction contribute to exertional dyspnea, fatigue, and palpitations. While this might ameliorate symptoms of mitral stenosis and allow fair exercise tolerance and survival for several decades, it is not without consequence. Pulmonary venous hypertension is prevented at the cost of earlier occurrence of pulmonary arterial hypertension and right-atrial enlargement. The latter eventually predisposes to AF with its deleterious effects on biventricular function and risk of thromboembolism. It is important to underscore the importance of a compliant right ventricle and pulmonary circuit, which offers this skewed advantage to the diseased mitral valve. The only disadvantage to a stenotic mitral valve from an ASD may be a further decline in the cardiac output.

To summarize, a patient with isolated mitral stenosis has features of pulmonary venous congestion and presents with exertional dyspnea, which might progress to orthopnea if unrecognized. Longstanding, severe mitral stenosis is accompanied by fatigue due to a reduction in cardiac output. Palpitations at rest point to atrial fibrillation. Thromoembolic sequelae are secondary to propagation of a thrombus in the left-atrial appendage.

A patient with an isolated atrial septal defect is usually asymptomatic until adulthood. Presentation is in the form of palpitations and fatigue due to volume overload of the right heart and relative decrease in the cardiac output. Pulmonary hypertension is uncommon and usually mild to moderate and exertional dyspnea is not often reported as the right heart is highly compliant.

A patient with Lutembacher will have features of an atrial septal defect, which are exaggerated and might appear early on. Palpitations and fatigue are the predominant symptoms, but exertional dyspnea is also seen due to the large shunt fraction. Orthopnea and paroxysmal nocturnal dyspnea are uncommon as pulmonary venous congestion is minimized by the large interatrial communication.

CLINICAL FINDINGS

The clinical signs of mitral stenosis are less conspicuous. In other words, a more severe mitral stenosis might still not produce characteristic signs in the presence of a large ASD. The signs of an atrial septal defect, on the contrary, are never masked; they only get more accentuated.

The jugular venous pulse may show a prominent a-wave even in the absence of significant pulmonary hypertension. A prominent a-wave in the absence of significant pulmonary hypertension in a patient with ASD should point to the possibility of Lutembacher syndrome. The a-wave in this instance is a reflection of elevated left-atrial pressure and is appreciated due to the large defect, which transmits the pressure to the right atrium and neck veins. In the presence of tricuspid regurgitation, a prominent v-wave is seen.

The apex is formed by the right ventricle as it is dilated and the left ventricle is underfilled. A parasternal heave may be present in patients with pulmonary hypertension. Pulsations in the second intercostal space are secondary to an enlarged pulmonary trunk. A systolic thrill is often palpated at the base of the heart at the upper-left sternal border. Prominent pulmonary artery pulsations and basal systolic thrill (and the basal ejection systolic murmur) are due to torrential flow across the right ventricular outflow tract. A diastolic thrill at the apex is uncommon as the mitral flow velocity is low.

A loud first heart sound may be appreciated between the lower-left sternal border and apex, as in a case of mitral stenosis. However, this loudness

is due to the tricuspid component. The second heart sound is wide and fixed. The pulmonary component may be loud and audible at the apex. An ejection systolic murmur across the pulmonary valve and mid-diastolic flow murmur across the tricuspid valve are more pronounced due to increased left-to-right shunt across the ASD. As little blood flows across the stenotic mitral orifice and left-atrial pressures are not very high, an opening snap is less often heard. An apical mid-diastolic murmur of mitral stenosis is less appreciable, but is essential to entertain a clinical diagnosis of Lutembacher syndrome. The length of the mid-diastolic murmur is shortened and does not correlate with the true degree of mitral stenosis. The mid-diastolic murmur due to increased flow across the tricuspid valve (from ASD) and the mid-diastolic murmur at the apex may be inseparable, resulting in a long diastolic murmur heard from the lower sternal border to the apex. In patients with coexistent mitral regurgitation, a pansystolic murmur may be heard at the apex. However, a pansystolic murmur is more often due to tricuspid regurgitation and is heard at the lower sternal border. In a few instances, where the atrial septal defect is restrictive and mitral stenosis is severe, transatrial pressure gradients exist throughout the cardiac cycle. The continuous murmur is best heard at the lower-right sternal border and corresponds to the site of the right atrium. A continuous murmur at this site has few differentials: Ruptured sinus of Valsalva to the right atrium and coronary cameral fistula to the right atrium. While the former is distinguished by its loud and harsh quality, the continuous murmur of a coronary cameral fistula draining to the right atrium is accentuated during systole.

ECG may show features of biatrial enlargement in patients with sinus rhythm. Atrial fibrillation is not uncommon. There is right-axis deviation with right-ventricular hypertrophy (qR or QR pattern in V1). Right-ventricular forces (complete or incomplete right bundle branch block) are more prominent in these patients compared to those with an isolated ASD.

Chest roentgenograms of atrial septal defect and mitral stenosis have quite a few similarities (Figure 17.1). There is cardiomegaly of varying degree. Left-atrial enlargement and pulmonary venous congestion serve to distinguish a patient of mitral stenosis with Lutembacher syndrome. Enlargement of the right heart and pulmonary artery is common to both. Pulmonary plethora reflects increased pulmonary blood flow from the pretricuspid shunt. Pulmonary venous congestion may be less conspicuous as compared to a patient with isolated mitral stenosis.

Echocardiographic features (Figures 17.2 and 17.3, Videos 17.1 and 17.2) of mitral valve involvement include leaflet and chordal thickening, chordal fusion, reduced mobility of the posterior mitral leaflet, diastolic doming of the anterior mitral leaflet, and reduced orifice area. Transmitral gradients are underestimated and cannot be used to assess the severity of mitral stenosis. Assessment of mitral valve area (MVA) using the Doppler pressure half-time method is inaccurate and tends to overestimate the MVA (in proportion to the magnitude of left-to-right shunt). Valve areas should be calculated by planimetry or by the continuity equation. The degree of pulmonary hypertension and orifice area help in assessing the severity of mitral stenosis. Associated mitral regurgitation may be present. The atrial septal defect should be profiled on two-dimensional echocardiography and color Doppler that shows left-to-right shunt, dilated right-sided chambers, and pulmonary hypertension. On rare occasions, sinus venosus defects have been associated with mitral stenosis. It is important to rule out pulmonary venous anomalies and cor triatriatum. Rheumatic involvement of other valves might coexist.

Cardiac catheterization is not performed to make a diagnosis, as the requisite information to diagnose and manage the condition is obtained on echocardiography. However, if transcatheter management is contemplated, several interesting features may be noted. The shunt fraction across the atrial septal defect could be obtained by oximetry. Pulmonary artery pressures are often elevated. Equalization of a- and v-wave amplitudes are demonstrated in right-atrial pressure tracings due to the large, non-restrictive atrial septal defect. The left- and right-atrial pressures are equal and usually not high, unless there is severe pulmonary hypertension. The increased pulmonary diastolic pressure would then translate into elevated right-ventricular end-diastolic and atrial pressures. Simultaneous pressure tracings of the left ventricle and left atrium should be obtained after the mitral valve has been crossed. The left-ventricular end-diastolic pressure and mean left-atrial pressure difference (transmitral gradient) is spuriously low due to decompression across the ASD.

MANAGEMENT

The size of ASD and severity of MS determine the management strategy in an individual case. The treatment has to be individualized. While MS with suitable valve morphology can easily be treated by PTMC, the size and morphology of ASD and its rims may contribute to decision-making. Failure to correctly assess the severity of MS can be catastrophic. If significant MS remains uncorrected at the time of closure of ASD, the patient will develop acute pulmonary edema in the immediate postoperative period.

Small restrictive ASD with moderate to severe MS

With suitable valve morphology, this is generally treated by PTMC alone. If a valve is not suitable for PTMC, open mitral valvotomy (OMV) or mitral valve replacement (MVR) with surgical ASD closure may be considered.

Moderate to large ASD with mild MS

This is treated by surgical closure with or without OMV.

Large ASD with moderate to severe MS

This could be managed as follows:

- OMV + surgical closure of ASD or
- PTMC + surgical closure of ASD or
- PTMC + device closure of ASD

Traditional approaches have included open or closed mitral commissurotomy with surgical closure of the atrial septal defect. Transcatheter treatment is an option, but PTMC has its own challenges in this setting, especially in a patient with large ASD. Crossing the mitral valve may be difficult due to the lack of support for an Inoue catheter system at the level of interatrial septum, especially if the atrioventricular or inferior venacaval rim is deficient. We may have to resort to an over-the-wire technique to track the balloon across the valve.[8] There is a high chance of the balloon prolapsing back into the left atrium due to the relatively smaller size of the left-ventricular cavity.

Although a large ASD with adequate rims could be closed by transcatheter techniques,[9,10] this option needs to be considered with caution when there has been only suboptimal relief of mitral stenosis. It is our practice to refer them for surgery, as device closure would preclude future transcatheter procedures for mitral restenosis.

Occasionally, PTMC may be life-saving in a critically ill patient with pulmonary edema as a bailout therapy, even in the presence of a large ASD. ASD could be closed electively, later. The dictum is not to close the atrial septal defect, unless the mitral stenosis has been relieved and has been followed up for gradual progression over several years. This is especially important in patients who have undergone percutaneous transmitral commissurotomy in the second decade of life, as there is a chance of progression and restenosis over subsequent years, necessitating a repeat procedure for mitral stenosis. On the same note, device closure of ASD and PTMC in patients with a favorable anatomy may be offered, if the patient chooses to have transcatheter treatment over surgery.

Pharmacological treatment with diuretics and β-blockers would be required in patients with symptoms of pulmonary venous congestion secondary to significant MS and in those with heart failure.

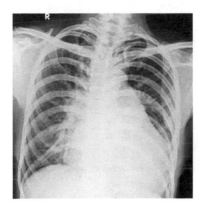

Figure 17.1 Chest X-ray PA view in a patient of Lutembacher's syndrome (rheumatic mitral stenosis and large atrial septal defect) showing right-atrial enlargement, prominent main pulmonary artery, straightening of the left heart border, mild cardiomegaly with a right-ventricular apical contour, and enlarged right pulmonary artery.

CONCLUSION

Lutembacher's syndrome, a combination of ASD with significant MS, is frequently encountered in developing countries with high prevalence of rheumatic heart disease. The size of ASD and severity of MS determine the hemodynamic effects and the management strategy in a given case. Suspicion of MS in a case of ASD arises in the presence of a systolic thrill at the upper-left sternal edge, an unusually long, loud, and widely transmitted delayed diastolic murmur, and ECG evidence of biatrial enlargement. Transmitral gradients are often underestimated and one has to rely on orifice area for assessing the severity of MS. Transcatheter

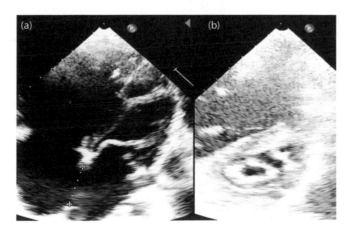

Figure 17.2 **(a)** 2D echo with Apical four-chamber view showing large fossa ovalis ASD, dilated right-sided chambers, and doming of the anterior mitral leaflet in diastole. **(b)** 2D echo with short-axis view at the level of the mitral valve showing narrow orifice (See Videos 17.1 and 17.2).

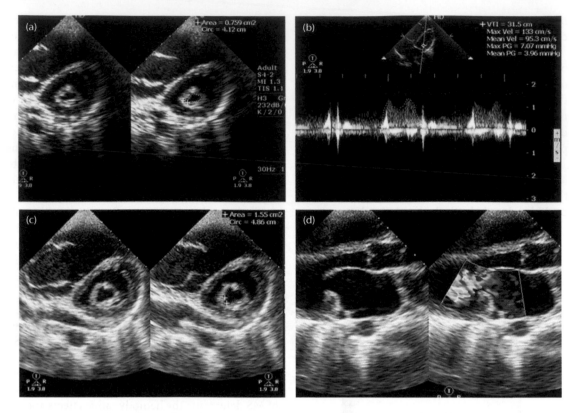

Figure 17.3 Panel **(a)** 2D echo short-axis view showing stenotic mitral orifice in a patient with Lutembacher's syndrome. Panel **(b)** Continuous-wave Doppler across the mitral valve showing under-estimated gradient in the same patient due to decompressive effect of ASD. Panel **(c)** Short-axis view after BMV showing increase in orifice area. Panel **(d)** Parasternal long-axis view in the same patient after BMV shows diastolic doming and laminar flow across the mitral orifice with mild submitral turbulence (See Videos 17.1 and 17.2).

PTMC is sufficient in a patient with significant MS with favorable valve morphology and a restrictive ASD. PTMC may be life-saving in a critically ill patient with pulmonary edema, as bailout therapy, irrespective of the size of ASD. A large ASD with insufficient rims is best treated by surgical closure along with OMV. Although not preferred by us, an ASD with sufficient rims could be closed by a device, after successful PTMC.

VIDEOS

Video 17.1 Apical four chamber view with colour Doppler showing severe mitral stenosis (MVA 0.7 cm²). https://youtu.be/EUt_3KMJG6k

Video 17.2 Apical four chamber view with colour Doppler showing large 21 mm ostium secundum atrial septal defect and moderate tricuspid regur-gitation. https://youtu.be/HZFem_QzpLA

REFERENCES

1. Lutembacher R. De la stenosemitrale avec communication interauriculaire. *Arch Mal Coeur* 1916;9:237–60.
2. Gueron M, Gussarsky J. Lutembacher's syndrome obsolete? A new concept of mitral valve disease and left to right shunt at the atrial level. *Am Heart J* 91(1976):535.
3. Bashi VV, Ravikumar E, Jairaj PS, Krishnaswami S, John S. Coexistent mitral valve disease with left to right shunt at atrial level: Clinical profile, hemodynamics and surgical considerations in 67 consecutive patients. *Am Heart J* 1987;114:406.

4. Craig RJ, Selzer A. Natural history and prognosis of atrial septal defect. *Circulation* 1968;37:805.

5. Steibrunn W, Cohn KE, Selzer A. Atrial septal defect associated with mitral stenosis: The Lutembacher syndrome revisited. *Am J Med* 1970;48:295.

6. CN Manjunath, A Panneerselvam, KH Srinivasa, Prabhavathi B, Kapil Rangan, KS Ravindranath. Incidence and predictors of atrial septal defect after percutaneous transvenous mitral commissurotomy – a transesophageal echocardiographic study of 209 cases. *Echocardiography* 2013;30:127–30.

7. Vaideeswar P, Marathe S. Lutembacher's syndrome: Is the mitral pathology always rheumatic? *Indian Heart J* 2017;69(1):20–3.

8. Manjunath CN, Srinivasa KH, Patil CB, Venkatesh HV, Bhoopal TS, Dhanalakshmi C. Balloon mitral valvuloplasty: Our experience with a modified technique of crossing the mitral valve in difficult cases. *Cathet Cardiovasc Diagn* 1998;44(1):23–6.

9. Ledesma M, Martinez P, Cazares MA, Feldman T. Transcatheter treatment of Lutembacher syndrome: Combined balloon mitral valvuloplasty and percutaneous atrial septal defect closure. *J Invasive Cardiol* 2004 Nov;16(11):678–9.

10. Arora R, Patted SV, Halkat PC, Amarked B, Sattur A, Joshi A. Definitive treatment of Lutembacher syndrome. *J Sci Soc* 2014;41:215–9.

18

Atrial fibrillation and other arrhythmias

NEERAJ PARAKH AND VIVEK CHATURVEDI

INTRODUCTION

Atrial fibrillation (AF) can occur as a complication of virtually any form of heart disease but its association with rheumatic mitral valve disease is most noteworthy. In the eighteenth century, French scientist Jean Baptiste De Senac described "rebellious palpitations" with mitral valve disease as the first description for AF. In 1902, James Mackenjie in his classic monogram "The analysis of the pulse" described the disappearance of a presystolic murmur and presystolic a-wave in a patient of mitral stenosis (MS) with development of irregular jugular venous pulsations. The first ECG description of AF in MS was reported by William Einthoven in 1906 as "pulsus inaequalis et irregularis"[1] (Figure 18.1). Development of AF in patients with MS leads to a significant increase in morbidity and mortality. These patients are at increased risk of thromboembolism and stroke, as well as complications of long term anticoagulation.[2] The loss of atrial kick because of AF leads to further deterioration in the already-compromised hemodynamics and subsequent worsening of symptoms. Other supraventricular tachycardias such as left-atrial flutter, ectopic atrial tachycardia, multifocal atrial tachycardia, and frequent atrial ectopics may occur in some cases (Figures 18.2 and 18.3). Occasionally, these arrhythmias are forerunners for the future development of AF.[3]

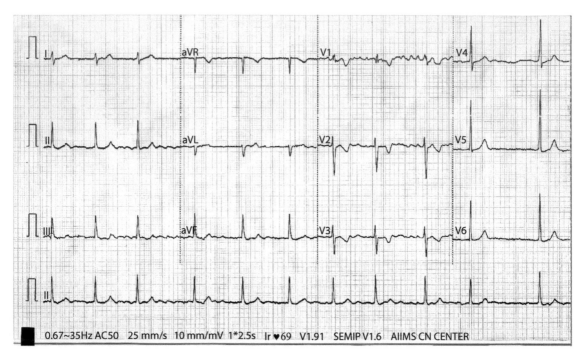

Figure 18.1 Mitral stenosis with atrial fibrillation and controlled ventricular rate.

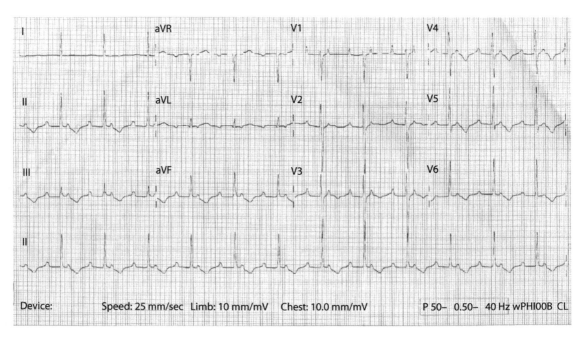

Figure 18.2 ECG of a patient with mitral stenosis showing ectopic atrial tachycardia from the left atrium with 2:1 AV conduction. See the negative p-waves in aVL and sharp peaked positive p-waves in V1.

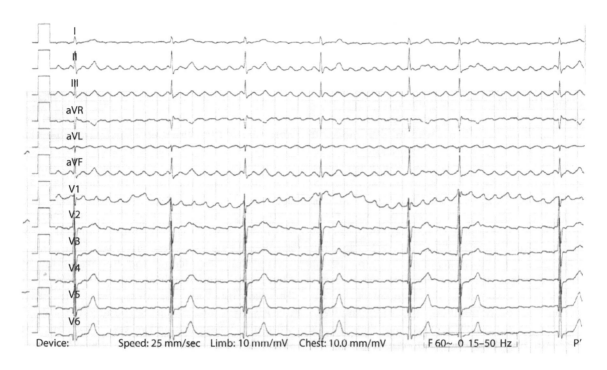

Figure 18.3 Mitral stenosis with left-atrial flutter and variable AV block (2:1 and 3:2). Lead V1 shows distinct flutter waves.

EPIDEMIOLOGY AND RISK FACTORS

The prevalence of AF in symptomatic MS is approximately 40%–75%.[4] In a historical series of MS, it was 17% in the third decade, 45% in the fourth decade, 60% in the fifth decade, and 80% in the sixth decade.[5] In a large global registry, the incidence of AF was 1.51 cases per 100 patient-years in patients with MS. Five-year survival in patients with AF and MS was 64% compared to 85% in those with sinus rhythm. Thus, the presence of AF was associated with a 40% increase in mortality.[6–8] In a retrospective study of MS in sinus rhythm, the incidence of AF was 3.5% per year, which increased to 6% per year if the left atrium (LA) size was 47 mm or more.[9]

Age and LA size are the most significant risk factors for the development of AF (Table 18.1). Various studies have reported mean LA size from 43–57 mm as risk factors for the development of AF.[5,10,11] The involvement of multiple valves is also an important risk factors. Left-atrial strain and flow velocities on echocardiography, LV ejection fraction, and right-atrial pressure have also been

Table 18.1 Risk factors for the development of atrial fibrillation in mitral stenosis

Established Risk Factors
- Age
- Left-atrial size
- Multivalvular involvement

Possible Risk Factors
- Severity of mitral stenosis
- LA appendage velocities
- Left-atrial strain
- A-VTI, A-VTI/VTI
- LV ejection fraction
- LV end-diastolic pressure
- Right-atrial pressure
- Pulmonary artery pressure

Associated Markers
- NT-ProBNP, BNP
- Hs CRP

Abbreviations: a-VTI, atrial velocity time integral; BNP, B natriuretic peptide, CRP, C reactive protein; LA, left atrium; LV, left ventricle.

reported to be associated with AF.[12] The relationship of AF with the severity of MS is not well established. In most of the studies, mitral valve area is not an independent risk factor for AF;[13-16] however, Moreyra et al. found that smaller valve area along with higher LA and pulmonary artery pressure are associated with greater prevalence of AF.[17] In asymptomatic patients with mild to moderate MS, peak LA strain on speckle tracking may predict future development of AF by detecting atrial dysfunction earlier than conventional 2D echocardiography.[18] A decrease in the atrial systolic component of mitral flow velocity time integral (A-VTI) has been found to be useful in predicting future development of AF in severe MS in sinus rhythm. A-VTI is a marker of atrial pump function and a decrease in atrial pump function is shown to be a precursor to the development of AF. The percentage contribution of A-VTI to the total VTI of 9% or less was 84% sensitive and 80% specific for predicting the development of AF at one year.[19] Certain biochemical markers such as NT-proBNP and CRP have also been found to be raised in AF, but their cause-effect association has not been established.[9]

PATHOLOGICAL CORRELATES OF AF IN MS

It is now well established that paroxysms of AF are initiated by trains of spontaneous activity arising from the pulmonary veins (PV) in the vast majority of the patients. AF begets AF by structural and electrophysiological changes that promote reentry.[20] Angiographic and autopsy studies of PVs in patients with rheumatic heart disease (RHD) have demonstrated almost similar morphologies of PVs, as shown in earlier studies of non-rheumatic AF. However, PV sizes are smaller than those reported for non-rheumatic AF and there is also an evidence of inflammation of PV tissue in RHD patients.[21-23]

Chronically raised atrial pressure and stretch leads to dilatation of the LA cavity, which in turn promotes fibrosis. Rheumatic inflammatory activity also contributes to myocardial disarray and fibrosis. Biopsy specimens of left atria from patients with rheumatic MS frequently reveal thickening of intima and lesions resembling Aschoff bodies in some cases. Though existence of specific changes related to rheumatic heart disease are questionable, the presence of AF is associated with more advanced forms of pathology in the form of myocyte degeneration, inflammation, fibrosis, and cellular hypertrophy in the LA tissue removed at the time of mitral valve surgery. Electron microscopic analysis of LA tissue removed at the time of surgery for mitral stenosis showed increased atrial natriuretic peptide (ANP)-containing granules in patients with AF compared to those without, despite similar atrial pressures in both the groups. In patients with AF, depletion of the contractile elements (Z-bands), glycogen particle accumulation, and an increase in mitochondria was much more common in the cardiomyocytes. In severe cases, extensive areas of sarcoplasmic vacuolation and presence of myelin figures and mitochondrial aggregates were seen. The majority of AF cases demonstrated extensive fibrosis in the form of collagen bundles in the interstitium.[24-26] Expression of receptors for advanced glycation end products (RAGE) is also increased in MS with AF. These receptors are thought to be responsible for increased fibrosis. The degree of their expression has been postulated to be directly proportional to the severity of MS. RAGE and renin-angiotensin (RAS) pathways have significant crosstalk at the tissue level and they may play a role in future targets for upstream therapy for AF or atrial fibrosis.[27] Late gadolinium-enhanced MRI (LGE-MRI) for the assessment of left-atrial substrate remodeling had shown a moderate agreement with the histological findings and may be used as a tool to assess LA substrate remodeling in AF patients. LGE-MRI has been used to assess fibrosis and it correlates well with deposition of collagen in the LA in the presence of AF.[28] Infiltration of LA tissue by mononuclear cells, especially M1 macrophages, and over-activation of NLRP3 inflammasomes may play an active role in atrial inflammation, which, in turn, promotes thrombosis. Various inflammatory markers such as neutrophil-lymphocyte ratio, C-reactive protein (CRP), tumor necrosis factor-α (TNF-α), interleukin (IL)-2, and IL-6 have been linked to embolism in AF.[29-32] A study of CD40:CD40 ligand ratio (a marker of platelet activation) in MS revealed that there is significant activation of platelets in MS irrespective of the underlying rhythm. This ratio was directly proportional to the severity of MS, thereby implicating stenotic mitral valve for the activation of platelets.[33]

ELECTROPHYSIOLOGICAL ABNORMALITIES

Pathological changes in atria results in marked alteration in their electrophysiological properties. Electrophysiological study of atria in patients undergoing percutaneous transvenous mitral commissurotomy (PTMC) revealed significant abnormalities. There are low-voltage and no-voltage signals indicating electrical scarring. Local and global conduction abnormalities in the form of fractionated electrograms, double potentials, and increased conduction time are present. The effective refractory period is either normal or increased. On electrical stimulation, these patients have a higher tendency to develop atrial fibrillation. These abnormalities were present in both atria, with the LA being affected more than the RA.[34] Chronic atrial stretch also leads to direction-dependent conduction slowing and anisotropy leading to a fertile substrate for the development of atrial fibrillation.[35] Mitral valvotomy in MS with AF reduces electrical anisotropy of the effective refractory period in the LA but atrial conduction properties remain unchanged.[36]

HEMODYNAMIC DISTURBANCES CAUSED BY AF

AF in MS results in the following hemodynamic disturbances:

- Increased mean atrial pressure, mean transmitral gradient, and larger LA size.
- Atrial contraction in severe MS raises transmitral gradient by 30%; loss of atrial kick due to AF leads to a decrease in cardiac output by approximately 20%.[37]
- Increased and irregular ventricular rate leading to reduction of diastolic filling period and tachycardia-induced decrease in left-ventricular function.

Hemodynamic changes with AF results in worsening of functional class, exercise capacity, and quality of life.[38]

THROMBOEMBOLISM AND STROKE

Systemic embolism, principally stroke, is the most serious complication of AF in the presence of mitral stenosis with RHD. The rate of embolism is significantly lower in RHD patients in sinus rhythm (0.7% patient-year) compared to those in AF (5% patient-year).[39] Mitral valve disease, LA size, presence of LA thrombus, left-ventricular dysfunction, and previous history of thromboembolism are associated with higher incidence of stroke in patients with AF.[17,40–42] In a study of 53 patients with rheumatic mitral stenosis, Akdemir et al. observed 25% incidence of silent brain infarction. The presence of LA enlargement and AF were associated with a higher (40%) incidence of silent brain infarction.[43] The incidence of Holter-detected transient subclinical AF (<30 sec) was 27% in a cohort of symptomatic MS patients with predominantly moderate to severe MS. In this study, subclinical AF was associated with a fivefold increase in the risk of stroke and systemic embolism.[44] The Framingham database has shown that AF with RHD carries 17 times more risk of stroke as compared to age-matched controls, with an annual incidence of 4.5% per year.[45]

Risk factors for stroke

In the presence of MS and AF, age and previous history of stroke are well-established risk factors for stroke.[46] About 12% of patients of MS with AF experience another stroke within 2 weeks of the index event.[47] Other less-well-established risk factors are severity of MS, LA size, spontaneous echo contrast (SEC), presence of LA thrombus, reduced LA appendage contractility, and concomitant aortic regurgitation (Table 18.2). SEC in some studies has been found to be an independent predictor for thromboembolism irrespective of rhythm or LA size.[48,49] In a prospective study of 534 patients, PTMC had a negative predictive value for stroke in MS with AF. For those in sinus rhythm-age, mitral valve area, LA thrombus, and aortic regurgitation were significant positive predictors for embolism.[46] Decreased contractility of the LA appendage (LAA) in MS may promote formation of LAA thrombus and is a risk factor for stroke. However, once the thrombus is formed, it is more likely to embolize with relatively preserved LAA flow velocities and contractility.[50] The CHADS$_2$ score is well-established for stroke risk prediction in the presence of AF but it is not validated for valvular heart disease. Data about utility of the CHADS$_2$ score in RHD is scarce. In RELY AF registry, the CHADS$_2$ score was a good predictor for stroke in RHD, suggesting conventional risk factors (heart

Table 18.2 Risk factors for thromboembolism in mitral stenosis

Established Risk Factors
- Age
- Previous thromboembolism
- Atrial fibrillation

Possible Risk Factors
- LA size >5.5 cm
- Severity of mitral stenosis
- Multivalvular involvement
- LA appendage clot
- Spontaneous echo contrast in LA
- LA appendage contractility
- Previous PTMC (negative predictor)

Associated Inflammatory Markers
- Hs CRP
- TNF – alpha
- IL-2, IL-6

Abbreviations: CRP, C reactive protein; LA, left atrium; PTMC, percutaneous transvenous mitral commissurotomy.

failure, hypertension, age >75 years, diabetes, and prior stroke or systemic thromboembolism) to be adequate in explaining stroke risk in RHD and AF.[51] However, another study of 130 patients with RHD and stroke (82% had AF) reported a higher recurrence rate of stroke of 13.6% per year. RHD was associated with twofold increased risk of death and 100% increased risk of recurrence in stroke patients.[52] It has been suggested that AF and RHD carries a risk of thromboembolism equivalent to $CHADS_2$ score 2 or 3.[53] The CHA_2DS_2VASc score incorporates more variables to calculate stroke risk but again it has not been validated in RHD. In a cross-sectional study of MS patients in sinus rhythm, a CHA_2DS_2VASc score of 2 or more predicted presence of left-atrial SEC (considered a marker for stroke risk) with a sensitivity of 71% and a specificity of 82%. The authors concluded that larger studies are needed to validate utility of the $CHADS_2$/CHA_2DS_2VASc scores in MS.[54] A couple of studies have reported the impact of ventricular rate control on thrombogenicity in MS with AF. These studies suggest that controlling ventricular rate attenuates a pro-thrombotic state in MS with AF and its benefit goes beyond mere hemodynamic improvement.[55,56]

DIAGNOSTIC EVALUATION

Symptoms

Palpitations and worsening of NYHA class are the most common presenting symptoms with the development of AF. Some patients may complain of fatigue, weakness, or light-headedness. It may also be picked up incidentally on a routine clinical workup. Sometimes, stroke or peripheral thromboembolism may be the first presentation of AF. Not uncommonly, a persistent high ventricular rate may lead to tachycardiomyopathy and heart failure. The development of AF in MS may precipitate or aggravate cardiac failure because of ineffective atrial contraction and poor heart rate control. A very fast ventricular rate may also cause dizziness or syncope.

Clinical examination and investigations

On clinical evaluation, irregular heart rate, significant pulse deficit (>10), beats per minute and variable heart sounds are indicators of AF. The ventricles are irregularly activated at a rate determined by the conduction properties of the AV node. The variable conduction produces the characteristic "irregularly irregular" pulse. ECG is diagnostic for AF (Figure 18.1). ECG shows normal but irregular QRS complexes; there are no p-waves but the baseline may show irregular fibrillation waves ("f-waves"). The f-waves have a rate of 300–600 beats/min and are variable in amplitude, shape, and timing. Sometimes, coarse or fine AF is defined depending upon the f-wave amplitude (>1 mm in V1 or II). Initially f-wave amplitude was thought to be a marker of LA enlargement but with current understanding of electrical activation of atria in AF, such distinction is of limited clinical utility and f-wave morphology may just reflect LA voltage map. Fine AF may indicate the presence of low-voltage areas in LA.[57,58] A very fast ventricular rate in AF (>170/min) may give an impression of regular heart rate since the beat-to-beat variability is attenuated. Sometimes, left-atrial flutter or ectopic atrial tachycardia from LA will be the presenting rhythm and can be identified from the ECG (Figures 18.2 and 18.3). Clinical features of these rhythms will be the same as that of AF. Paroxysmal AF will require 24-hour Holter or event recorder for confirmation.

Echocardiographic evaluation for the assessment of mitral valve, atrial thrombus, and other features of valve involvement is also required for comprehensive evaluation of these patients. Large atrial thrombus is not uncommon in AF with MS and requires early surgery.

TREATMENT

Anticoagulation to prevent thromboembolic complications is an important consideration in these patients. Heart rate needs to be controlled and conversion to sinus rhythm in some selected patients is a reasonable option.

Prevention of thromboembolism

Oral anticoagulants (vitamin K antagonists; VKA) are mainstay of therapy for preventing thromboembolism in rheumatic AF. Randomized trials regarding the role of anticoagulation in rheumatic AF are lacking, but evidence from observational studies and extrapolation from non-valvular AF trials support their use in rheumatic AF. Recent focused ACC/AHA guidelines have given class I recommendation with level of evidence B-NR for use of VKA in patients of MS with AF.[59] The use of warfarin reduces the risk of thromboembolism in rheumatic AF from 5.5% per year to 0.7% per year.[11,40,60,61] The use of anticoagulation in MS with normal sinus rhythm (NSR) is much more controversial. Previous stroke, increasing age, LA/LAA thrombus, large LA (>55 mm) and SEC have been proposed as risk factors for stroke but OAC has only been recommended for LA/LAA thrombus and previous stroke. In other conditions, the use of VKA is debatable.[62–64] A major issue with VKA treatment in rheumatic AF is poor INR monitoring due to socioeconomic and access constraints. This leads to poor efficacy and increased bleeding risk with VKA. The percentage of INR value in the therapeutic range is also poor (<40%).[51] As rheumatic MS is predominantly a disease of young women, teratogenicity due to warfarin in childbearing females is also an area of concern. Newer oral anticoagulants (NOACS) have a proven safety and efficacy record in non-valvular AF, but valvular AF has selectively been excluded from NOACS trials. Retrospective analysis from a large database of more than 20,000 patients showed no difference in bleeding in MS

patients treated with NOACs or warfarin.[65] The role of rivaroxaban in rheumatic AF is being studied in INVICTUS trial.[66] As of now, NOACs are not recommended for rheumatic AF due to moderately or severe mitral stenosis. The role of antiplatelets alone or in conjunction with VKAs is not proven. In a sub-analysis of the NASPEAF study by Pérez-Gómez et al. there was a trend towards the beneficial effect of antiplatelet therapy when administered with anticoagulant treatment in the subgroup of patients with MS and AF. This effect might have been caused by a reduction in sudden death and myocardial infarction. Use of antiplatelet therapy for stroke prevention in rheumatic AF needs further evaluation.[67]

Rhythm versus rate control

Results from most of the large trials in non-rheumatic AF, comparing the rhythm control versus rate control strategy, suggest that the rhythm control strategy offers no survival advantage over the rate control strategy. Although exercise tolerance was better with rhythm control, there were more frequent hospital admissions and an increase in non-cardiovascular mortality in the rhythm control group. This data pertains mainly to non-rheumatic AF and very few patients were subjected to non-pharmacological interventions.[68–70] This data cannot be extrapolated to the rheumatic population, wherein patients are much younger and have associated structural heart disease and a very high risk of embolism and stroke. Sinus rhythm is difficult to achieve and maintain in MS with AF. Limited data on these populations suggest rhythm control to be superior.[71] Although direct current cardioversion can restore normal sinus rhythm at least transiently in most patients with AF, the recurrence rate is very high, especially when maintenance anti-arrhythmic therapy or non-pharmacological interventions are not used.[72] Furthermore, in the presence of large LA (>55–60 mm), cardioversion is less likely to succeed.[73] Currently available anti-arrhythmic drugs are far from ideal and some of the studies have reported an increase in overall mortality.[74] PTMC or surgical correction results in increased mitral valve area, decreased transmitral gradient, and decreased LA pressure, but as a standalone therapy these are not found to be effective in restoring sinus rhythm in patients with AF. However, these interventions may lead to a higher rate of successful cardioversion and maintenance of sinus rhythm.[75] The role of PTMC or surgery in preventing the future development of AF in patients with NSR is also variable.[76]

The rhythm control strategy for rheumatic AF has largely been confined to the interventions done valvular surgeries and the results have so far been encouraging. With continuing refinement and advances in catheter-based techniques, curative strategies for rheumatic AF are focused on catheter-based ablation with satisfactory short-term results, when accompanied with PTMC.[77,78] If AF is of more than 24-hour duration, then anticoagulation for 3 weeks is usually required before cardioversion. Alternatively, after ruling out the presence of atrial thrombus on transesophageal echocardiography, immediate cardioversion can be carried out after intravenous heparin anticoagulation.

Rhythm control in rheumatic AF: The surgical approach

In 1987, Cox et al.[79] introduced the MAZE procedure for the treatment of AF. Kosakai et al.[80] reported that the MAZE procedure was also effective in controlling AF in association with mitral valve disease. Combined mitral valve surgery and maze procedure and/or its modifications have a reported success rate of 75% at one year for restoring sinus rhythm as compared to 26% for those without MAZE.[81] There was no difference in 30-day mortality, pacemaker implantation, stroke, and embolic episodes. The conventional maze procedure requires large LA incisions and sutures, and prolongs bypass time. Therefore, the conventional full maze procedure carries a potential risk of postoperative complications, such as bleeding, low-output syndrome, and sick sinus syndrome. The substitution of conventional incisions by sutureless techniques such as cryoablation or radiofrequency ablation has significantly decreased the bypass time and helped in preserving the mechanical function of the atria. These modifications are equally effective in restoring sinus rhythm. Surgical catheter ablation using saline-irrigated catheter ablation (SICTRA) was effective in restoring sinus rhythm at the time of MVR. In a comparative study of Cox MAZE operation using SICTRA at the time of MVR to that of RF circumferential PVI at six

months after surgery, Cox MAZE with SICTRA was more effective in restoring sinus rhythm.[82] Patients who have an indication for mitral valve surgery and have chronic AF should be considered for concurrent AF surgery. Large LA size (>60 mm), longer duration of AF, advanced LA fibrosis, early postoperative AF, and postoperative mitral valve dysfunction are negative predictors for long-term procedural success.[83,84] Recent technical improvements such as radiofrequency catheters and cryoablation have significantly shortened the additional time required for AF surgery. The early success of less extensive procedures like PVI has evoked considerable enthusiasm regarding ablation of AF and further investigations are required in this field.

Rhythm control in rheumatic AF: The pharmacological approach

Amiodarone, used in conjunction with PTMC, can safely convert rheumatic AF in about 40% of patients. The addition of electrical cardioversion improves the success rate to 87%. AF duration remains the most important predictor of long-term success.[71,72,85] The CRAAFT study investigators concluded that electrical cardioversion will restore and maintain sinus rhythm in 36% of patients of AF due to RHD at 1 year. The addition of amiodarone increases the success rate to 69%. They suggested that restoring and maintaining the sinus rhythm might be beneficial because it improves the symptoms, QOL scores, effort tolerance, and possibly lowers the mortality rate when compared to patients treated in rate control group. Amiodarone is well known for its "cardiac" safety profile but its organ effects make it a poor alternative for the rheumatic MS population, who are younger (predominantly <40 years old) and will need therapy for long durations with unacceptable adverse effects.

Though the pharmacological approach appears satisfactory in short-term studies, the result may not be sustained in long term. As shown in various large trials of non-rheumatic AF, all anti-arrhythmic drugs have potentially serious side effects and even a trend towards higher mortality with their use. Data on class IC drugs in AF with RHD is lacking, because of poor availability, higher cost, and fear of proarrhythmias. Proarrhythmia with these drugs may be less likely in patients with RHD as there is very or no ischemia substrate, which is the major reason for pro-arrhythmia.

Rhythm control in rheumatic AF: The catheter-based approach

Radiofrequency isolation of PVs (PVI) is now an established treatment modality for the treatment of nonrheumatic AF, but experience with the catheter-based ablation of rheumatic AF is very limited. Nair et al. in 2001 showed that the region near the coronary sinus os is the site of earliest atrial activation and ablation of this region is successful in suppressing the arrhythmia in most of the patients.[78] Small observational studies have shown favorable outcomes with catheter-based PVI in rheumatic AF following PTMC/MVR.[77,86] Derejko et al. performed 25 procedures in 14 patients after mitral valve procedures, which included PTMC, surgical valvotomy, and MVR. AF and atrial tachycardias were the most common arrhythmias. The mainstay of therapy was PVI for AF. Atrial flutter and atrial tachycardias were treated on the basis of activation and entrainment mapping. While the efficacy of a single procedure was 35%, nearly three-quarters of patients were in sinus rhythm at 2 years after repeat procedure(s).[87] Machino et al. demonstrated the feasibility and safety of combined PTMC and RFA for AF as a hybrid procedure with a 90% success rate at one year.[88]

In view of the success of catheter-based PVI for restoring sinus rhythm in non-rheumatic AF and encouraging results of surgical PVI concomitant with valve surgery, the role of catheter-based PVI for maintaining the sinus rhythm in patients of rheumatic mitral stenosis with chronic AF undergoing PTMC appears to be a promising tool and needs further evaluation.

Rate control

Adequate ventricular rate control ameliorates the negative hemodynamic effect of fast heart rate. Guidelines regarding heart rate management in patients with permanent AF are not well defined. Even though there have been no prospective studies of appropriate rate control, it is generally appreciated that the control of ventricular response of AF is important in improving patients' symptoms, especially fatigue and dyspnea. Prolonged periods of rapid ventricular rate can lead to tachyarrhythmic

cardiomyopathy and contribute to the worsening of clinical congestive heart failure. Optimal rate control should consider the patient's heart rate at rest, during normal activity, and during significant exercise. At rest, the heart rate would ideally be below 70 bpm. A reasonable Holter definition of heart rate during normal activity should be ≤80 bpm and certainly none of the hour-averaging rates ≥90 bpm. Heart rate during moderate exercise should be between 90 and 115 bpm and at peak exercise 20%–30% less than the specific age-predicted maximum heart rate.[89] B-blockers, non-dihydropyridine calcium channel blockers, and digoxin are commonly used AV node blockers to control heart rate in AF with MS. β-blockers are the most effective agents. Digoxin has synergistic action with CCBs and β-blockers but offers poor exercise rate control in isolation. Intravenous diltiazem, verapamil, or β-blockers are effective in controlling heart rate more rapidly and are used in severely symptomatic patients. Rarely, AV node ablation with pacing may be required to control the heart rate.

CONCLUSIONS

AF in MS results in significant mortality and morbidity. Anticoagulation remains the mainstay for preventing thromboembolic complications. Rate control with AV nodal blocking agents is the current practice of choice; however, rhythm control is emerging as an upcoming strategy in a selected subgroup of patients.

REFERENCES

1. Fazekas T, Liszkai G, Bielik H, Lüderitz B. History of atrial fibrillation. *Z Kardiol* 2003;92:122–7.
2. Zühlke L, Karthikeyan G, Engel ME et al. Clinical outcomes in 3343 children and adults with rheumatic heart disease from 14 low- and middle-income countries: Two-year follow-up of the Global Rheumatic Heart Disease Registry (the REMEDY Study). *Circulation* 2016;134:1456–66.
3. Ramsdale DR, Arumugam N, Singh SS, Pearson J, Charles RG. Holter monitoring in patients with mitral stenosis and sinus rhythm. *Eur Heart J* 1987;8:164–70.
4. Chandrashekhar Y, Westaby S, Narula J. Mitral stenosis. *Lancet* 2009;374:1271–83.

5. Otto CM, Bonow RO. Valvular heart disease. In Bonow RO, Mann DL, Zipes DP, Libby P, Braunwald E, eds. *Braunwald's Heart Disease: A Textbook of Cardiovascular Medicine.* 9th ed. St. Louis, MO: WB Saunders; 2011: chap 66.

6. Diker E, Aydogdu S, Ozdemir M et al. Prevalence and predictors of atrial fibrillation in rheumatic valvular heart disease. *Am J Cardiol* 1996;77:96–8.

7. Rowe JC, Bland EF, Sprague HB, White PD. The course of mitral stenosis without surgery: Ten- and twenty-year perspectives. *Ann Intern Med* 1960;52:741–9.

8. Olesen KH. The natural history of 271 patients with mitral stenosis under medical treatment. *Br Heart J* 1962;24:349–57.

9. Kim HJ, Cho GY, Kim YJ et al. Development of atrial fibrillation in patients with rheumatic mitral valve disease in sinus rhythm. *Int J Cardiovasc Imaging* 2015;31:735–42.

10. Ozaydin M, Turker Y, Varol E et al. Factors associated with the development of atrial fibrillation in patients with rheumatic mitral stenosis. *Int J Cardiovasc Imaging* 2010;26:547–52.

11. Wood JC, Cohn HL Jr. Prevention of systemic arterial embolism in chronic rheumatic heart disease by means of protracted anticoagulant therapy. *Circulation* 1954;10:517–23.

12. Pourafkari L, Ghaffari S, Bancroft GR, Tajlil A, Nader ND. Factors associated with atrial fibrillation in rheumatic mitral stenosis. *Asian Cardiovasc Thorac Ann* 2015;23:17–23.

13. Fraser HRL, Turner RW. Auricular fibrillation with special reference to rheumatic heart disease. *Br Med J* 1955;2:1414–8.

14. Probst P, Goldschlager N, Selzer A. Left atrial size and atrial fibrillation in mitral stenosis. Factors influencing their relationship. *Circulation* 1973;48:1282–7.

15. Unverferth DV, Fertel RH, Unverferth BJ, Leier CV. Atrial fibrillation in mitral stenosis: Histologic, hemodynamic and metabolic factors. *Int J Cardiol* 1984;5:143–54.

16. Kabukcu M, Arslantas E, Ates I, Demircioglu F, Ersel F. Clinical, echocardiographic, and hemodynamic characteristics of rheumatic mitral valve stenosis and atrial fibrillation. *Angiology* 2005;56:159–63.

17. Moreyra AE, Wilson AC, Deac R et al. Factors associated with atrial fibrillation in patients with mitral stenosis: A cardiac catheterization study. *Am Heart J* 1998;135:138–45.

18. Ancona R, Comenale Pinto S, Caso P et al. Two-dimensional atrial systolic strain imaging predicts atrial fibrillation at 4-year follow-up in asymptomatic rheumatic mitral stenosis. *J Am Soc Echocardiogr* 2013;26:270–7.

19. Krishnamoorthy KM, Dash PK. Prediction of atrial fibrillation in patients with severe mitral stenosis: Role of atrial contribution to ventricular filling. *Scand Cardiovasc J* 2003;37:344–8.

20. Haissaguerre M, Jais P, Shah DC et al. Spontaneous initiation of atrial fibrillation by ectopic beats originating in the pulmonary veins. *N Engl J Med* 1998;339:659–66.

21. Nathan H, Eliakim M. The junction between the left atrium and the pulmonary veins. An anatomic study of human hearts. *Circulation* 1966;34:412–22.

22. Rajdev S, Sutrale A, Wani S et al. Angiographic and histomorphometric study of pulmonary veins in rheumatic heart disease. *Indian Heart J* 2004;229 abs.

23. Rajdev S, Narula D, Bajaj H et al. Angiographic study of pulmonary venous anatomy in patients with rheumatic heart disease with mitral stenosis undergoing balloon mitral valvotomy. *Indian Heart J* 2004;209 abs.

24. Enticknap JB. Biopsy of left auricle in mitral stenosis. *Brit Heart J* 1953;15:37–46.

25. Sharma S, Sharma G, Hote M et al. Light and electron microscopic features of surgically excised left atrial appendage in rheumatic heart disease patients with atrial fibrillation and sinus rhythm. *Cardiovasc Pathol* 2014;23:319–26.

26. Doubell AF, Greef MP, Rossouw DJ, Weich HF. Electron microscopic analysis of the specific granule content of human atria. An investigation of the role of atrial pressure and atrial rhythm in release of atrial natriuretic peptide. *South African Med J* 1990;78:207–11.

27. Yang PS, Lee SH, Park J et al. Atrial tissue expression of receptor for advanced glycation end-products (RAGE) and atrial fibrosis in patients with mitral valve disease. *Int J Cardiol* 2016;220:1–6.

28. Zhu D, Wu Z, van der Geest RJ et al. Accuracy of late gadolinium enhancement - magnetic resonance imaging in the measurement of left atrial substrate remodeling in patients with rheumatic mitral valve disease and persistent atrial fibrillation. *Int Heart J* 2015;56:505–10.

29. Kaya MG, Akpek M, Elcik D et al. Relation of left atrial spontaneous echocardiographic contrast in patients with mitral stenosis to inflammatory markers. *Am J Cardiol* 2012;109:851–5.

30. He G, Tan W, Wang B et al. Increased M1 Macrophages infiltration is associated with thrombogenesis in rheumatic mitral stenosis patients with atrial fibrillation. *PLoS One* 2016;11:e0149910.

31. Cianfrocca C, Loricchio ML, Pelliccia F et al. C-reactive protein and left-atrial appendage velocity are independent determinants of the risk of thrombogenesis in patients with atrial fibrillation. *Int J Cardiol* 2010;142:22–8.

32. Patel P, Dokainish H, Tsai P, Lakkis N. Update on the association of inflammation and atrial fibrillation. *J Cardiovasc Electrophysiol* 2010;21:1064–70.

33. Azzam H, Abousamra NK, Wafa AA, Hafez MM, El-Gilany AH. Upregulation of CD40/CD40L system in rheumatic mitral stenosis with or without atrial fibrillation. *Platelets* 2013;24:516–20.

34. John B, Stiles MK, Kuklik P et al. Electrical remodelling of the left and right atria due to rheumatic mitral stenosis. *Eur Heart J* 2008;29:2234–43.

35. Wong CX, John B, Brooks AG et al. Direction-dependent conduction abnormalities in the chronically stretched atria. *Europace* 2012;14:954–61.

36. Fan K, Lee KL, Chow WH, Chau E, Lau CP. Internal cardioversion of chronic atrial fibrillation during percutaneous mitral commissurotomy: Insight into reversal of chronic stretch-induced atrial remodeling. *Circulation* 2002;105:2746–52.

37. Wood P. An appreciation of mitral stenosis. I. Clinical features. *Br Med J* 1954;1:1051–63.

38. Karthikeyan G. The value of rhythm control in mitral stenosis. *Heart* 2006;92:1013–16.

39. Szekely P, Farmer MB. Rheumatic fever and rheumatic heart disease; natural history and preventive aspects. *Public Health* 1964;78:78–84.

40. Szekely P. Systemic embolism and anticoagulant prophylaxis in rheumatic heart disease. *Br Med J* 1964;1:1209–12.

41. The stroke prevention in atrial fibrillation investigators. Predictors of thromboembolism in atrial fibrillation: II. Echocardiographic features of patients at risk. *Ann Intern Med* 1992;116:6–12.

42. Benjamin EJ, D'Agostino RB, Belanger AJ et al. Left atrial size and risk of stroke and death. The Framingham Heart Study. *Circulation* 1995;92:835–41.

43. Akdemir I, Dagdelen S, Yuce M et al. Silent brain infarction in patients with rheumatic mitral stenosis. *Jpn Heart J* 2002;43:137–44.

44. Karthikeyan G, Ananthakrishnan R, Devasenapathy N et al. Transient, subclinical AF and risk of systemic embolism in patients with rheumatic mitral stenosis in sinus rhythm. *Am J Cardiol* 2014;114:869–74.

45. Wolf PA, Dawber TR, Thomas HE Jr, Kannel WB. Epidemiologic assessment of chronic atrial fibrillation and risk of stroke: The Framingham study. *Neurology* 1978;28:973–7.

46. Chiang CW, Lo SK, Ko YS, Cheng NJ, Lin PJ, Chang CH. Predictors of systemic embolism in patients with mitral stenosis: A prospective study. *Ann Intern Med* 1998;128:885–9.

47. Cerebral Embolism Task Force. Cardiogenic brain embolism. *Arch Neurol* 1986;43:71–84.

48. Acartürk E, Usal A, Demir M, Akgül F, Ozeren A. Thromboembolism risk in patients with mitral stenosis. *Jpn Heart J* 1997;38:669–75.

49. Chimowitz MI, DeGeorgia MA, Poole RM, Hepner A, Armstrong WM. Left atrial spontaneous echo contrast is highly associated with previous stroke in patients with atrial fibrillation or mitral stenosis. *Stroke* 1993;24:1015–19.

50. Kavlak ES, Kucukoglu H, Yigit Z et al. Clinical and echocardiographic risk factors for embolization in the presence of left atrial thrombus. *Echocardiography* 2007;24:515–21.

51. Oldgren J, Healey JS, Ezekowitz M. RE-LY Atrial Fibrillation Registry Investigators. Variations in cause and management of atrial fibrillation in a prospective registry of 15,400 emergency department patients in 46 countries: The RE-LY Atrial Fibrillation Registry. *Circulation* 2014;129:1568 76.

52. Wang D, Liu M, Hao Z et al. Features of acute ischaemic stroke with rheumatic heart disease in a hospitalised Chinese population. *Stroke* 2012;43:2853–7.
53. Chin A. Management of rheumatic atrial fibrillation. *SA Heart* 2015;12:152–5.
54. Belen E, Ozal E, Pusuroglu H. Association of the CHA2DS2-VASc score with left atrial spontaneous echo contrast: A cross-sectional study of patients with rheumatic mitral stenosis in sinus rhythm. *Heart Vessels* 2016;31:1537–43.
55. Atak R, Turhan H, Senen K et al. Relationship between control of ventricular rate in atrial fibrillation and systemic coagulation activation in patients with mitral stenosis. *J Heart Valve Dis* 2004;13:159–64.
56. Yusuf J, Goyal M, Mukhopadhyay S et al. Effect of heart rate control on coagulation status in patients of rheumatic mitral stenosis with atrial fibrillation: A pilot study. *Indian Heart J* 2015;67 Suppl 2:S40–5.
57. Mutlu B, Karabulut M, Eroglu E et al. Fibrillatory wave amplitude as a marker of left atrial and left atrial appendage function, and a predictor of thromboembolic risk in patients with rheumatic mitral stenosis. *Int J Cardiol* 2003;91:179–86.
58. Yin R, Fu Y, Yang Z, Li B, Pen J, Zheng Z. Fibrillatory wave amplitude on transesophageal ECG as a marker of left atrial low-voltage areas in patients with persistent atrial fibrillation. *Ann Noninvasive Electrocardiol* 2017. doi:10.1111/anec.12421 [Epub ahead of print].
59. Nishimura RA, Otto CM, Bonow RO et al. 2017 AHA/ACC Focused Update of the 2014 AHA/ACC Guideline for the Management of Patients with Valvular Heart Disease: A Report of the American College of Cardiology/American Heart Association Task Force on Clinical Practice Guidelines. *J Am Coll Cardiol* 2017. doi:10.1016/j.jacc.2017.03.011 [Epub ahead of print].
60. Fleming HA. Anticoagulants in rheumatic heart-disease. *Lancet* 1971;2:486.
61. Roy D, Marchand E, Gagné P, Chabot M, Cartier R. Usefulness of anticoagulant therapy in the prevention of embolic complications of atrial fibrillation. *Am Heart J* 1986;112:1039–43.
62. January CT, Wann LS, Alpert JS et al. 2014 AHA/ACC/HRS guideline for the management of patients with atrial fibrillation: Executive summary: A report of the American College of Cardiology/American Heart Association task force on practice guidelines and the Heart Rhythm Society. *Circulation* 2014;130(23):2071–2104.
63. Camm AJ, Kirchhof P, Lip GY et al. Guidelines for the management of atrial fibrillation: The Task Force for the Management of Atrial Fibrillation of the European Society of Cardiology (ESC). *Eur Heart J* 2011;31:2369–2429.
64. Nishimura RA, Otto CM, Bonow RO et al. 2014 AHA/ACC Guideline for the management of patients with valvular heart disease: A report of the American College of Cardiology/American Heart Association task force on practice guidelines. *Circulation* 2014;129:521–643.
65. Noseworthy PA, Yao X, Shah ND, Gersh BJ. Comparative effectiveness and safety of non-vitamin K antagonist oral anticoagulants versus warfarin in patients with atrial fibrillation and valvular heart disease. *Int J Cardiol* 2016;209:181–3.
66. Investigation of rheumatic AF treatment using vitamin K antagonists, rivaroxaban or aspirin studies, Non-Inferiority (INVICTUS-VKA). 2016. Available at https://clinicaltrials.gov/ct2/show/NCT02832544.
67. Pérez-Gómez, Salvador A, Zumade J et al. Effect of antithrombotic therapy in patients with mitral stenosis and atrial fibrillation: A sub-analysis of NASPEAF randomized trial. *Eur Heart J* 2006;27:960–7.
68. Hohnloser SH, Kuck KH, Lillienthel J. Rhythm or rate control in atrial fibrillation – Pharmacological Intervention in Atrial Fibrillation (PIAF): A randomised trial. *Lancet* 2000:356;1789–94.
69. Wyse DG, Waldo AL, DiMarco JP et al. The Atrial Fibrillation Follow-up Investigation of Rhythm Management (AFFIRM) Investigators. A comparison of rate control and rhythm control in patients with atrial fibrillation. *N Engl J Med* 2002;347:1825–33.
70. Denis R, Mario T, Paul D et al. Amiodarone to prevent recurrence of atrial fibrillation. The Canadian Trial of Atrial Fibrillation (CTAF) Investigators. *N Engl J Med* 2000;342:913–20.
71. Vora A, Karnad D, Goyal V et al. Control of rate versus rhythm in rheumatic atrial fibrillation: A randomized study. *Indian Heart J* 2004;56:110–16.

72. Liu TJ, Hsueh CW, Lee WL et al. Conversion of rheumatic atrial fibrillation by amiodarone after percutaneous balloon mitral commissurotomy. *Am J Cardiol* 2003; 92:1244–6.

73. Krittayaphong R, Chotinaiwatarakul C, Phankingthongkum R et al. One-year outcome of cardioversion of atrial fibrillation in patients with mitral stenosis after percutaneous balloon mitral valvuloplasty. *Am J Cardiol* 2006;97:1045–50.

74. Jonathan SS, Ara S, Jack K et al. Analysis of cause specific mortality in the AFFIRM study. *Circulation* 2004;109:1973–80.

75. Langerveld J, van Hemel NM, Kelder JC et al. Long-term follow-up of cardiac rhythm after percutaneous mitral balloon valvotomy. Does AF persist? *Europace* 2003;5:47–53.

76. Krasuki RA, Asar MD, Kisslo KB et al. Usefulness of percutaneous balloon mitral commissurotomy in preventing the development of AF in patients with mitral stenosis. *Am J Cardiol* 2004;93:936–9.

77. Adragao P, Machado FP, Aguiar C, Parreira L, Cavaco D, Ribeiras R, Bonhorst D, Queiroz e Melo J, Seabra-Gomes R. Ablation of atrial fibrillation in mitral valve disease patients: Five year follow-up after percutaneous pulmonary vein isolation and mitral balloon valvuloplasty. *Rev Port Cardiol* 2003 Sep; 22(9):1025–36.

78. Nair M, Shah P, Batra R et al. Chronic atrial fibrillation in patients with rheumatic heart disease. *Circulation* 2001;104:802–9.

79. Cox JL, Schuessler LB, D'Agostino HJ Jr et al. The surgical treatment of atrial fibrillation. III. Development of a definitive surgical procedure. *J Thorac Cardiovasc Surg* 1991;101:569–83.

80. Kosakai Y, Kawagushi A, Isobe F et al. Cox maze procedure for chronic atrial fibrillation associated with mitral valve disease. *J Thorac Cardiovasc Surg* 1994;108:1049–55.

81. Phan K, Xie A, Tian DH, Shaikhrezai K, Yan TD. Systematic review and meta-analysis of surgical ablation for atrial fibrillation during mitral valve surgery. *Ann Cardiothorac Surg* 2014;3:3–14.

82. Liu X, Tan HW, Wang XH et al. Efficacy of catheter ablation and surgical CryoMaze procedure in patients with long-lasting persistent atrial fibrillation and rheumatic heart disease: A randomized trial. *Eur Heart J* 2010;31:2633–41.

83. Kainuma S, Masai T, Yoshitatsu M et al. Advanced left-atrial fibrosis is associated with unsuccessful maze operation for valvular atrial fibrillation. *Eur J Cardiothorac Surg* 2011;40:61–9.

84. Kim JB, Lee SH, Jung SH et al. The influence of postoperative mitral valve function on the late recurrence of atrial fibrillation after the maze procedure combined with mitral valvuloplasty. *J Thorac Cardiovasc Surg* 2010;139:1170–6.

85. Kapoor A, Kumar S, Singh RK et al. Management of persistent atrial fibrillation following balloon mitral commissurotomy: Safety and efficacy of low-dose amiodarone. *J Heart Valve Dis* 2002;11:802–9.

86. Lang CC, Santinelli V, Augello G et al. Transcatheter radiofrequency ablation of atrial fibrillation in patients with mitral valve prostheses and enlarged atria. *J Am Coll Cardiol* 2005;45:868–72.

87. Derejko P, Walczak F, Chmielak Z et al. Catheter ablation of complex left atrial arrhythmias in patients after percutaneous or surgical mitral valve procedures. *Kardiol Pol* 2013;71:818–26.

88. Machino T, Tada H, Sekiguchi Y et al. Hybrid therapy of radiofrequency catheter ablation and percutaneous transvenous mitral commissurotomy in patients with atrial fibrillation and mitral stenosis. *J Cardiovasc Electrophysiol* 2010;21:284–9.

89. Camm AJ, Kirchof P, Lip GYH et al. Guidelines for the management of atrial fibrillation. *Europace* 2010;12:1360–1420.

19

Congenital mitral stenosis

DANNY MANGLANI AND SAURABH KUMAR GUPTA

INTRODUCTION

Congenital malformations of the mitral valve represent a heterogeneous group of anomalies. They are often associated with other congenital heart disease (CHD). Clinically significant abnormalities are rare and affect 0.4% of patients with CHD.[1,2] Minor mitral valve abnormalities, however, are not uncommon, with 0.5%–1% of healthy school-age children having altered morphology or function.[3,4] The discrepancy in the prevalence of mitral valve anomalies is possibly related to variable reporting of milder forms. Combined regurgitation and stenosis is more common than isolated regurgitation or stenosis.[5] In this chapter, we focus on mitral valve abnormalities with dominant mitral stenosis (MS).

EMBRYOLOGY AND MORPHOLOGY OF THE MITRAL VALVE

A detailed discussion of the development and morphology of the mitral valve is beyond the scope of this chapter. A brief discussion, however, is important for understanding the pathology and management of congenital MS.

Normal mitral valve

The mitral valve derives its name from its resemblance to an episcopal "miter." The mitral valve apparatus is comprised of an annulus, anterior and posterior leaflets, chordae tendineae, and papillary muscles. The annulus is saddle-shaped. The lateral and medial hinge points are lower than the anterior and posterior hinge points. Of the two leaflets, the anterior (aortic) leaflet is broader than the posterior (mural) leaflet. Both anterior and posterior leaflets are divided into three scallops. The leaflets close along a curvilinear line of apposition. Each end of this closure line, located anterolaterally and posteromedially, is known as a commissure. Hence, the two commissures of the mitral valve are anterolateral and posteromedial. Some authors, however, argue that being bileaflet, the mitral valve can have only one commissure, i.e., the curvilinear line of apposition.[5,6] These leaflets are attached to two papillary muscles, usually located in anterolateral and posteromedial location via chordae tendineae. Unlike the tricuspid valve, the mitral valve is free from an attachment to ventricular septum.

Embryology

A faulty development of the mitral valve apparatus underlies congenital MS. Mitral valve formation begins during the fourth week of gestation. During the sixth week, fusion of endocardial cushions divides the atrioventricular canal into the right- and left-atrioventricular junction.[7] Normally, the aortic or anterior leaflet is derived from the apposition of the left part of the superior and inferior cushions and has no attachment to the ventricular myocardium except through the papillary muscles. The mural or posterior leaflet, on the other hand, is formed by the protrusion and growth of a sheet of atrioventricular myocardium into the ventricular lumen, with the subsequent formation of valvular mesenchyme on its surface.[8,29] During the eighth week, the shape of the orifice looks like a crescent, the two ends of which are connected to compacting columns in the trabecular muscle of the left ventricle. These columns form a muscular ridge, the anterior and posterior parts of which become the papillary muscles.[7] The transformation of the ridge into papillary muscles is by delamination, a process of gradual loosening of muscle. Simultaneously, the cushion tissue loses contact with the myocardium of the ridge, except at the insertion of the future tendinous cords. As substantiated by immuno-histochemical analysis, both leaflets and chordae originate from the cushion tissue, whereas papillary muscles are derived from the ventricular myocardium.[7,8]

Changes in the inflow pattern across the mitral valve alter the development of mitral valve by altered hemodynamic patterning[9] and local gene expression.[10] As a result, congenital anomalies of the mitral valve are common, with malformations of the left ventricle, ventricular septum, and ventricular outflow.[5]

CLASSIFICATION OF CONGENITAL MITRAL VALVE DISEASE

It is tempting to classify mitral valve pathologies into stenotic and regurgitant lesions. This approach, however, is impractical as most anomalies result in combined stenosis and regurgitation. Morphological variations add to the complexity. A combined use of physiologic and morphologic abnormalities permits a more relevant descriptive classification. Mitral regurgitation is more common than mitral stenosis and is present in three-quarters of cases with congenital anomalies of the mitral valve.[11]

Morphologic classification

The first classification was proposed by Davachi and colleagues in 1971.[12] The first few classifications were complicated by attempts of including both stenotic and regurgitant lesions. Ruckman and Van Praagh, for the first time, classified congenital MS separately.[13] They classified congenital MS in four subtypes: typical congenital mitral stenosis, hypoplastic mitral stenosis, supramitral ring, and parachute mitral valve. In 1994, Moore and colleagues modified Ruckman's classification and categorized hypoplastic mitral valve into typical with symmetrical papillary muscles and atypical with asymmetrical papillary muscles.[14] They also added double orifice mitral valve. Hypoplastic type is the most common type, seen in 74% of patients, while double orifice mitral valve is the least common.[11]

Surgical classification

While morphologic classifications help in detailed description of mitral valve pathology, they offer little guidance for surgical repair. In 1998, Carpentier et al. classified congenital MS, based on the location of obstruction, into predominant valvular lesion with normal papillary muscle and predominant subvalvular lesion with abnormal papillary muscle.[15] This classification, despite its simple approach, provides insights into pathological anatomy and guides surgical repair.

Clinically, a more relevant approach is to combine morphologic and surgical aspects to classify congenital mitral stenosis (Table 19.1). In some cases, however, the obstruction is at multiple levels and exact classification is not possible. In such cases, a descriptive analysis is much more appropriate.

Table 19.1 Clinical classification of congenital mitral stenosis

Location of obstruction	Morphologic variant
1. Leaflets	Supramitral ring
	Double-orifice mitral valve
2. Annulus	Hypoplastic and dysplastic mitral valve
3. Tensor apparatus	Mitral valve arcade or Hammock mitral valve
4. Papillary muscles	Parachute mitral valve
	Parachute-like mitral valve

CLINICAL PRESENTATION

Congenital mitral stenosis is more common in males (male:female ratio of 1.5:1).[16,17] The clinical presentation is highly variable and is not only related to the degree of coexisting regurgitation but is also affected by the presence and severity of associated malformations. The spectrum ranges from an incidentally detected mitral valve disease in an asymptomatic child to an infant presenting early in life with poor feeding, failure to thrive, heart failure, and recurrent respiratory tract infections. Cardiogenic shock is seldom due to isolated MS. Its presence necessitates a search for associated cardiac malformation(s) causing ventricular outflow obstruction.

Although physiologic alterations are similar to rheumatic MS, physical findings are different (Table 19.2). These differences stem from almost universal involvement of subvalvular apparatus in congenital MS. Restricted motion of valve leaflets preclude loud first heart sound and opening

Table 19.2 Differences in rheumatic and congenital mitral stenosis

	Rheumatic MS	Congenital MS
Pathology		
Commissural fusion	Yes	No
Subvalvular pathology	+	++
Calcification	Common	Rare
Associated CHDs	Rare	Common
Clinical presentation		
Age group	Adolescents and adults	Children
Male/female	More common in females	More common in males
Opening snap	+	−
Loud S1	+	−
Presystolic accentuation	Present	Absent
ECG		
Atrial fibrillation	Common (infrequent in juvenile MS)	Rare
Echocardiography		
M-mode assessment	Reliable	Not reliable in majority
Pressure half-time	Reliable	Not reliable
Mitral valve planimetry	Reliable	Difficult (eccentric orifice)
Treatment		
BMV	First-line	High complication rate, low success
Surgical commissurotomy	Good results	Performed only as part of valvuloplasty
Surgical valvuloplasty	Rare	Preferred
Mitral valve replacement	Annular	Annular or supra-annular

snap. Physical examination includes a low-pitched, mid-diastolic murmur at the apex but with no or minimal presystolic accentuation. In the presence of pulmonary hypertension, the pulmonary component of the second heart sound is loud.

The interpretation of clinical findings is complicated by the presence of associated lesions. An associated post-tricuspid left-to-right shunt result in increased transmitral flow and cause overestimation of mitral stenosis. If diastolic murmur is louder than expected in a child with left-to-right shunt, then associated MS should be suspected. Similarly, symptoms or pulmonary hypertension out of proportion to the adjudged severity of left-to-right shunt should prompt an evaluation for MS.[17,18]

DIAGNOSTIC EVALUATION

Electrocardiogram

The electrocardiogram (ECG) may be completely normal in mild stenosis, while left-atrial enlargement may be the only clue towards moderate stenosis. Pulmonary hypertension secondary to severe MS reflects as right-ventricular hypertrophy, right-axis deviation and right-atrial enlargement. Unlike rheumatic MS in adolescents and adults, atrial fibrillation is rare in children with congenital MS.[17,18] This is possibly related to shorter duration of illness compared to adolescents and adults with rheumatic MS.

Chest x-ray

Chest radiograph has limited utility in the diagnosis of mild or moderate MS and, therefore, should not be routinely performed. Even in children with severe MS, chest x-ray is not a sensitive tool. Hemodynamically significant MS may present with radiologic signs of left-atrial enlargement and pulmonary venous hypertension. Cardiomegaly and right-atrial enlargement indicate pulmonary hypertension and right-ventricular dysfunction.

Echocardiography

Echocardiography, by providing both morphological and physiological information, permits complete assessment of mitral valve pathology. It provides almost all hemodynamic and morphologic information necessary to make a clinical decision about timing and type of intervention.

Prolonged EF slope and paradoxical anterior motion of posterior mitral leaflet, well-known M-mode hallmarks of rheumatic MS, have limited utility in congenital MS.[17,19]

Cross-sectional echocardiography provides a unique opportunity to understand the pathophysiology of congenital MS. More importantly, echocardiography allows the detection of otherwise milder forms that assume significance in the presence of associated CHD. All children with CHD, particularly those with cono-truncal anomalies and obstruction to left-ventricular inflow and outflow (Shone's complex), should undergo a mitral valve evaluation. Once preliminary echocardiographic assessment suggests MS, the focus should be on defining its hemodynamic and morphologic severity.

ASSESSMENT OF SEVERITY

Unlike rheumatic MS in adults, the assessment of severity is not based on planimetry, as in most cases the valve orifice is eccentric and stenosis is not at the zone of leaflet coaptation. An overall appearance of mitral valve apparatus, including the interchordal space, determines the severity. Pulse-wave Doppler helps in localizing the site of maximum obstruction. The pressure gradient across the mitral valve mandates careful interpretation when associated with left-to-right shunt or mitral regurgitation. Higher heart rates in children and associated lesions limit the diagnostic utility of pressure half-time.[19] Tricuspid and pulmonary regurgitation jets provides an estimate of right-ventricular and pulmonary artery pressure, which in turn helps in assessing the hemodynamic significance of mitral stenosis.

MORPHOLOGIC ASSESSMENT

This is the most important aspect of echocardiographic evaluation in congenital MS. The complex anatomy of the mitral valve apparatus necessitates the careful assessment of each of its components. A systematic approach of examining from "base to apex" or "apex to base" should be followed, at least in the operator's mind, as it is not often possible to follow a standard imaging sequence in children. The importance of a segmental approach in determining the abnormalities of veno-atrial, atrioventricular, and ventriculo-arterial connections and defining associated malformations cannot be overemphasized.

Two-dimensional (2D) echocardiography allows optimal evaluation in majority. However, complete assessment of all aspects of abnormality remains challenging in some. An inability to demonstrate surgical perspective adds to the limitations of 2D echocardiography. Three-dimensional (3D) echocardiography by providing "surgical views" and 3D perspectives of the mitral valve and adjacent cardiac structures permits improved visualization. This in turn results in a better understanding of patho-anatomy. Three-dimensional color Doppler aids in localizing the site of obstruction. Biplane echocardiography using 3D echo probe and 3D reconstruction, particularly in multiplanar reformation (MPR) mode, allows the localization of the true short axis of the mitral valve and permits the accurate measurement of valve area by planimetry. Rapid online and offline processing capabilities in currently available echocardiography machines has further improved the acceptability of 3D echocardiography in clinical practice.[11,17,19–21]

A rapid improvement and change in surgical techniques demands a detailed morphologic assessment. Classic terminologies, although used often in clinical practice, are grossly insufficient to direct modern surgical repair. A descriptive analysis of each component of mitral valve apparatus, on the other hand, enables the surgeon to craft an individualized repair technique.[11,22–25]

Magnetic resonance imaging

Magnetic resonance imaging (MRI) has a limited role in the assessment of congenital MS, as a good-quality echocardiography provides almost all the relevant information. Long study time and the need for general anesthesia in children also makes it less attractive. Nevertheless, MRI provides invaluable hemodynamic information in the presence of coexisting malformations. A flow and volumetric analysis of the mitral valve and the LV provides crucial information about the suitability of biventricular repair in cases with suspected LV hypoplasia.[22]

Cardiac catheterization and angiocardiography

In the current era of advances in echocardiography and non-invasive cardiac imaging, routine cardiac catheterization is no longer performed. Cardiac catheterization is rather performed as a part of percutaneous intervention. Invasive hemodynamic evaluation, however, remains necessary to assess operability in children with associated VSD or PDA presenting beyond infancy. The presence of MS, by causing post-capillary pulmonary hypertension, appears to protect these patients from developing irreversible pulmonary vascular disease.[26,27]

INDIVIDUAL LESIONS CAUSING CONGENITAL MITRAL STENOSIS

The pathologic abnormalities in congenital MS are heterogenous and complex. There is a great deal of ambiguity in various pathologic forms, with different authors using different terminologies for conditions with similar morphologic abnormality. The differences in the descriptions by the surgeons and the cardiologists also adds to the complexity.

Hypoplastic and dysplastic mitral valve

In this form of congenital MS, all components of mitral valve apparatus are malformed when the valve is dysplastic and hypoplastic. The leaflets are thickened, interchordal space is obliterated, and papillary muscles are deformed (Figure 19.1).[13,14,16,28–29] This is the most common lesion causing congenital MS, both as an isolated malformation or more frequently in the setting of hypoplasia of the left heart. Thickened and rolled free edges of leaflets leave a zone of non-coaptation accounting for coexisting regurgitation.

Supramitral ring

This represents a fibrous membrane close to the mitral valve annulus. The fibrous ring is located distal to the left-atrial appendage, differentiating it from cor-triatriatum. The extent of circumferential involvement determines the onset and severity of symptoms.[30] Based on the location of the ring, two distinct subtypes can be identified—a more common "intramitral ring" with coexisting valve pathology and worse outcome and a "supramitral ring" with normal mitral valve and good outcome.[30] In the intramitral subtype the membrane is attached to the leaflets while in the supramitral ring type it is attached to the mitral annulus.

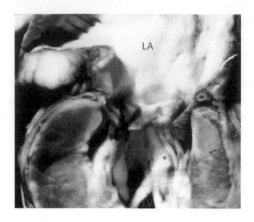

Figure 19.1 Typical congenital MS: Hypoplastic, dysplastic, and thickened mitral valve with thickened, deformed papillary muscles and obliterated interchordal spaces (*) in the setting of hypoplastic left ventricle. (Courtesy of Prof. Robert H Anderson, Institute of Genetic Medicine, Newcastle University, UK.)

Echocardiography provides an excellent view of the membrane, enabling diagnosis of even milder forms of supramitral ring (Figure 19.2). Occasionally, a non-circumferential ring may be too close to the leaflets, making the detection challenging. Once the diagnosis is made, surgical excision of the ring in the supramitral variant is sufficient. On the other hand, an intramitral variant necessitates the repair of other abnormalities of mitral valve apparatus in addition to the excision of the fibrous ring.[17,30] Failure to diagnose and treat additional causes of obstruction result in residual MS, despite surgical resection of the ring. Fortunately, residual MS from associated lesions is generally not severe and most children enjoy freedom from reoperation.[17]

Mitral valve arcade (hammock mitral valve)

This rare entity results from faulty muscularization of the chordal apparatus. Classically, the chordae are fused, making it difficult to differentiate chordae and papillary muscles (Figure 19.3). There are often more than two papillary muscles, with additional papillary muscle attaching to the posterior leaflet. Secondary chords arising from the posterior free wall of the LV also attach to the midportion of the leaflet. This combination of faulty chordae and papillary muscles results in immobile leaflet and diminutive interchordal space. The result is mitral regurgitation with a variable degree of stenosis. While pathologists describe it as an arcade, the surgeon's view from the left atrium has earned it the label of hammock mitral valve.[11,17,29,31]

Echocardiographically, it is characterized by a normal mitral valve orifice; short, thick, and poorly differentiated chordae connecting directly to the papillary muscles with narrow or nearly nonexistent interchordal space (Figure 19.4). The arcade mitral valve represents the most difficult mitral valve anatomy for surgical reconstruction.[32] The surgical techniques include fenestration in the chordal apparatus, resection of secondary chordae, and/or accessory papillary muscle.

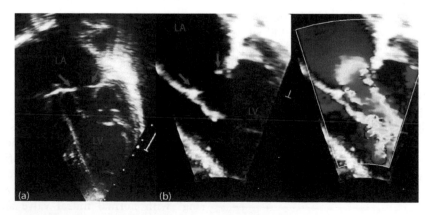

Figure 19.2 Transthoracic echocardiogram showing supramitral ring. (a) typical supramitral ring; (b) intramitral variant. Note that the turbulence in panel b starts proximal to the line of coaptation (see Video 19.1).

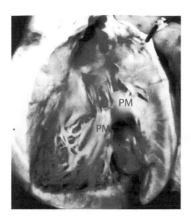

Figure 19.3 Heart specimen from a child with hammock mitral valve seen through the incision made in the free wall of the left ventricle. Chordae are fused with diminutive interchordal space. (Courtesy of Prof. Robert H Anderson, Institute of Genetic Medicine, Newcastle University, UK.)

Parachute mitral valve or parachute-like mitral valve

Parachute mitral valve (PMV) results from both leaflets attaching to a single mass of papillary muscle(s). The initial description by Shone and colleagues included hearts with a solitary papillary muscle.[33] More often, however, the appearance results from fusion of two closely placed papillary muscles (Figure 19.5). Generally, the anterolateral

muscle is hypoplastic and the posteromedial papillary muscle is dominant. There has been considerable controversy in defining what constitutes PMV. Rosenquist[34] and Carpentier[15] et al. included those with fused papillary muscles while Ruckman and Van Praagh[13] excluded them from the label of PMV. From a practical viewpoint, both these variants have similar appearance and hemodynamic impact. Generally, children with typical single papillary muscle variant are labeled "PMV," while others with two fused papillary

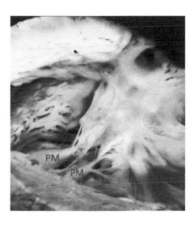

Figure 19.5 Heart specimen from an infant with parachute-like mitral valve (PLMV). Note two closely placed papillary muscles (PM) attached to the chordae tendineae. (Courtesy of Prof. Robert H Anderson, Institute of Genetic Medicine, Newcastle University, UK.)

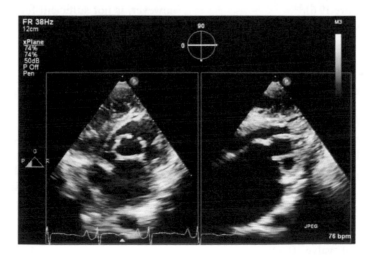

Figure 19.4 Biplane echocardiogram showing normal mitral valve orifice (left panel) with short, thick chordae attaching directly to the papillary muscle (right panel). (Courtesy of Prof. Shyam S Kothari, All India Institute of Medical Sciences, New Delhi, India.)

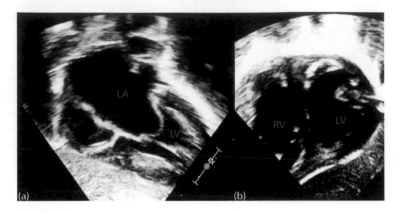

Figure 19.6 Transthoracic echocardiogram in subcostal long-axis (panel a) view demonstrating the appearance of a pear (see Video 19.2). (Panel b) shows single mass of papillary muscle(s) (*) attached to the lateral wall of the left ventricle.

muscles, symmetric or asymmetric, are said to have "parachute-like mitral valve (PLMV)."[35] This distinction is important for valve reconstruction surgery (see later).

Echocardiography, especially 3D reconstruction, provides all relevant morphologic details. The parasternal short-axis view at mid-cavity level demonstrates a single or two fused papillary muscle(s). In the apical or subcostal long-axis view, symmetric doming of both the leaflets with a central connection to papillary muscle(s) gives a "pear-like" appearance, with the left atrium forming the base, the mitral leaflets occupying the apex, and the connection to papillary muscle(s) forming the central stalk (Figure 19.6).[36]

Fortunately, despite remarkable echocardiographic and pathologic abnormalities, the majority of children have no or only mild symptoms and do not require surgical intervention in their first decade.[37,38] Depending upon the extent of associated lesions, surgical repair may include chordal fenestration, splitting of papillary muscles, and commissurotomy.[22–25,38] An associated hypoplasia of the left ventricle, seen more with PMV than PLMV, may preclude biventricular repair.

Double-orifice mitral valve

Double-orifice mitral valve (DOMV) is common with atrioventricular septal defects. It is occasionally seen in an otherwise-normal heart. In the setting of normal atrioventricular connections, each orifice is supported by chordal apparatus and papillary muscles of their own. Trowitzsch and colleagues categorized DOMV into complete bridge type, incomplete bridge type, and hole type, based on the extent of division of the subvalvular apparatus.[39] The two orifices are unequal in the majority of cases and equal orifices are seen in only 15% of cases.[40] Two orifices of DOMV are seen clearly in parasternal or subcostal short-axis view. Rather than the ellipsoid shape of a normal mitral valve, DOMV opens as two circles in diastole (Figure 19.7).[6] The mere appearance of two orifices, however, is not sufficient for diagnosis of DOMV, which requires antegrade flow across both orifices. Mitral regurgitation is seen in 43%, mitral stenosis in 13%, and combined stenosis and regurgitation in 6.5% of cases. DOMV has no hemodynamic implications in the remaining 37% of cases.[40,41]

MANAGEMENT

When associated with other lesions, the management of MS is influenced by the severity and complexity of coexisting malformations. In other patients with isolated congenital MS, the severity and mechanism of the obstruction defines the management strategy. As indicated before, not all mitral valve abnormalities are hemodynamically significant and a careful follow-up may be

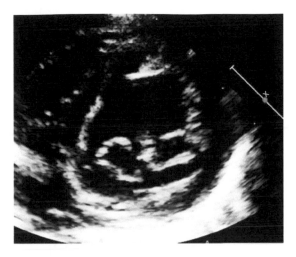

Figure 19.7 Transthoracic echocardiogram in parasternal short-axis view showing two equal-sized orifices of the mitral valve.

sufficient. Patients with mild to moderate stenosis do not warrant intervention and may benefit from heart rate control and titrated use of diuretics. Aggressive diuresis and heart rate control, however, must be avoided. Congenital MS is a progressive disease and, therefore, all patients should be on regular follow-up to monitor progression of obstruction and mitral regurgitation, and to look for other possible complications such as failure to thrive, recurrent lower respiratory tract infections, and development of pulmonary hypertension.[17]

Patients with severe MS require relief of obstruction by percutaneous balloon mitral valvuloplasty or surgical mitral valvuloplasty or mitral valve replacement. Understandably, all efforts must be made to avoid a prosthetic mitral valve. Before any management strategy is chosen it is imperative to carefully assess the feasibility of valvuloplasty and biventricular repair. A grossly hypoplastic mitral valve with a z score of less than −3, LV volume index <25 mL/m², the presence of more than mild endocardial fibroelastosis, and associated hypoplasia of ascending aorta precludes biventricular repair.[22] The impact of associated lesions on the assessment of MS severity must be carefully interpreted while determining the severity of congenital MS. Figure 19.8 provides an algorithm for the management of congenital MS.

Percutaneous balloon mitral valvuloplasty

Percutaneous transvenous mitral commissurotomy (PTMC) is an established treatment modality for rheumatic MS and is well known to predictably relieve the obstruction in MS. While commissurotomy relieves stenosis in rheumatic MS, the mechanism of relief in congenital MS is not clear. It possibly results from leaflet tear and disruption of the tension apparatus. As a result, the term "balloon mitral valvuloplasty" (BMV) should be preferred over PTMC in the context of congenital MS. Also, unlike rheumatic MS where BMV is definitive, it only defers definitive surgical repair in congenital MS.

McElhinney and colleagues reported successful deferral of re-intervention in more than half of 64 children undergoing BMV. The procedure allowed five-year freedom from intervention in 40% of cases.[42] However, 28% of children developed significant MR requiring mitral valve replacement. The results of BMV are suboptimal in infants and with complex mitral valve anatomy. In addition, BMV entails risk of uncontrolled disruption of mitral valve apparatus, leaving the valve unrepairable surgically. Generally, considering the high rate of complications and the need of re-interventions, BMV is not preferred by most of the pediatric cardiologists.[17]

Surgical management

The heterogeneous nature of congenital MS, the presence of associated lesions, and its rarity make the surgical management challenging. Severe hypoplasia of the left ventricle and mitral valve mandates careful assessment of the feasibility of biventricular repair. The aggressive approach of mitral valve repair in borderline cases may result in significant residual MS and pulmonary hypertension, making the child a poor candidate for univentricular palliation or cardiac transplantation in future. Therefore, it is important to identify such high-risk cases who have a high likelihood of surgical repair failure. If recognized in the neonatal period, an alternative strategy of early atrial septectomy with pulmonary artery banding can prepare them for univentricular palliation in the future.[17,22]

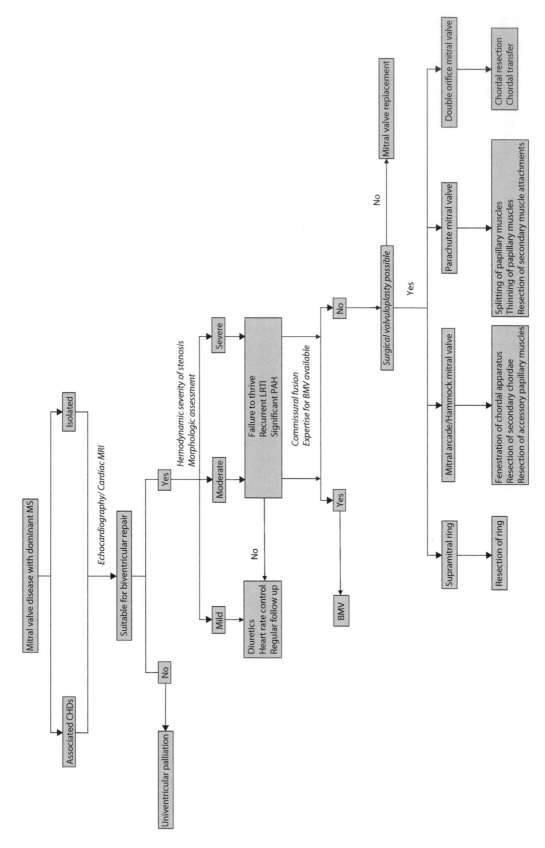

Figure 19.8 Algorithm for management of congenital mitral stenosis.

Those with a suitable anatomy for biventricular repair and a mitral valve amenable to valvuloplasty should be offered timely surgical repair. The mechanism of stenosis determines the surgical technique and outcomes in others. A valve deemed not amenable to surgical repair should be replaced by a prosthetic valve. Unlike MV replacement with annular placement of prosthesis in adults, the prosthesis in children is often placed in a supra-annular position.[43] The supra-annular position of prosthesis limits LA compliance and causes pulmonary hypertension even in the absence of prosthetic valve dysfunction.[43,44] This results in greater morbidity and mortality than annular implantation.[44] Tierney and colleagues, in their report on mitral valve replacement in 118 children younger than 5 years of age, had 32% supramitral placement of valve prosthesis. The survival was worse in children with supra-annular mitral valve replacement, with 56% requiring redo mitral valve replacement.[45] Currently, most of the prosthetic mitral valves are placed at the annular position.

Recent reports suggest improving surgical outcomes with a 60% to 70% reduction in transmitral gradient and in-hospital mortality of approximately 10%.[46] Survival and freedom from re intervention is steadily improving, with some centers reporting 98% and 95.7% survival at 1 year and 5 years follow-up, respectively. A repeat surgical mitral valvuloplasty or mitral valve repair is indicated in 10%–25% of patients. The best surgical outcomes are seen in those with an isolated supramitral ring placed well above the leaflets while PMV has the worst surgical outcomes.[46] In addition to associated cardiac malformations and pathologic involvement of the mitral valve, younger age at intervention predisposes to greater risk of reintervention. Compared to surgical valvuloplasty, reinterventions are more common following BMV.

SUMMARY

A variety of malformations result in congenital MS either in isolation or in association with other cardiac anomalies. A detailed assessment of morphology and hemodynamic alteration by echocardiography is crucial to decide the timing and management strategy. Surgical repair is preferred. Mitral valve replacement should be performed only if valve repair is not possible.

VIDEOS

Video 19.1 Colour compare echocardiography showing intramitral ring and the flow turbulence starting from the ring. https://youtu.be/Y9wTkvoXMDU

Video 19.2 Single papillary muscle. https://youtu.be/ge1136bSrXk

REFERENCES

1. Nadas AS, Fyler DC. *Pedatric Cardiology*. 3rd ed. Philadelphia: WB Saunders Co.; 1972:683–7.
2. Mitchell SC, Korones SB, Berendes HW. Congenital heart disease in 56100 births: Incidence and natural history. *Circulation* 1971;43:323–32.
3. Banerjee A, Kohl T, Silverman NH. Echocardiographic evaluation of congenital mitral valve anomalies in children. *Am J Cardiol* 1995;76:1284–91.
4. Webb RH, Wilson NJ, Lennon DR, Wilson EM, Nicholson RW, Gentles TL, O'Donnell CP, Stirling JW, Zeng I, Trenholme AA. Optimising echocardiographic screening for rheumatic heart disease in New Zealand: Not all valve disease is rheumatic. *Cardiol Young* 2011;21:436–43.
5. Seguela PE, Houyel L, Acar P. Congenital malformations of the mitral valve. *Arch Cardiovasc Dis* 2011;104:465–79.
6. Asante- Korang A, O'Leary PW, Anderson RH. Anatomy and echocardiography of the normal and abnormal mitral valve. *Cardiol Young* 2006;16:27–34.
7. Oosthoek PW, Wenink AC, Wisse LJ, Gittenberger-de Groot AC. Development of the papillary muscles of the mitral valve: Morphogenetic background of parachute-like asymmetric mitral valves and other mitral valve anomalies. *J Thorac Cardiovasc Surg* 1998;116:36–46.
8. DeLange FJ, Moorman AF, Anderson RH, Manner J, Soufan AT, de Gier-de Vries C, Schneider MD, Webb S, van den Hoff MJ, Christoffels VM. Lineage and morphogenetic analysis of the cardiac valves. *Circ Res* 2004;95:645–54.

9. Yalcin HC, Shekhar A, McQuinn TC, Butcher JT. Hemodynamic patterning of the avian atrioventricular valve. *Dev Dyn* 2011;240:23–35.

10. Groenendijk BC, Hierck BP, Vrolijk J, Baiker M, Pourquie MJ, Gittenberger-de Groot AC, Poelmann RE. Changes in shear stress-related gene expression after experimentally altered venous return in the chicken embryo. *Circ Res* 2005;96:1291–8.

11. Remenyi B, Gentles TL. Congenital mitral valve lesions: Correlation between morphology and imaging. *Ann Pediatr Cardiol* 2012;5:3–12.

12. Davachi F, Moller JH, Edwards JE. Diseases of the mitral valve in infancy. An anatomic analysis of 55 cases. *Circulation* 1971;43:565–79.

13. Ruckman RN, van Praagh R. Anatomic types of congenital mitral stenosis: Report of 49 autopsy cases with consideration of diagnosis and surgical implications. *Am J Cardiol* 1978;42:592–601.

14. Moore P, Adatia I, Spevak PJ, Keane JF, Perry SB, Castaneda AR, Lock J. Severe congenital mitral stenosis in infants. *Circulation* 1994;89:2099–2106.

15. Carpentier A, Branchini B, Cour JC et al. Congenital malformations of the mitral valve in children. Pathology and surgical treatment. *J Thorac Cardiovasc Surg* 1976;72:854–66.

16. Collins- Nakai RL, Rosenthal A, Castaneda AR, Bernhard WF, Nadas AS. Congenital mitral stenosis. A review of 20 years' experience. *Circulation* 1977;56:1039–47.

17. Mackie AS, Smallhorn JF. Anatomical and functional mitral valve abnormalities in the pediatric population. In *Moss and Adams' Heart Disease in Infants, Children, and Adolescents*, 8th ed. Philadelphia: Wolter Kluwer Health-Lippincott Williams & Wilkins; 2013:1003–22.

18. Perloff JK. Congenital obstruction to left atrial flow: Mitral stenosis, cor triatriatum, pulmonary vein stenosis. In *Clinical Recognition of Congenital Heart Disease*, 6th ed. Perloff JK, Marelli A, eds. Philadelphia: Elsevier Saunders;2012:129–40.

19. Banerjee A, Kohl T, Silverman NH. Echocardiographic evaluation of congenital mitral valve anomalies in children. *Am J Cardiol* 1995;76:1284–91.

20. Garcia-Orta R, Moreno E, Vidal M, Ruiz-Lopez F, Oyonarte JM, Lara J, Moreno T, Garcia-Fernandezd MA, Azpitarte J. Three-dimensional versus two-dimensional transesophageal echocardiography in mitral valve repair. *J Am Soc Echocardiogr* 2007;20:4–12.

21. Balestrini L, Fleishman C, Lanzoni L, Kisslo J, Resat Bengur A, Sanders SP, Li JS. Real-time 3-diemensional echocardiography evaluation of congenital heart disease. *J Am Soc Echocardiogr* 2000;13;171–6.

22. Alghamdi AA, Yadava M, Arsdell GSV. Surgical management of congenital mitral stenosis. *Oper Tech Thorac Cardiovasc Surg* 2010;15:273–81.

23. del Nido PJ, Baird C. Congenital mitral valve stenosis: Anatomic variants and surgical reconstruction. *Semin Thorac Cardiovasc Surg Pediatr Card Surg Ann* 2012;15:69–74.

24. Hoashi T, Bove EL, Devaney EJ, Hirsch JC, Ohye RG. Mitral valve repair for congenital mitral valve stenosis in pediatric population. *Ann Thoarc Surg* 2010;90:36–41.

25. Baird CW, Mark GR, Borisuk M, Emani S, del Nido PJ. Review of congenital mitral valve stenosis: Analysis, repair technique and outcomes. *Cardiovasc Engeering and Technology* 2015;6:167–73.

26. Talwar S, Upadhyay M, Ramakrishnan S, Gharade P, Choudhary SK, Airan B. Window-type patent ductus arteriosus with acquired rheumatic mitral stenosis. *Congenit Heart Dis* 2013;8:E10–12.

27. Gupta A, Kothari SS. Operable patent ductus arteriosus even with differential cyanosis: A case of patent ductus arteriosus and mitral stenosis. *Cardiol Young* 2017. doi: https://doi.org/10.1017/S1047951117001275.

28. Daliento L, Thiene G, Chirillo F, Milanesi O, Stellin G, Caneve F, Dalla Volta S. Congenital malformations of the mitral valve: Clinical and morphological aspects. *G Ital Cardiol* 1991;21:1205–16.

29. Smallhorn JF, Anderson RH. Anomalies of the morphologically mitral valve. In: *Pediatric Cardiology* 3rd ed. Anderson RH, Baker EJ, Penny D, Redington AN, Rigby ML, Wernovsky G, eds. Philadelphia: Churchil Livingstone Elsevier; 2010: 731–51. ISBN 978-0-7020-3064-2.

30. Toscano A, Pasquini L, Iacobelli R, Di Donato RM, Raimondi F, Carotti A, Di Ciommo V, Sanders SP. Congenital supravalvular mitral ring: An underestimated anomaly. *J Thorac Cardiovasc Surg* 2009;137:538–42.

31. Perez JA, Herzberg AJ, Reimer KA, Bashore TM. Congenital mitral insufficiency secondary to anomalous mitral arcade in an adult. *Am Heart J* 1987;114:894–5.

32. Deepti S, Devagourou V, Kothari SS. Repair of anomalous mitral arcade in a child. *Ann Pediatr Card* 2017;10:200–202.

33. Shone JD, Sellers RD, Anderson RC, Adams P Jr, Lillehei CW, Edwards JE. The developmental complex of "parachute mitral valve" supravalvular ring of left atrium, subaortic stenosis, and coarctation of aorta. *Am J Cardiol* 1963;11:714–25.

34. Rosenquist GC. Congenital mitral valve disease associated with coarctation of the aorta. A spectrum that includes parachute deformity of the mitral valve. *Circulation* 1974;49:985–93.

35. Oosthoek PW, Wenink AC, Macedo AJ, Gittenberger-de Groot AC. The parachute-like asymmetric mitral valve and its two papillary muscles. *J Thorac Cardiovasc Surg* 1997;114:9–15.

36. Purvis JA, Smyth S, Barr SH. Multimodality imaging of an adult parachute mitral valve. *J Am Soc Echocardiogr* 2011;24:351.

37. Marino BS, Kruge LE, Cho CJ, Tominson RS, Shera D, Weinberg PM, Gaynor JW, Rychik J. Parachute mitral valve: Morphologic descriptors, associated lesions, and outcomes after biventricular repair. *J Thorac Cardiovasc Surg* 2009;137:385–93.

38. Schaverien MV, Freedom RM, McCrindle BW. Independent factors associated with outcomes of parachute mitral valve in 84 patients. *Circulation* 2004; 109:2309–13.

39. Trowitzsch E, Bano-Rodrigo A, Burger BM, Colan SD, Sanders SP. Two dimensional echocardiographic findings in double orifice mitral valve. *J Am Coll Cardiol* 1985;6:383–7.

40. Bano-Rodrigo A, Van Praagh S, Trowitzsch E, Van Praagh R. Double orifice mitral valve: A study of 27 postmortem cases with developmental, diagnostic and surgical considerations. *Am J Cardiol* 1988;61:152–60.

41. Zalzstein E, Hamilton R, Zucker N, Levitas A, Gross GJ. Presentation, natural history, and outcome in children and adolescents with double orifice mitral valve. *Am J Cardiol* 2004;93:1067–9.

42. McElhinney DB, Sherwood MC, Keane JF, del Nido PJ, Almond CS, Lock JE. Current management of severe congenital mitral stenosis: Outcomes of transcatheter and surgical therapy in 108 infants and children.

43. Adatia I, Moore PM, Jonas RA, Colan SD, Lock JE, Keane JF. Clinical course and hemodynamic observations after supraannular mitral valve replacement in infants and children. *J Am Coll Cardiol* 1997;29:1089–94.

44. van Doorn C, Yates R, Tsang V, deLeval M, Elliott M. Mitral valve replacement in children: Mortality, morbidity, and haemodynamic status up to medium term follow up. *Heart* 2000;84:636–42.

45. Tierney ESS, Pigula FA, Berul CI, Lock JE, del Nido PJ, McElhinney DB. Mitral valve replacement in infants and children 5 years of age or younger: Evolution in practice and outcome over three decades with a focus on supra-annular prosthesis implantation. *J Thorac Cardiovasc Surg* 2008;136:954–61.

46. Stellin G, Padalino MA, Vida VL, Boccuzzo G, Orru E, Biffanti R, Milanesi O. Surgical repair of congenital mitral valve malformations in infancy and childhood: A single-center 36-year experience. *J Thorac Cardiovasc Surg* 2010;140:1238–44.

20

Degenerative mitral stenosis

NEERAJ PARAKH

INTRODUCTION

Degenerative mitral stenosis (MS) is a chronic degenerative process of mitral annulus resulting in mitral annular calcification (MAC) and mitral stenosis in the elderly. With a growing aging population and increasing risk factors such as hypertension, radiation, and left-ventricular hypertrophy (especially in developed countries), the prevalence of degenerative MS is increasing. The basic pathology of degenerative MS is slowly progressive calcification of the fibrous annulus of the mitral valve. With severe annular calcification, MS and/or mitral regurgitation (MR) may develop.[1]

EPIDEMIOLOGY AND RISK FACTORS

The prevalence of MAC and degenerative MS has varied depending on the population characteristics, the imaging modality used, and the definition used. The prevalence of MAC in unselected adults (45–84 years of age) without CAD was 9% in a community-based study.[2] In elderly patients (>62–65 years of age), the prevalence increased to 42%–55%.[3,4] However, severe MAC resulting in MS is relatively uncommon and occurs in 6%–8% of

patients with MAC.[5] In a Japanese echocardiography study, the prevalence of degenerative MS was 0.22% and in the elderly population of >90 years of age, its prevalence was 2.5%.[6] In the Euro Heart survey, degenerative MS accounted for 12.5% of all MS cases detected by echocardiography. When age was taken into account, degenerative MS was responsible for ~10%, 20%, and 30% of all MS cases in the age groups 60–70, 70–80, and >80 years of age, respectively.[7] Other studies have reported that degenerative MS may account for up to 26% of all MS cases.[8,9]

Advanced age, female gender, chronic kidney disease, diabetes mellitus, hypertension, dyslipidemia, increased body mass index, aortic stenosis, and left-ventricular hypertrophy have been identified as risk factors for MAC.[2,10] Chest wall radiation also predisposes for MAC. Other associations include white race, smoking, high C reactive protein, and polymorphisms related to the proinflammatory gene *IL1F9*.[11–14]

Degenerative MS is a slowly progressive disease. The rate of progression of mitral valve gradient in degenerative MS was 0.8 ± 2.4 mmHg/year in one study.[15] A lower initial valve area and absence of β-blocker use was associated with faster progression. In another study, the mean increase in the mitral valve gradient was 2.0 mmHg/year.[16] Unlike aortic valve calcification, long-term prospective studies of degenerative MS are not available. Only one large retrospective study assessed the outcomes of 1004 degenerative MS patients over a mean follow-up of 3.5 ± 2.8 years.[17] The mean age was 73 ± 14 years. The one, five, and ten-year survival rates were 78%, 47%, and 25%, respectively. Five-year mortality was three times higher than expected mortality in the US general population. Higher grades of degenerative MS had lower survival rates. Thus, the prognosis of degenerative MS is poor.

MAC may be a marker of atherosclerosis as it is commonly associated with coronary and aortic calcification. MAC had a 92% positive predictive value for severe coronary artery disease in one study.[18] In another study of patients >65 years of age, 27% had combined aortic calcification and MAC.[3] MAC has been described as an independent risk factor for future cardiovascular events such as cardiovascular mortality, stroke, myocardial infarction, and atrial fibrillation.[19-21]

PATHOPHYSIOLOGY

MAC is a multifactorial process involving abnormal calcium and phosphorus hemostasis. Atherosclerosis and hemodynamic stress may further contribute to the calcification process. MAC typically involves the mitral fibrous annulus, with the posterior annulus being affected more than the anterior annulus. The entire circumference is involved in only 1.5% of cases.[22] The mitral annulus is a saddle-shaped structure and it provides important structural support to the atrial and ventricular myocardium. Annular movement in turn is determined by atrial and ventricular contraction and relaxation. Three types of annular movement have been identified: (1) translation movement, towards and away from the left-ventricular (LV) apex; (2) circumferential contraction; and (3) folding movement across the intercommissural axis. At the time of LV contraction, the folding motion prevents leaflet distortion during leaflet coaptation. Thus, the folding motion decreases leaflet closure stress as the LV systolic pressure increases. The mitral valve orifice and the LV systolic pressure are the two main determinants of mitral annular stress. Excessive stress on the mitral annulus as a result of increased LV systolic pressure (which in turn causes increased mitral valve closing pressure) results in tension and trauma to this fibrous structure. The sites of annular trauma are the nidus for dystrophic calcification resulting in MAC.[23] The calcification process may extend into the base of the valve leaflets and rarely may extend further into the leaflets, especially the anterior leaflet, restricting its mobility. The ventricular myocardium and papillary muscles may rarely be involved. Unlike rheumatic MS, commissural fusion is not seen in degenerative MS.[24]

Geometric distortion of the mitral apparatus, protruding calcification, reduction of normal mitral annular dilatation during diastole, and impaired anterior mitral leaflet mobility are possible mechanisms responsible for the development of MS by MAC.[25-27]

Caseous calcification is a rare variant of MAC. It is seen as a large, round echodense soft mass with a central echolucent area that may lead to exploratory cardiotomy. It consists of an admixture of calcium, fatty acids, and cholesterol, with a "toothpaste-like consistency" and may be mistaken for a tumor.[28,29] Caseous annular calcifications are less echo-dense and can be well distinguished on non-contrast-enhanced CT.

CLINICAL FEATURES

Exertional dyspnea, fatigue, and exercise intolerance are common presenting complaints. Pulmonary hypertension and atrial fibrillation are also common. Mid-diastolic murmur is the hallmark of MS, although a little more difficult to appreciate than that of rheumatic MS.

DIAGNOSIS

Echocardiography remains the main imaging modality for the diagnosis of degenerative MS.[30] Calcification of the mitral annulus and base of the leaflets are prominent findings. Calcification can be identified on echocardiography due to its echo-dense appearance and acoustic shadowing. However, echocardiography cannot discriminate calcium from dense collagen as it has poor tissue characterization. Valve leaflets are thickened and there may be decreased excursion of the anterior mitral leaflet. Commissural fusion is not seen. The estimation of mitral valve area and mean transmitral gradient forms the basis of estimation of MS severity.[30] Various echocardiographic methods are available for the assessment of mitral valve area, namely planimetery, pressure half-time, continuity equation, and proximal isovelocity surface area. While these methods have been evaluated and validated in rheumatic MS, their application in degenerative MS has not been corroborated by invasive hemodynamic study or surgically excised valves. Planimetry may be performed by two-dimensional or three-dimensional examination of the mitral orifice. The distorted mitral valve anatomy and the presence of calcium pose significant difficulty in getting a good parasternal short-axis view and accurate estimation of the mitral valve area. To some extent, this may be overcome by three-dimensional echocardiography. Pressure half-time may overestimate valve area due to the decreased LV compliance in elderly patients. While the continuity equation is best suited for degenerative MS, it is time-consuming. Further, it may be unreliable in the presence of coexistent regurgitant lesions.

The mean transmitral gradient is an easily derived parameter from Doppler echocardiography that helps quantify the severity of MS. In rheumatic MS, a mean gradient of <5 mmHg supports mild MS, whereas a mean gradient of >10 mmHg suggests severe MS. Similar criteria have been used for degenerative MS, although they have not been validated in this setting.[30] It must be noted that the transmitral gradient is affected by heart rate, mitral valve flow, presence of MR, and atrioventricular compliance.

Echocardiographic assessment should include visual appearance, calcification, thickening, leaflet mobility, adequacy of coaptation, mitral valve area, gradients, and severity of MR. The degree of calcification is best viewed in parasternal short-axis (or equivalent TEE) view.

Cardiac catheterization is the gold standard whenever echocardiographic assessment is inconclusive. Coronary evaluation is an additional advantage of cardiac catheterization. Fluoroscopic examination also provides a good estimate of calcification (Figure 20.1).

Computed tomography (CT) is ideal for evaluating the degree and extent of calcification. It provides complementary data to echocardiography. ECG gated CT can also be used to calculate mitral valve area by planimetry. CT also provides information about coronary arteries, cardiac anatomy, cardiac chamber volumes, intracardiac thrombus, ejection fraction, and wall motion abnormalities.

Advanced imaging techniques such as three-dimensional intracardiac echocardiography or fusion imaging with CT may be the answer to the limitations of MAC evaluation with conventional echocardiography and CT.

MANAGEMENT

The mainstay of treatment of degenerative MS is medical treatment with diuretics and heart rate control (usually with β-blockers).[31] Currently, no

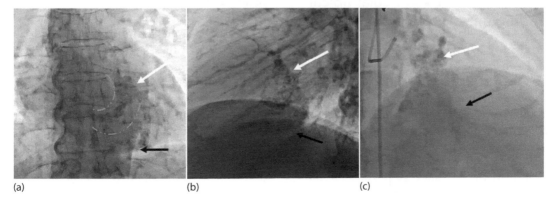

(a)   (b)   (c)

Figure 20.1 Fluroscopic imaging for mitral annular calcification (white arrow and between dotted lines) with myocardial extension (black arrow). **(a)** Anteroposterior view, **(b)** lateral view and **(c)** right oblique view.

therapy is available for preventing the progression of MAC. For those who are symptomatic despite medical therapy, the options are difficult. Percutaneous or surgical commissurotomies are not helpful in degenerative MS. Mitral valve replacement is an option, although technically challenging and difficult.[31,32]

Mitral valve replacement

The presence of annular calcium and associated multiple comorbities in the elderly population makes surgical treatment more challenging. MAC prevents reconstruction, reduction, and realignment of the mitral annulus during surgery. Further, the placement of valve sutures is difficult. Annular debridement with reconstruction is the standard surgical procedure for degenerative MS. Debridement of the annular calcium may result in ventricular rupture, injury to the left circumflex coronary artery or separation of the atrium and ventricle.[33,34] Ultrasonic pulverization has been used by some surgeons for decalcification in MAC.[35] Deep periannular sutures around the calcific annular bar can be used for anchoring the prosthetic mitral valve but it increases the chance of injury to the circumflex artery and paravalvular leak.[36] Paravalvular leak is an important complication and can be seen in up to 10% of cases after MVR for degenerative MS.[37] Patients with very high surgical risk should be offered palliative care or novel therapies such as transcatheter MVR (TMVR) or mitral valve bypass.

Left-atrial to left-ventricular apical conduit (mitral valve bypass)

Mitral valve bypass is an experimental treatment for degenerative MS that involves the placement of a valved conduit between the left atrium (LA) and LV without manipulating the calcified mitral annulus. The LA side of the conduit is sewn to the LA appendage and LV side at the apex. This provides the shortest path for the conduit. A bioprosthetic or mechanical valve is placed in the conduit as close to the LV apex as possible. If the LA appendage has been ligated previously or is very friable, the conduit is sewn to the left atriotomy site. Mitral valve bypass appears to be a less morbid and safer technique than standard MVR in this high-risk group of patients. However, long-term results are not available. Cardiopulmonary bypass and the aortic cross clamp times are shorter with this technique. Conduit thrombosis and kinking are some uncommon complications with this technique.[38]

Transcatheter mitral valve replacement (TMVR)

Transcatheter aortic valve devices are being used at the mitral valve, giving rise to the concept of TMVR. Both the SAPIEN XT valve and Direct Flow valve are being used for this purpose with reasonable success. In a global registry of TMVR[39] for degenerative MS with the balloon-expandable valves (N = 64), the prosthetic mitral valve was implanted via transatrial (15.6%), transapical (43.8%), antegrade (transvenous-transseptal), or modified antegrade (40.6%) approaches. The modified antegrade approach involved deploying the valve via the typical antegrade approach with a wire externalized through a sheath percutaneously placed in the left ventricle. Technical success was achieved in 72% of cases with 30-day all-cause mortality of 29.7%. Mean mitral valve gradient decreased from 11.4 ± 4.4 mmHg to 4 ± 2.2 mmHg. A second valve was required in 17.2% of cases, while LV outflow obstruction occurred in 9.3% of cases. Surprisingly, there were no incidence of significant paravalvular leak. Other complications of TMVR are valve embolization, left-ventricular perforation and pulmonary vein perforation.[31] The ongoing MITRAL (Mitral Implantation of Transcatheter Valves) trial will determine the feasibility and safety of this approach.[40]

A number of dedicated TMVR systems are available and some are in the process of development. However, these systems have been designed for severe native valve MR. Specifically designed devices will need to be developed for the treatment of degenerative MS. Special challenges in the development of such devices include anchoring devices in calcific annulus, difficulty in grasping leaflets, and the inability to place screws into the annulus. More recently, septal reduction in the setting of TMVR is an important consideration as LVOT obstruction is a common occurrence and degenerative MS usually occurs in the setting of LV hypertrophy. Surgical resection or alcohol septal ablation can be done to achieve an adequate LV outflow tract.[41]

Eleild and colleagues have proposed a treatment scheme on the basis of degree of MAC.[41]

1. *Grade 1 (mild)*. Focal noncontiguous calcification involving less than half of the total annular circumference, without any extra-annular calcification. Medical therapy and standard MVR are reasonable treatment options.
2. *Grade 2 (moderate)*. Dense continuous calcification involving more than half but less than three-quarters of the total annular circumference with/without posterior and/or anterior leaflet calcification. Standard MVR is reasonable if leaflets are not involved. Otherwise, TMVR or LA-LV conduit (if < moderate MR) can be considered.
3. *Grade 3 (severe)*. Dense continuous calcification extending past the commissures into the anterior annulus or complete circumferential calcification involving more than three-quarters of annulus. Calcification may extend into valve leaflets, papillary muscles, or ventricular myocardial. TMVR or LA-LV conduit (if < moderate MR) are reasonable therapeutic options.

CONCLUSION

Degenerative MS remains a difficult subset to treat. Emerging treatment options such as TMVR are promising modalities. Future research is needed to develop therapies for preventing the progression of mitral annular calcification.

REFERENCES

1. Korn D, Desanctis RW, Sell S. Massive calcification of the mitral annulus. A clinicopathological study of fourteen cases. *N Engl J Med* 1962;267:900–9.
2. Kanjanauthai S, Nasir K, Katz R et al. Relationships of mitral annular calcification to cardiovascular risk factors: The Multi-Ethnic Study of Atherosclerosis (MESA). *Atherosclerosis* 2010;213:558–62.
3. Barasch E, Gottdiener JS, Larsen EK, Chaves PH, Newman AB, Manolio TA. Clinical significance of calcification of the fibrous skeleton of the heart and aortosclerosis in community dwelling elderly: The Cardiovascular Health Study (CHS). *Am Heart J* 2006;151:39–47.
4. Aronow WS, Schwartz KS, Koenigsberg M. Correlation of murmurs of mitral stenosis and mitral regurgitation with presence or absence of mitral anular calcium in persons older than 62 years in a long-term health care facility. *Am J Cardiol* 1987;59:181–2.
5. Labovitz AJ, Nelson JG, Windhorst DM, Kennedy HL, Williams GA. Frequency of mitral valve dysfunction from mitral annular calcium as detected by Doppler echocardiography. *Am J Cardiol* 1985;55:133–7.
6. Ukita Y, Yuda S, Sugio H et al. Prevalence and clinical characteristics of degenerative mitral stenosis. *J Cardiol* 2016;68:248–52.
7. Iung B, Baron G, Butchart EG et al. A prospective survey of patients with valvular heart disease in Europe: The Euro Heart Survey on Valvular Heart Disease. *Eur Heart J* 2003;24:1231–43.
8. Akram MR, Chan T, McAuliffe S, Chenzbraun A. Non-rheumatic annular mitral stenosis: Prevalence and characteristics. *Eur J Echocardiogr* 2009;10:103–5.
9. Toufan M, Javadrashid R, Paak N, Gojazadeh M, Khalili M. Relationship between incidentally detected calcification of the mitral valve on 64-row multidetector computed tomography and mitral valve disease on echocardiography. *Int J Gen Med* 2012;5:839–43.
10. Abramowitz Y, Jilaihawi H, Chakravarty T, Mack MJ, Makkar RR. Mitral annulus calcification. *J Am Coll Cardiol* 2015;66:1934–41.
11. Kurtoğlu E, Korkmaz H, Aktürk E, Yılmaz M, Altaş Y, Uçkan A. Association of mitral annulus calcification with high-sensitivity C-reactive protein, which is a marker of inflammation. *Mediators Inflamm* 2012;606:207.
12. Bhatt H, Sanghani D, Julliard K, Fernaine G. Is mitral annular calcification associated with atherosclerotic risk factors and severity and complexity of coronary artery disease? *Angiology* 2015;66:659–66.
13. Forman MB, Virmani R, Robertson RM, Stone WJ. Mitral annular calcification in chronic renal failure. *Chest* 1984;85:367–71.
14. Thanassoulis G, Campbell CY, Owens DS et al. CHARGE Extracoronary Calcium Working Group. Genetic associations with valvular calcification and aortic stenosis. *N Engl J Med* 2013;368:503–12.

15. Tyagi G, Dang P, Pasca I, Patel R, Pai RG. Progression of degenerative mitral stenosis: Insights from a cohort of 254 patients. *J Heart Valve Dis* 2014;23:707–12.

16. Pressman GS, Agarwal A, Braitman LE, Muddassir SM. Mitral annular calcium causing mitral stenosis. *Am J Cardiol* 2010;105:389–91.

17. Pasca I, Dang P, Tyagi G, Pai RG. Survival in patients with degenerative mitral stenosis: Results from a large retrospective cohort study. *J Am Soc Echocardiogr* 2016;29:461–9.

18. Atar S, Jeon DS, Luo H, Siegel RJ. Mitral annular calcification: A marker of severe coronary artery disease in patients under 65 years old. *Heart* 2003;89:161–4.

19. Potpara TS, Vasiljevic ZM, Vujisic-Tesic BD et al. Mitral annular calcification predicts cardiovascular morbidity and mortality in middle aged patients with atrial fibrillation: The Belgrade Atrial Fibrillation Study. *Chest* 2011;140:902–10.

20. De Marco M, Gerdts E, Casalnuovo G et al. Mitral annular calcification and incident ischemic stroke in treated hypertensive patients: The LIFE study. *Am J Hypertens* 2013;26:567–73.

21. Kizer JR, Wiebers DO, Whisnant JP et al. Mitral annular calcification, aortic valve sclerosis, and incident stroke in adults free of clinical cardiovascular disease: The Strong Heart Study. *Stroke* 2005;36:2533–7.

22. Carpentier AF, Pellerin M, Fuzellier JF, Relland JY. Extensive calcification of the mitral valve anulus: Pathology and surgical management. *J Thoracic Cardiovasc Surg* 1996;111:718–29; discussion 729–30.

23. Silbiger JJ. Anatomy, mechanics, and pathophysiology of the mitral annulus. *Am Heart J* 2012;164:163–76.

24. Nestico PF, Depace NL, Morganroth J, Kotler MN, Ross J. Mitral annular calcification: Clinical, pathophysiology, and echocardiographic review. *Am Heart J* 1984;107:989–96.

25. Ramirez J, Flowers NC. Severe mitral stenosis secondary to massive calcification of the mitral annulus with unusual echocardiographic manifestations. *Clin Cardiol* 1980;3:284–7.

26. Osterberger LE, Goldstein S, Khaja F, Lakier JB. Functional mitral stenosis in patients with massive mitral annular calcification. *Circulation* 1981;64:472–6.

27. Muddassir SM, Pressman GS. Mitral annular calcification as a cause of mitral valve gradients. *Int J Cardiol* 2007;123:58–62.

28. Harpaz D, Auerbach I, Vered Z et al. Caseous calcification of the mitral annulus: A neglected, unrecognized diagnosis. *J Am Soc Echocardiogr* 2001;14:825–31.

29. Deluca G, Correale M, Ieva R et al. The incidence and clinical course of caseous calcification of the mitral annulus: A prospective echocardiographic study. *J Am Soc Echocardiogr* 2008;21:828–33.

30. Oktay AA, Gilliland YE, Lavie CJ et al. Echocardiographic assessment of degenerative mitral stenosis: A diagnostic challenge of an emerging cardiac disease. *Curr Probl Cardiol* 2017;42:71–100.

31. Sud K, Agarwal S, Parashar A et al. Degenerative mitral stenosis: Unmet need for percutaneous interventions. *Circulation* 2016;133:1594–1604.

32. Hellgren L, Kvidal P, Hörte LG, Krusemo UB, Ståhle E. Survival after mitral valve replacement: Rationale for surgery before occurrence of severe symptoms. *Ann Thorac Surg* 2004;78:1241–7.

33. Spencer FC, Galloway AC, Colvin SB. A clinical evaluation of the hypothesis that rupture of the left ventricle following mitral valve replacement can be prevented by preservation of the chordae of the mural leaflet. *Ann Surg* 1985;202:673–80.

34. MacVaugh H 3rd, Joyner CR, Johnson J. Unusual complications during mitral valve replacement in the presence of calcification of the annulus. *Ann Thorac Surg* 1971;11:336–42.

35. Baumgartner FJ, Pandya A, Omari BO, Turner C, Milliken JC, Robertson JM. Ultrasonic debridement of mitral calcification. *J Cardiac Surg* 1997;12:240–2.

36. Cammack PL, Edie RN, Edmunds LH Jr. Bar calcification of the mitral anulus. A risk factor in mitral valve operations. *J Thoracic Cardiovasc Surg* 1987;94:399–404.

37. Genoni M, Franzen D, Vogt P, Seifert B, Jenni R, Künzli A, Niederhäuser U, Turina M. Paravalvular leakage after mitral valve replacement: Improved long-term survival with aggressive surgery? *Eur J Cardiothorac Surg* 2000;17:14–9.

38. Said SM, Schaff HV. An alternate approach to valve replacement in patients with mitral stenosis and severely calcified annulus. *J Thoracic Cardiovasc Surg* 2014;147:e76–8.

39. Guerrero M, Dvir D, Himbert D et al. Transcatheter mitral valve replacement in native mitral valve disease with severe mitral annular calcification: Results from the first multicenter global registry. *J Am Coll Cardiol Intv* 2016;9:1361–71.

40. Guerrero M. Mitral implantation of transcatheter valves (MITRAL). Available at: https://clinicaltrials.gov/ct2/show/NCT02370511.

41. Eleid MF, Foley TA, Said SM, Pislaru SV, Rihal CS. Severe mitral annular calcification: Multimodality imaging for therapeutic strategies and interventions. *JACC Cardiovasc Imaging* 2016;9:1318–37.

21

Mitral bioprosthetic valve dysfunction

NEERAJ PARAKH

INTRODUCTION

There has been a significant increase in the use of bioprosthetic valves over the last few years. The main reasons for this change in clinical practice are an increase in the number of elderly population undergoing valve replacement, an improvement in the performance of newer-generation bioprosthetic valves, and the inherent problems of thromboembolic events and anticoagulation-related bleeding associated with the use of mechanical valves.[1] Increased use of bioprosthetic valves, combined with their relatively shorter durability and the increasing life expectancy of the population requiring valve replacements, has resulted in a major increase in the incidence of bioprosthetic valve dysfunction/failure.[2,3]

BIOPROSTHETIC VALVES

These are either aortic valves of porcine origin or prepared from bovine pericardium, that are mounted on a metallic stent for use as mitral bioprosthetic valves. These valves are fixed in glutaraldehyde to crosslink collagen fibers and reduce their antigenicity and cell viability. This results in improved valve durability. The advantage of bioprosthesis is that anticoagulation is not required after a period of 3 to 6 months post-implantation. However, depending upon the age at implantation, bioprosthetic valves start degenerating after 5 to 7 years and the average life span of the valve is 10 to 12 years. Earlier-generation bioprosthetic valves were fixed in glutaraldehyde at a higher pressure, which destroyed the normal architecture of the tissue. This resulted in early degeneration of these valves. Later-generation valves were fixed in zero or lower pressure, resulting in enhanced durability of these valves.[4] Improved valve design, anti-mineralization, and surfactant treatment have further contributed to the improvement in the durability of the bioprosthetic valves.[5] (Commonly used bioprostheses are listed in Table 14.6, Chapter 14.) More than 20 years' worth of follow-up data is available for Hancock II porcine and Carpentier-Edwards Perimount valves,[6] whereas data on Carpentier-Edwards Magna valves, Mosaic porcine valves, and Carbomedics Mitroflow pericardial valves spans 10–15 years.[7,8]

DEFINING VALVE DYSFUNCTION AND DURABILITY

Various definitions have been proposed for defining valve dysfunction. However, the most accepted definition as per guidelines for reporting mortality and morbidity after cardiac valve interventions is "Dysfunction or deterioration involving operated valve as determined by reoperation, autopsy or clinical investigations." This excludes reoperation because of infection or thrombosis. Durability of a valve is best defined as reoperation-free survival within their lifetime or actual freedom from reoperation before death.[9] The durability of bioprosthetic valves depends on three main factors: (1) intrinsic durability of the valve; (2) age of the patient at the time of implantation; and (3) life expectancy of the patient. The timing of reoperation also depends on patient- and physician-related factors. Comparative assessment of the durability of various bioprosthetic valves is difficult to determine as randomized studies for the same are not available. The observational studies have their inherent limitations as they are heterogeneous in nature, used different definitions for valve durability, substantial lost to follow-up, and a relatively small sample size with poorly defined statistical methods.[10] Grunkemeier et al. compiled 70 studies comprising more than 24,000 tissue valves and 132,000 years of follow-up. They concluded that "it cannot be known for certain from this information whether the newer valves have extended variability," and the current view is that decisions to choose a particular second- or third-generation bioprosthesis should be based on surgeon preference in the absence of outcome data favoring one valve over the other.[8] The lifetime risk of reoperation for a 50-year-old patient undergoing bioprosthetic valve replacement is approximately 45%, which decreases by approximately 10% for every five-year increment in the age of the patient at the time of surgery, and approximately 5% at 75 years of age.[10]

RISK FACTORS AND MECHANISMS OF BIOPROSTHETIC VALVE DYSFUNCTION

The most important risk factor for the failure of bioprosthetic valves is the age of the patient.[8] Besides younger age at implantation, renal failure, hyperparathyroidism, left-ventricular hypertrophy, left-ventricular dysfunction, hypertension, higher post-operative gradients, prosthesis-patient mismatch, and mitral valve position are associated with a higher risk of tissue valve deterioration.[11,12] A higher degeneration rate for mitral valve bioprosthesis as compared to aortic valve bioprosthesis may be partially related to the higher close-off pressure in the mitral position (usually >100 mmHg vs. <100 mmHg in the aortic position). Another factor is greater closure time with mitral prosthesis as compared with an aortic prosthesis, which possibly contributes to a greater degeneration rate of mitral bioprosthesis.[13]

Progressive degeneration of the valve tissue leads to structural dysfunction and bioprosthetic valve failure. The main pathophysiological mechanisms[13] leading to bioprosthetic valve dysfunction are described below:

1. *Calcification.* Calcification of the valve cusp is modulated by altered calcium-phosphorus hemostasis, lipid-mediated inflammation, and immune reactions. Besides intrinsic calcification of the leaflet tissue, extrinsic calcification can occur in the thrombi or vegetations attached to the valve tissue. Leaflet calcification decreases its mobility and promotes secondary tears. Calcification starts at the commissure and basal area of the cusps and may extend further into the leaflet.
2. *Collagen deterioration.* Bioprosthetic design-related tears due to progressive collagen deterioration are one possible mechanism for pericardial valve failure. Besides tears, perforation, stretching, thickening, stiffening, and prolapse of valve cusps also contribute to valve dysfunction. Microscopic examination of degenerated tissue valve leaflets show plasma fluid and lipid insudation, tissue swelling, tissue loss, fraying of collagen fibres, and distortion of the architecture of the leaflet.
3. Pannus formation, thrombus, and paravalvular leaks are other factors that are not related to intrinsic leaflet failure.

Valve stenosis as a result of bioprosthetic valve dysfunction occurs as a consequence to calcification, thickening, thrombus, or pannus formation, whereas valve regurgitation is because of leaflet tear, perforation, and paravalvular leak. In mitral bioprostheses, regurgitation is the predominant mechanism of valve dysfunction (49%), followed by stenosis (21%) and combined mechanisms (30%).[14]

DIAGNOSIS

Echocardiographic assessment is the most important investigation for the assessment of mitral valve bioprosthetic dysfunction. Although principles of echocardiographic examination remain the same as in the native valve, it poses more challenge for the examiner in the case of bioprosthetic valves. Echocardiography should determine the type of prosthesis, evaluate the valve leaflet morphology and mobility (thickness, calcification, prolapse, etc.), check the integrity and stability of the sewing ring, and assess the size of cardiac chambers, left-ventricular (LV) hypertrophy, LV function, and the pulmonary arterial systolic pressure (PASP). Transesophageal echocardiography (TEE) is more often required for the assessment of bioprosthetic valves as acoustic windows may not be optimal and Doppler alignment is difficult to achieve with transthoracic echocardiography (TTE).[15]

Normal echocardiographic appearance of bioprosthetic valves

Mitral bioprosthetic valves have three leaflets. Leaflets are thin structures with unrestricted movement. Two-dimensional echocardiography reveals a box-like appearance in diastole. The sewing ring and the three struts are more echogenic and hamper proper evaluation of leaflets. Sometimes thin, mildly echogenic, filamentous structures are several millimeters long (up to 30 mm in length) and move independently from the prosthetic valve can be seen intermittently during cardiac cycles. These strands are present in 6%–45% of cases. These are fibrinous or collagenous structures and their clinical or therapeutic implication is not clear.[16] A small central jet (<1 mL) of mitral regurgitation (at the point of apposition or close to the commissures) is normally present in "bioprosthetic valves" and is more frequently seen in bovine pericardial valves. The pressure half-time (PHT) method has not been validated for calculating valve area of a stenotic mitral prostheses. Other than the prosthetic valve area, PHT also depends on the pressure gradient at the start of diastole and to LV and left-atrial compliance.[17] However, the PHT may be useful if it is significantly delayed or shows significant lengthening on serial measurements, despite similar heart rates. Because of their design, prosthetic valves are inherently stenotic. The normal reference values for various bioprosthetic valves at mitral position are mentioned in Table 21.1.

Pathological valve obstruction

Restricted leaflet movements along with thickening and calcification are commonly occurring changes encountered with degenerative bioprosthetic valves and can be identified on 2D and 3D echocardiography (Figure 21.1). An increase in mean gradient of greater than 5 mmHg with similar heart rates is suggestive of pathological valve stenosis. Other Doppler parameters that indicate prosthetic mitral valve obstruction are PHT >130, peak velocity >1.9 m/s and increase in mean gradient of >5 mmHg on stress echocardiography (Figure 21.2). Indicators of pathological valve stenosis on effective orifice area are valve area <2 cm^2 or less than one standard deviation from the reference value or a decrease of >0.25 cm^2 from the reference value.[15] Criteria for definitive valve stenosis are PHT >200, peak velocity >2.5 m/s, mean gradient >10 mmHg, effective orifice area <1.0 cm^2 or <2 standard deviation from the reference value or a decrease of >0.35 cm^2 from the reference value. Patient prosthesis mismatch can sometimes give the impression of bioprosthesis stenosis. Comparison from immediate postoperative values can help in differentiating between the two conditions.

Table 21.1 Normal reference values of effective orifice areas in mm$_2$ for bioprosthetic valves at mitral position[18]

Valve size (mm)	25	27	29	31	33
Medtronic mosaic	1.5 ± 0.4	1.7 ± 0.5	1.9 ± 0.5	1.9 ± 0.5	–
Hancock II	1.5 ± 0.4	1.8 ± 0.5	1.9 ± 0.5	2.6 ± 0.5	2.6 ± 0.7
Carpentier-Edwards Perimount	1.6 ± 0.4	1.8 ± 0.4	2.1 ± 0.5	–	–

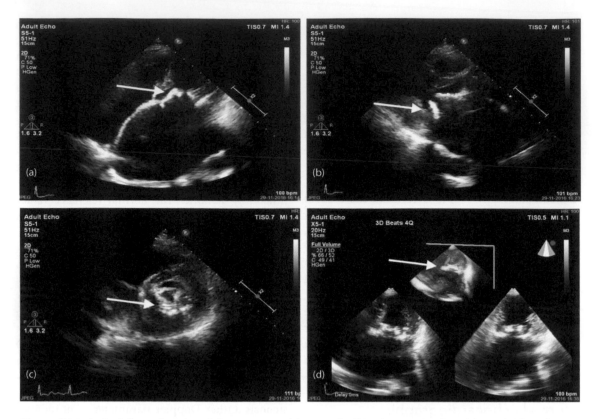

Figure 21.1 Apical four-chamber **(a)**, parasternal long-axis **(b)**, short-axis view **(c)**, and 3D echocardiography view **(d)** of bioprosthetic valve showing hyperechoic annulus and struts (arrow) with early degenerative changes.

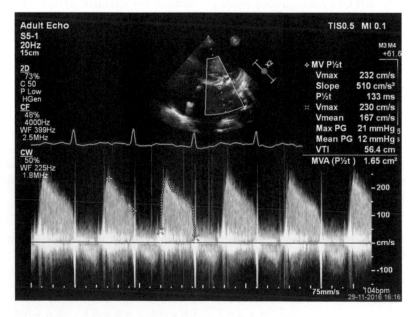

Figure 21.2 Pressure half-time and gradients across the bioprosthetic valve suggestive of early degenerative changes.

Computed tomography (CT) could be considered for imaging the cusps of tissue valves (leaflet thickening, calcification, or thrombus) if TEE is not conclusive. CT may help in differentiating between thrombus and pannus. Cardiac magnetic resonance may be helpful in showing leaflet restriction and calculating valve orifice area.[19]

TREATMENT

Repeat mitral valve replacement (MVR) is the standard-of-care treatment for mitral bioprosthetic valve dysfunction. Given the challenges of repeat operation, especially in elderly and high-surgical-risk populations, novel methods such as transcatheter mitral valve replacement (TMVR) are increasingly being used. Percutaneous balloon mitral valvuloplasty (BMV) has occasionally been tried in those with suitable valve morphology[20] (Figure 21.3, Video 21.1). Some studies have suggested that BMV for mitral bioprosthesis stenosis carries significant risk of leaflet tear and rupture.[21] However, BMV may be a suitable palliative procedure in appropriately selected patients, who have commissural fusion but without marked cusp degeneration and calcification.

Transcatheter mitral valve replacement or mitral valve in valve

Transcatheter mitral valve replacement (TMVR) has emerged as a less invasive procedure to redo MVR for high-surgical-risk patients. It provides acceptable outcomes in high-risk patients with degenerated bioprosthesis. Originally used for aortic valves, these devices are being used for the mitral valve as an off-label indication. For a retrograde (transapical) TMVR approach, the Sapien aortic valve has to be inversely mounted onto the balloon catheter.[22]

In a recently published TMVR registry[23] of 248 patients with a mean Society of Thoracic Surgeons score of 8.9 ± 6.8%, 176 patients underwent mitral valve in valve (ViV) and 72 patients underwent valve in ring (ViR) between 2009 to 2017. In the ViV group, 36% had pure MR, 36% had pure MS, and 28% had combined lesions. MS was uncommon in the ViR group, with 4% having pure MS and 18% having combined lesions. Transseptal access and the balloon-expandable valve were used in 33.1% and 89.9% of cases, respectively. Since MS is not an issue for previous ring repair, here we will only focus on the results of ViV. However, in general, results and complications were better with ViV than ViR. The technical success rate for the ViV group was 96%, as second valve implantation was required in 2.8%. The device success rate was 89.2% due to repeat intervention in 7.4% of cases. The post-procedural mitral valve gradient was 5.8 ± 2.7 mmHg. Significant MR was present in 6.8%, life-threatening bleeding in 2.3%, acute kidney injury in 4.0%, and LVOT obstruction in 2.3% of cases. Thirty-day and one-year all-cause mortality was 5.75% and 12.6%, respectively. A frequent concern related to the transseptal ViV procedure is the presence of a large atrial septal defect at the end of the transcatheter procedure, requiring the placement of a percutaneous closure device in

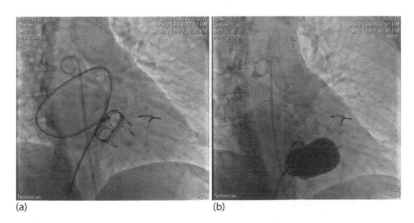

(a) (b)

Figure 21.3 Balloon mitral valvotomy for stenotic mitral bioprosthesis. **(a)** Left-ventricular entry with reverse loop; **(b)** balloon inflation across the valve (see Video 21.1). (Courtesy of Dr. Sunil K Verma, Department of Cardiology, AIIMS, New Delhi, India.)

12.2% of cases. On univariable analysis, the factors associated with one-year all-cause mortality were age, predominant MR at baseline, LV ejection fraction, failed annuloplasty ring, and more than moderate post-procedural MR. After multivariable analysis, only age and failed annuloplasty ring were independently associated with one-year all-cause mortality. The authors of this registry concluded that the procedural and clinical outcomes of TMVR for patients with degenerated mitral bioprostheses were acceptable in the study subjects despite high surgical risk and presence of multiple comorbidities.

Onorati et al. analyzed 260 patients (who were potential candidates for TMVR) undergoing redo-surgery in an observational, retrospective study. They identified advanced age, very high EuroSCORE-II or STS-score, preoperative severe left-ventricular systolic dysfunction, severe pulmonary hypertension, renal failure on dialysis, and previous CABG as extremely high-risk factors for redo MVR. These patients might possibly benefit from TMVR.[24]

Overall, TMVR is still an evolving technology and more experience and innovation are required for using this technology as a definitive therapeutic option. There is a need for dedicated mitral devices for TMVR, the standardization of technique and patient selection criteria, appropriate experience and training for the procedure, and evaluation of need for antithrombotic therapy after TMVR.

CONCLUSIONS

Mitral bioprosthetic valvular dysfunction is emerging as an important cause of mitral stenosis in developed countries, owing to the increased usage of bioprosthetic valves and an aging population with greater life expectancy. As of now, redo MVR is the standard of care for this high-surgical-risk population but transcatheter mitral valve replacement is rapidly evolving as a promising therapeutic option.

VIDEO

Video 21.1 Balloon dilatation of stenotic bioprosthetic valve (corresponds to Figure 21.3). https://youtu.be/eJ0PyffdLZU (Courtesy of Dr. Sunil K. Verma, AIIMS, New Delhi.)

REFERENCES

1. Brown JM, O'Brien SM, Wu C et al. Isolated aortic valve replacement in North America comprising 108,687 patients in 10 years: Changes in risks, valve types, and outcomes in the Society of Thoracic Surgeons National Database. J Thorac Cardiovasc Surg 1990;137:82–90.
2. Bonow RO, Carabello BA, Kanu C et al. ACC/AHA 2006 guidelines for the management of patients with valvular heart disease: A report of the American College of Cardiology/American Heart Association Task Force on Practice Guidelines (writing committee to revise the 1998 Guidelines for the Management of Patients with valvular Heart Disease): Developed in collaboration with the Society of Cardiovascular Anesthesiologists: Endorsed by the Society for Cardiovascular Angiography and Interventions and the Society of Thoracic Surgeons. Circulation 2006;114:e84–231.
3. Carpentier A. Lasker Clinical Research Award. The surprising rise of nonthrombogenic valvular surgery. Nat Med 2007;13:1165–8.
4. Eric Jamieson WR, Marchand MA, Pelletier CL et al. Structural valve deterioration in mitral replacement surgery: Comparison of Carpentier-Edwards supra-annular porcine and perimount pericardial bioprostheses. J Thorac Cardiovasc Surg 1999;118:297–304.
5. Chikwe J, Filsoufi F, Carpentier A. Prosthetic Heart Valves, in Fuster V, Walsh RA, O'Rourke RA et al. Hurst's the Heart. New York, McGraw-Hill Medical, 2011:1757–3.
6. Chan V, Kulik A, Tran A et al. Long-term clinical and hemodynamic performance of the Hancock II versus the perimount aortic bioprostheses. Circulation 2010;122:S10–S16.
7. Dalmau MJ, González-Santos JM, Blázquez JA et al. Hemodynamic performance of the Medtronic Mosaic and perimount Magna aortic bioprostheses: Five-year results of a prospectively randomized study. Eur J Cardiothorac Surg 2011;39:844–52.
8. Grunkemeier GL, Li HH, Naftel DC et al. Long-term performance of heart valve prostheses. Curr Probl Cardiol 2000;25:73–154.

9. Akins CW, Miller DC, Turina MI et al. Guidelines for reporting mortality and morbidity after cardiac valve interventions. *J Thorac Cardiovasc Surg* 2008;135:732–8.

10. Chikwe J, Filsoufi F. Durability of tissue valves. *Semin Thorac Cardiovasc Surg* 2011;23(1):18–23.

11. Poirer NC, Pelletier LC, Pellerin M et al. 15 year experience with the Carpentier-Edwards pericardial bioprosthesis. *Ann Thorac Surg* 1998;66:S57–61.

12. Ruel M, Kulik A, Rubens FD et al. Late incidence and determinants of reoperation in patients with prosthetic heart valves. *Eur J Cardiothorac Surg* 2004;25:364–70.

13. Schoen FJ, Levy RJ. Calcification of tissue heart valve substitutes: Progress toward understanding and prevention. *Ann Thorac Surg* 2005;79:1072–80.

14. Ribeiro AHS, Wender OCB, de Almeida AS et al. Comparison of clinical outcomes in patients undergoing mitral valve replacement with mechanical or biological substitutes: A 20 years cohort. *BMC Cardiovasc Disord* 2014;14:146–58.

15. Lancellotti P, Pibarot P, Chambers J et al. Recommendations for the imaging assessment of prosthetic heart valves: A report from the European Association of Cardiovascular Imaging endorsed by the Chinese Society of Echocardiography, the Inter-American Society of Echocardiography, and the Brazilian Department of Cardiovascular Imaging. *Eur Heart J Cardiovasc Imaging* 2016;17:589–90.

16. Rozich JD, Edwards WD, Hanna RD, Laffey DM, Johnson GH, Klarich KW. Mechanical prosthetic valve-associated strands: Pathologic correlates to transesophageal echocardiography. *J Am Soc Echocardiogr* 2003;16:97–100.

17. Baumgartner H, Hung J, Bermejo J et al. Echocardiographic assessment of valve stenosis: EAE/ASE recommendations for clinical practice. *Eur J Echocardiogr* 2009;10:1–25.

18. Pibarot P, Dumesnil JG. Prosthetic heart valves: Selection of the optimal prosthesis and long-term management. *Circulation* 2009;119:1034–48.

19. von Knobelsdorff-Brenkenhoff F, Rudolph A, Wassmuth R et al. Feasibility of cardiovascular magnetic resonance to assess the orifice area of aortic bioprostheses. *Circ Cardiovasc Imaging* 2009;2:397–404.

20. Calvo OL, Sobrino N, Gamallo C, Oliver J, Dominguez F, Iglesias A. Balloon percutaneous valvuloplasty for stenotic bioprosthetic valves in the mitral position. *Am J Cardiol* 1987;60:736–7.

21. Lin PJ, Chang JP, Chu JJ, Chang CH. Balloon valvuloplasty is contraindicated in stenotic mitral bioprosthesis. *Am Heart J* 1994;127:724–6.

22. Cheung A, Webb JG, Barbanti M, Freeman M, Binder RK, Thompson C, Wood DA, Ye J. 5-year experience with transcatheter transapical mitral valve-in-valve implantation for bioprosthetic valve dysfunction. *J Am Coll Cardiol* 2013;61:1759–66.

23. Yoon SII, Whisenant BK, Bleiziffer S et al. Transcatheter mitral valve replacement for degenerated bioprosthetic valves and failed annuloplasty rings. *J Am Coll Cardiol* 2017;70:1121–31.

24. Onorati F, Mariscalco G, Reichart D et al. Hospital outcome and risk-indices of mortality after redo-mitral valve surgery in potential candidates to transcatheter procedures: Results from a European registry. *J Cardiothorac Vasc Anesth* (Accepted manuscript). https://doi.org/10.1053/j.jvca.2017.09.039.

Miscellaneous

22

Pulmonary hypertension in mitral stenosis

RAVI S. MATH

INTRODUCTION

Pulmonary hypertension (PH) often complicates the course of mitral stenosis (MS). It significantly affects the clinical scenario and the long-term prognosis of MS. The PH is frequently out of proportion to the degree of elevation of left-atrial pressure (LAP), indicating a rise in pulmonary vascular resistance (PVR). In the words of Paul Wood: "The behavior of the pulmonary vascular resistance is perhaps the most important physiological event in mitral stenosis and, to a large extent, determines the course and pattern of the disease."[1]

DEFINITION

PH is defined as a mean pulmonary artery pressure (PAP) of ≥25 mmHg at rest as measured by right-heart catheterization.[2,3] PH associated with valvular heart disease (including MS) is classified as group 2 PH in the WHO classification of PH.[2] In this group, the mean pulmonary capillary wedge pressure (PCWP) is elevated (>15 mmHg). (Technically speaking, the term pulmonary artery hypertension is reserved for group 1 PH. In this review, the term PH is deemed to indicate group 2 PH unless specified otherwise.) PVR forms an important part of the assessment of PH in MS. The upper limit of normal PVR is 2 Wood Units (WU) and a cutoff of 3 WU is used as part of the hemodynamic definition of PH.[3,4] However, PVR is not a part of the general definition of pulmonary artery hypertension (PAH).[4]

MECHANISM

The mechanism of PH secondary to MS may be passive or reactive.[5-7] In the former, the elevated PH is due to passive retrograde transmission of the elevated left-atrial and pulmonary venous pressures into the pulmonary arterial vasculature. Here, the mean PAP and mean PCWP are elevated while the PVR is within normal limits (<3 WU).[3] The transpulmonary gradient (TPG = mean PAP minus mean PCWP) and the diastolic pulmonary gradient

(DPG = diastolic PAP minus mean PAWP) are not elevated (<12 and <7 mmHg, respectively).[3] The rise in PAP runs parallel to the rise in left-atrial pressure; the latter may reach extremely high levels. This type of PH is also described as isolated post-capillary PH and is immediately reversed by relief of mitral obstruction (by valvotomy or valve replacement).

The reactive PH is due to two mechanisms: (1) pulmonary arteriolar vasoconstriction induced by pulmonary venous hypertension; and (2) morphologic changes in pulmonary vasculature. The mean PAP and mean PCWP are elevated. The PVR is elevated to >3 WU.[3] The elevation of PAP is out of proportion to that of PCWP (or left-atrial pressure).[5] The TPG and DPG are also elevated (>12 and >7 mmHg, respectively).[3] This form of PH is described as combined/mixed post-capillary and pre-capillary PH.[3] The first component of reactive PH (i.e., vasoconstriction) is reversible and slowly reduces over weeks to months after relief of obstruction. The second component (morphologic change) is often described as the "fixed" component and tends to persist after relief of MS and may or may not reverse over years.[8]

PREVALENCE AND NATURAL HISTORY

The prevalence of PH has varied depending on the severity of MS, the symptomatic status of patients, and the time period during which these studies have been published. Over the decades, the cutoffs used to demarcate moderate and severe degrees of PH have changed with a progressive lowering of the values. In approximately 10%–20% of patients with severe MS, PA pressure is normal.[9-11] Fifty to sixty percent of patients have mild degrees of PH[10,12] (mean PAP 25–40 mmHg, PASP <50 mmHg), whereas moderate elevation of PAP is noted in another 20%–30% of patients[10,12] (mean PAP 41–55 mmHg, PASP 50–79 mmHg). Severe and extreme PH is noted in 5%–10% of patients[12-14] (mean PAP >55 mmHg, PASP >80 mmHg). As mentioned earlier, the prevalence of severe PH is sensitive to the definition used. When a lower cutoff for PASP (>50–60 mmHg) is used, the proportion of severe PH jumps to 23%–40%.[9,11] An elevated PVR of >4 WU is seen in 28% of patients.[15] Moderately high PVR (6–10 WU) was seen in 16% of cases and extremely high PVR (>10 WU) was noted in 12% of cases, among a series of 500 patients with

severe MS.[16] Patients with juvenile MS develop PH more frequently and rapidly.[17] Two-thirds of these patients have moderate to severe PH and an equal number of patients have grossly abnormal PVR.[17]

Patients with PH have poor survival. Ward and Hancock[13] followed up 48 patients with mitral valve disease with severe PH (PASP >80 mmHg and PVR >10 WU). The mean survival among patients who did not undergo surgery was 2.9 ± 0.5 years. One quarter of these patients died within six months and half by 12 months after catheterization. Olesen[18] noted that unoperated patients with right-axis deviation on ECG and/or increased hilar markings (suggestive of pulmonary hypertension) had markedly poor survival rates as compared to those without these signs (ten-year survival of 14% and 5%, respectively, vs. 38% and 49% for patients without these signs). It has been shown that the PVR may rise four- to tenfold within a span of 2 to 3 years.[19] Further, this increase in PVR could occur abruptly at any time within the course of the disease and this rise does not necessarily coincide with increase in the severity of MS or a rise in LAP. On the other hand, in many patients with advanced MS and elevated LAP, elevated PVR never develops. Thus, while left-atrial hypertension is required for sustaining high PVR, other factors are needed to trigger this abnormal reaction.[19]

ETIOLOGY

The severity of MS (in terms of mitral valve area and transmitral gradient) is an important factor for the development of reactive PH.[20] Reactive PH is not seen in cases of mild MS.[5] Varying degrees of PH develop only when MS is moderate or severe.[12,21] It must be noted that not all patients with severe MS develop severe degrees of elevation of PAP. There is a group of patients with severe MS where the PAP is either normal or only mildly elevated (from passive PH alone and no reactive PH).[5,9-12] Thus, there is a marked variability in the pulmonary vascular reactivity to chronic LAP elevation.

Patients developing severe PH are more often female[22,23] (the male:female ratio is even more skewed than in usual MS), with a tendency to be in sinus rhythm,[22,24] are more symptomatic,[14,23] with more severe subvalvular fibrosis,[14] higher transmitral gradient and lower mitral valve area.[14,23] No significant relation has been noted between left-atrial size and PAP. Rather, left-atrial enlargement may serve to "cushion" the effects of increased LAP.[20]

The time frame as to when the passive form of PH transits to the reactive form is highly variable[25] and is not related to either the degree or chronicity of LAP elevation.[25] Thus, neither the patient's age nor the duration of symptoms are important factors.[16,19] Whether ethnic, congenital, or environmental factors are involved is unknown. Roy et al. noted that PH and extreme PVR is common and frequently seen before the age of 20 years in India. He postulated that the severe PH with severe pulmonary vascular changes at such a young age may be due to a hypersensitive reaction of the pulmonary vasculature to a fulminant rheumatic process or a tissue response to recurrent attacks of rheumatic fever or ongoing low-grade rheumatic activity.[17] However, conclusive experimental evidence for this theory is currently lacking.

Jordan proposed that once the LAP exceeds the plasma colloid osmotic pressure (25 mmHg), fluid passes into the alveolar walls, causing them to become thickened due to edema and fibrosis.[26] This initially affects the lower zones more than the upper zones due to greater hydrostatic pressure. This leads to a difference in compliance between adjacent alveoli, a reduction in ventilation:perfusion ratio, and alveolar hypoxia. The reduced oxygen tension in the pulmonary venous blood leaving these alveoli is sensed by chemoreceptors, which leads to reflex constriction of the small muscular pulmonary arteries. This process diverts much of the pulmonary blood flow to the mid- and upper zones without an overall increase in PVR initially. However, eventually, the alveolar thickening spreads upwards to involve the whole lung, leading to an increase in PVR.

Wood had initially postulated the existence of a vasoconstrictive factor that was responsible for reactive PH.[1] He demonstrated a significant fall in the PAP and PVR along with a rise in LAP and cardiac output after intrapulmonary injection of acetylcholine.[16] A similar fall in TPG, PAP, and PVR was demonstrated after inhalation of nitric oxide in women with severe MS with PH,[27] thereby demonstrating that endothelium-dependent vascular tone plays a major role in the elevated PVR in MS patients. Finally, levels of endothelin-1 have been shown to be increased in patients with MS with PH[28,29] and correlated with mean PAP, mean PCWP, and PVR. Endothelin-1 is a potent vasoconstrictor and mitogen that is involved in vasoconstriction and vascular remodeling in PH. Endothelin-1 levels from pulmonary capillaries were an independent predictor of regression of PCWP after correction of mitral stenosis.[29]

PATHOLOGY[5,30,31]

Morphologic changes are noted in the pulmonary vasculature and lung parenchyma in patients with reactive PH. These are responsible for the "fixed" component of the reactive PH. The large pulmonary arteries (main trunk and branch PA) demonstrate fatty streaks and uncomplicated atheromas. The most important changes are seen in the small muscular arteries, arterioles, and venules. The muscular arteries show intimal thickening and hypertrophy of the media along with fragmentation of elastic lamina. The arterial lumen is severely narrowed and sometimes occluded with thrombi. This thickening of pulmonary artery walls has been demonstrated in-vivo using optical coherence tomography.[32] Pulmonary vascular changes beyond grade III (Heath-Edwards' classification) are not commonly seen.[33] Dilatation lesions (Heath-Edwards grade 5, vein like branches of hypertrophied pulmonary artery and angiomatoid lesions) were reported from 4% of cases from India.[31] Rarely, necrotizing arteritis (Heath-Edwards Grade 6) is seen.[5] Plexiform lesions (Heath Edwards Grade 4) have not been described in MS with severe PH.[34] Arterioles show muscularization and intimal proliferation. The main veins are dilated while the small veins show medial hypertrophy. Lymphatics are dilated. Alveolar walls show thickening and fibrosis along with intimal proliferation of alveolar capillaries. Importantly, hypertrophy of the musculature of the bronchiolo-alveolar system was noted in a majority of cases from India.[31] Hemosiderosis was noted in 70% of cases. There was a lack of correlation between the degree of elevation of PVR and the magnitude of pathologic changes in lungs suggesting that vasoconstriction plays an important role in producing PH in MS.[30] However, the degree of medial hypertrophy was proportional to the level of PAP.[31]

HEMODYNAMICS

As the mitral valve (MV) narrows, a stage is reached where the LAP is elevated. Initially this elevation occurs during exercise alone, but subsequently, as the MV narrows further, the LAP is elevated even at rest. This increased LAP is transmitted to the pulmonary veins, then further back to pulmonary capillaries (leading to an increase in PCWP) and finally the pulmonary artery, as these are all serially connected. In the initial stage, the rise in PAP is due to passive transmission of the elevated LAP and the normal pressure gradient across the lungs is maintained. The degree of elevation of PAP is concordant to the degree of elevation of LAP. As a result, the TPG, DPG, and PVR are all within normal limits. This form of passive PH is completely reversible with relief of MS. This phase of passive elevation in the PAP has been thought to be maintained until the LAP is chronically elevated to 20–25 mmHg (approximately equal to the plasma colloid osmotic pressure). Once the LAP rises above 20–25 mmHg,[20,26] a disproportionate rise in the PAP pressure occurs along with an increase in TPG, DPG, and PVR. It needs to be emphasized that this "reactive" rise in PAP is variable and, as mentioned earlier, is not uniformly seen in all patients with the same degree of elevation of LAP. This reactive form of PH may be reversible or fixed. What triggers this disproportionate rise in some patients has been a matter of research and great debate.

An important aspect is the relationship of elevated PAP and PVR. In the original Wood study,[1] when the PASP was above 100 mmHg, the PVR was always raised, whereas when the PASP was <50 mmHg, the PVR was rarely raised. Between PASP of 50–100 mmHg, the PVR varied significantly. When the TPG was >25 mmHg, the PVR was always more than 6 WU. Further, the PVR was linearly related to TPG; a PVR of 6–10 WU was seen when the TPG was between 20 and 30 mmHg, whereas the PVR was between 10 and 30 WU when the TPG ranged between 30 and 70 mmHg[1].

The right ventricle (RV) bears the brunt of all these processes. Chronically, the RV adapts to increased afterload by means of hypertrophy.[24] In severe MS, massive RV hypertrophy enables the RV to function against tremendous pressures (even suprasystemic PAP) over sustained periods of time. The RV pressure increases in consort with the PASP. Over time, the RV begins to dilate and loses its normal crescent shape to become more spherical. This leads to functional tricuspid regurgitation (TR). Initially, the dilated RV maintains cardiac output through the Frank-Starling mechanism. Once all mechanisms of contractile reserve are exhausted, the RV begins to fail. As the RV and LV are in series, reduction in RV output will lead to reduced LV filling (already aggravated by MS) and low cardiac output with a fall in systemic pressure. Thus, with the onset of PH, a "secondary" stenosis develops at the pulmonary bed-level that further leads to a decline in cardiac output. As the RV fails, the PAP may become relatively low, leading to underestimation of the extent of pulmonary vascular disease.[24] In such cases, despite the relatively low PAP, PVR is markedly elevated, thereby reflecting the true extent of pulmonary vascular disease. It has been suggested that this increased PVR protects the pulmonary capillary bed at the expense of the RV.[1] The high PVR saves the patient from drowning in pulmonary edema at the expense of a low cardiac output. This is unlikely to be a protective mechanism in the long term, given the rapidity with which death occurs from congestive heart failure in these patients. The RV hypertrophy leads to reduced subendocardial perfusion, whereas RV dilatation leads to increased wall stress, both of which lead to mismatch in oxygen demand and supply, provoking ischemia and symptoms of effort angina.

SYMPTOMS AND SIGNS IN MS WITH PULMONARY HYPERTENSION[1,5,24,35,36]

When the PH is passive, the symptoms expected in MS predominate, namely, exertional dyspnea, orthopnea, paroxysmal nocturnal dyspnea, hemoptysis, etc. When the PH becomes reactive, these symptoms are overshadowed by symptoms of low cardiac output and right-heart failure. Thus, fatigue, angina, exertional syncope, pedal edema, and abdominal distension predominate when the PVR becomes extreme. Wood[1] had suggested that this is protective to the patient as it saves the patient from drowning in pulmonary edema at the expense of low cardiac output. This has been contested by other authors,[24,35] who demonstrated that patients with reactive PH continue to have nocturnal dyspnea and hemoptysis.

The classic physical signs of MS with passive PH are modified in the presence of elevated PVR. The low cardiac output leads to cold cyanosed peripheries, malar flush (mitral facies), low volume pulse, and low arterial BP.[1,5,35] The jugular venous pressure (JVP) is raised with a prominent *a* wave in patients with sinus rhythm. A prominent *v* wave may be seen in the presence of TR. A left parasternal heave indicative of RV hypertrophy and palpable second heart sound is seen in moderate to severe PH. Auscultation is often modified. The first heart sound may be soft and the opening snap absent as the MV is often calcified. The pulmonary component of the second heart sound is loud and may be delayed in the presence of RV failure. A pulmonary ejection click may be heard in some cases. The characteristic murmur of MS is modified. The mid-diastolic murmur is often soft or entirely absent ("silent" MS[19]) due to the low volume of blood flowing across the tightly stenosed MV. Similarly, the presystolic accentuation is often not appreciated. The functional TR leads to a systolic murmur, which is often widely heard. Owing to the rotation of the heart and the increased RV size, its differentiation from the murmur of mitral regurgitation may be difficult. A Graham-Steell murmur (pulmonary diastolic murmur) may be heard at the left sternal border. Other signs of right-heart failure such as hepatomegaly, ascites, and pedal edema may be evident.

DIAGNOSIS

Right-heart catheterization is the gold standard for confirming the diagnosis of PH.[2,3] In the current era, a commonly used classification based on mean PAP and PASP is as follows:[10,11] (1) Mild PAH, mean PAP 25–40 mmHg, PASP 35–44 mmHg; (2) Moderate PAH, mean PAP 41–55 mmHg, PASP 45–59 mmHg; and (3) Severe PAH, mean PAP >55 mmHg, PASP ≥60 mmHg. Being invasive, right-heart catheterization is performed only at the time of intervention or when non-invasive methods are non-diagnostic.

The ECG and chest X-ray are helpful in the diagnosis of PH, although they have low sensitivity. The ECG findings of severe PH include right-ventricular hypertrophy (tall R-wave, with or without a small s-wave, followed by T-wave inversion in lead V1), right-atrial enlargement, and right-axis deviation. The chest X-ray reveals dilatation of the main PA and its branches along with the other classical findings of MS.

Echocardiography is the non-invasive imaging modality of choice for the assessment of PH. It needs to be emphasized that the correlation between echocardiography and catheterization is

modest (r ≈ 0.7)[25] and the PASP may be over- or underestimated by TR velocity. The TR jet velocity enables assessment of PASP, whereas the mean PAP can be estimated using various formulae.[37] Detailed evaluation is covered in the chapter on echocardiography. Findings in reactive PH include moderate to severe elevation of PAP, dilatation of right-sided chambers, significant TR, RV dysfunction, systolic flattening of interventricular septum, reduced acceleration time (<100 ms), and systolic RV outflow tract Doppler notching.[36,37] The absence of RV outflow Doppler notching predicts a PVR of ≤3 WU, whereas systolic notching strongly corresponds with a PVR >3 WU (mid- and late systolic notching correspond to a PVR >6 WU and 3–6 WU, respectively).[38]

Differentiation between the reversible and fixed types of PH before relief of MS is difficult although a response to vasodilator challenge (inhaled nitric oxide, intrapulmonary acetylcholine)[16,27] in normalizing TPG has been used to suggest that the functional abnormality predominates over structural abnormality.

OUTCOMES OF SURGERY/ PERCUTANEOUS INTERVENTION IN PH

The presence of PH leads to higher surgical mortality owing to right-heart failure and low cardiac output. The mortality for surgical valvotomy increased fourfold to 11%–13%[8,13] when the PVR was >10 WU. These studies were conducted more than four to five decades ago. Over the years, surgical techniques have improved, with better myocardial preservation, preservation of subvalvular apparatus, and improved postoperative care. Yet, the mortality for mitral valve replacement with severe PAH remains elevated even in the current era. The operative mortality of severe MS with severe PH is around 5%–10%.[11,33,39,40] The mortality is even greater in patients with suprasystemic PAH, at 28.5%.[33] Following MVR, the long-term survival of patients with MS with moderate to severe PH is reduced. In this group, ten-year survival ranges from 58% to 64%[11,40] as compared to 83% for patients with normal to mild PH.[11] As such, early intervention has been recommended before "fixed" PVR sets in.

The performance of percutaneous transvenous mitral commissurotomy (PTMC) in patients with severe PH has its own set of challenges.[14,41]

The dilated right-heart chambers make transseptal puncture more challenging, whereas the tightly stenosed MV makes the balloon crossing technically difficult. As these patients have a higher Wilkins score and more subvalvular disease, there is a greater risk of development of severe MR. Finally, the precarious pre-procedural hemodynamics in this subset leads to diminished tolerance to the stress of the procedure and any complications thereof. Despite these shortcomings, PTMC has been successfully performed among patients with severe PH and systemic and suprasystemic PAP. Mortality rates of 0%–1%[14,15,41–43] and success rates of 86%–98% have been reported.[14,41–43] Even among patients with systemic or suprasystemic PAP the success rate was 95% without any mortality.[14] One study noted an increase in MR grade of >1 (out of 4) in one-third of patients.[41] However, none of these patients needed emergency MVR. Thus, in suitable valves, PTMC is preferred over surgery among patients with severe PH. PTMC may also be considered in patients with suboptimal valve anatomy who are otherwise high risk for surgery. In such cases, PTMC can allow a temporary improvement in hemodynamic status, thereby reducing the risk of subsequent surgery.

REGRESSION OF PH AFTER RELIEF OF MS

In the early era of closed mitral valvotomy (during the 1950s and 1960s, before the advent of MVR), surgery often failed to correct the elevated PVR. It was presumed that this was due to "fixed" obstructive changes in the pulmonary vasculature. This led to a skepticism among surgeons to offer closed mitral valvotomy (CMV) in patients with severe or extreme elevation in PVR, given the high surgical mortality in this subgroup. It was subsequently realized that this lack of regression of PH could also be due to ineffective correction of MS or due to the development of significant MR.

With the availability of the prosthetic valves, it was possible to completely or nearly completely abolish both obstruction and regurgitation, thereby enabling a relook at the question as to how much of the elevated PH in MS is reversible. By serial daily hemodynamic evaluations, Dalen et al.[44] demonstrated that the total pulmonary resistance fell by 78% and PAP by 51% over 8 to 10 days following MVR. Braunwald et al.[45]

and Zener et al.[22] performed pre and postoperative catheterization studies in patients with severe and extreme PH. The postoperative study was performed 7 and 29 months after MVR, respectively. The PASP, mean PAP, and PVR reduced by 44%–62%, 40%–63%, and 52%–80%, respectively, at follow-up. The greatest reduction in PAP and PVR occurred in those with the highest preoperative values. Further, the reduction in PAP and PVR was 31% and 62% more in the MVR group as compared to those who had undergone open mitral valvotomy.[22] This proved that the more complete the relief of MS, the more likely it is that the PVR will return to normal. It is important to note that although the PVR fell drastically, it had not normalized in many patients (average PVR at follow-up was 3 WU).[22,44] An interesting case was reported by Ramirez et al.[46] A 28-year-old female patient underwent CMV for severe MS and suprasystemic PH (PASP 160, mean 95). At the time of CMV, her lingular biopsy revealed Harris-Heath Grade 3 pulmonary vascular changes. A catheterization 6 years later revealed a PAP of 30/15 mmHg with MVA of 3.2 cm². Five years later (11 years after CMV), her autopsy revealed marked regression of the pulmonary vascular changes corresponding to Harris-Heath Grade 0–1. There was marked regression of medial hypertrophy in the small pulmonary arteries (<100 microns). Thus, they demonstrated both hemodynamic and anatomic regression of PH in MS.

With the advent of PTMC, it was possible to assess the results of the relief of MS immediately without the confounding factors of cardiopulmonary bypass. Further, the availability of echocardiography enabled the assessment of PAP noninvasively at multiple time intervals over a long period. These studies have shown that immediately after PTMC, the mean PAP fell significantly.[7,14,15,41–43,47,48] The fall in PVR immediately after PTMC is variable. Some studies did not show a significant immediate fall in PVR,[7,23,42,47] whereas studies that evaluated patients with severe to extreme PH did note an immediate fall in PVR after PTMC.[12,14,41,43] Thus, the passive increase in PAP associated with MS falls immediately after successful PTMC. Subsequently, over the next week there is a further fall in PAP along with a significant drop in PVR.[47] This second phase of regression of PH with reduction in PVR is likely due to resolution of pulmonary artery vasoconstriction. Subsequent hemodynamic evaluation at 7–12 months[7,42,47] after PTMC revealed a further improvement in PH with a continued fall in both PAP and PVR. This phase indicates the regression of the fixed portion of PH. In some of the patients the PVR had normalized by follow-up, whereas in others the PVR had reduced but was still abnormal. Whether this latter group would have further resolution of PVR is unclear. However, in patients with development of restenosis, PH returns to predilatation values.

As mentioned earlier, despite a marked regression of PH, a complete normalization of PVR does not always occur. Using a strict criterion of 1.5 WU, Gamra et al.[6] found that 43% of patients failed to return to normal when restudied at 22 ± 13 months after PTMC. Using the same criteria (1.5 WU), none of the patients in the Braunwald[45] or Zener[22] study had normal PVR at follow-up. This can be attributed to fixed PVR. Predictors of failure of normalization of PVR were older age, atrial fibrillation, higher echo score, smaller MVA, higher mean PAP and PVR before procedure, and higher TPG after procedure.[6] Patients with a normal LAP and maintenance of normal rhythm postoperatively were the ones who experienced the most benefit after MVR.[22] Patients with optimal PTMC results (MVA >1.5 cm[2] with no or mild MR) were more likely to have a normal PAP and PVR.[42]

To summarize, PH in MS is reversible to a great extent. The greater the relief of MS, the greater the fall in PAP and PVR. The magnitude of decline in PVR and PAP is a function of the preoperative level, i.e., the higher the preoperative level, the greater the fall. The rapid reduction in PAP and PVR after relief of mitral stenosis indicates a predominant role of passive transmission of elevated left-atrial pressures and concomitant pulmonary arteriolar vasoconstriction. The organic element of pulmonary vascular disease may or may not regress completely after intervention. However, the threat of irreversible PH is not as serious in mitral valve disease as in congenital heart disease. As such, severe pulmonary vascular disease should not be a contraindication to surgery, although the risk of surgery is increased. Following successful surgery, a striking improvement is noted in the functional class among survivors, with a majority (>90%) being in NYHA class I–II.[39]

An early intervention is recommended before the fixed "PH" sets in. The ESC 2012 guidelines give a class IIa indication for intervention in asymptomatic severe MS patients with PASP >50 mmHg.[49] The 2006 ACC/AHA guidelines for valvular heart disease had given a class I recommendation for PTMC in asymptomatic patients with a MVA <1.5 cm[2] and pulmonary hypertension (PASP >50 mmHg at rest or >60 mmHg with exercise).[50] However, the latest 2014 ACC/AHA guidelines do not make any recommendations regarding intervention for PH in MS patients.[51] This is surprising as the same guidelines have recommended early surgery for asymptomatic severe MR with resting PASP >50 mmHg.

The contrast between PH in MS as compared to that in shunt lesions is interesting. The former, even if longstanding, is usually reversible after relief of MS, whereas the latter is often fixed or even progressive after repair. The reason for this difference is not clear. One possibility is that the PH associated with shunt lesions (ventricular septal defect or patent ductus arteriosus) exposes the immature pulmonary vasculature to high pressure right from birth, thereby preventing the normal regression of pulmonary vascular musculature and maturation from occurring.[52] Another important difference is that shunt lesions, unlike MS, lead to increased pulmonary blood flow, which may lead to vascular injury and fixed anatomic changes.

PERSISTENT PH AFTER RELIEF OF MS

Persistent PH despite relief of MS may be due to a number of factors. These include inadequate valve dilatation, development of significant mitral regurgitation, development of mitral restenosis, iatrogenic ASD after PTMC with significant left-to-right shunt, chronic lung disease, "fixed" component of PH, and, rarely, due to the coexistence of primary pulmonary hypertension (PPH).[34] The first four factors are related to valvotomy and are probably not relevant when the valve has been replaced. Differentiation between PH complicating MS and PPH is difficult except by means of lung biopsy, which reveals plexiform lesions in PPH (plexiform lesions have not been reported in MS).[34]

The prevalence of persistent PH varies and is most likely related to the completeness of the relief of MS (Figure 22.1, Videos 22.1–22.6). The more complete the relief, the more likely the PVR will return to normal. In one study, using a criterion of PASP >40 mmHg one year after successful PTMC, the

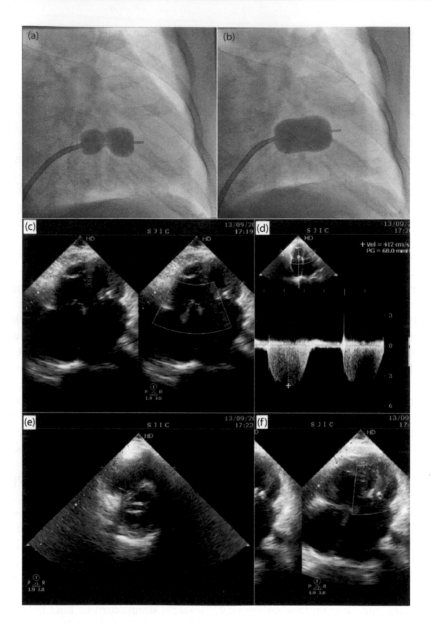

Figure 22.1 Persistent PH in MS. A 41-year-old male post-CMV, post-PTMC underwent redo-PTMC for severe mitral restenosis (MVA 1.1 cm²) and severe PH (PASP 80). Successful PTMC performed with Accura 24 mm-sized balloon with splitting of both commissures **(a, b)**. Follow-up echo at 1, 3, and 12 months after PTMC revealed persistent PH. Echo at 12 months after PTMC. **(c)** Dilated right atrium and right ventricle with mild tricuspid regurgitation; **(d)** TR jet gradient of 68 mmHg; **(e)** short-axis view of mitral valve showing bilateral split commissures; **(f)** laminar flow across mitral valve. A contrast-enhanced CT chest and CT pulmonary angiogram were normal (see Videos 22.1 through 22.6).

prevalence was 41%.[53] Another study noted a prevalence of 43% using a criterion of PVR >1.5 WU at follow-up.[6] These patients are older, more often have AF, have a higher Wilkins score, and have a larger LA.[53] The MVA is lower with higher TPG, higher LAP and PAP (PASP and mean). Post-procedure, these patients had lesser gain in MVA, and the TPG, LAP, and PAP were higher as compared to those with no persistent PH.[53] Patients with persistent PH have a worse prognosis. They have a greater incidence of strokes, new-onset heart failure, restenosis, and need for reintervention.[53] This is most likely related to the advanced stage of the disease in these patients. Thus, patients with persistent PH need close frequent follow-up.

TREATMENT OF PERSISTENT PH

It is important to identify the remediable conditions mentioned earlier (namely inadequate relief of MS, development of significant MR, mitral restenosis, or, rarely, significant ASD) before labeling a patient as persistent PH. Overestimation of MVA following PTMC, underestimation of the degree of postprocedural MR, or a lack of appreciation of the severity of subvalvular disease are common errors on echocardiography that may lead to a diagnosis of persistent PH while the primary pathology remains uncorrected. In doubtful cases, a complete hemodynamic assessment by cardiac catheterization may be needed. The persistence of moderate to severe PH in association with inadequate MVA or significant MR following PTMC should lead to a strong consideration for MVR. An attempt at repeat PTMC may be resorted to if the first procedure was technically inadequate (e.g., undersized balloon). Finally, as the reduction in PVR secondary to the fixed component takes time to resolve, it is pertinent to wait for at least one year before a diagnosis of persistent PH is entertained.

Correctable medical conditions that lead to PH should be sought for and corrected. These include anemia, thyroid disorders, chronic lung diseases, etc. Volume overload and atrial arrhythmias are common causes of elevated PAP in the postoperative period. Other factors such as pain, anxiety, and hypoxia are often contributory. Intravenous diuretics and the management of atrial arrhythmias (control of ventricular rate or electric/chemical cardioversion to restore sinus rhythm) are extremely important, both in the immediate postoperative period and in the long term. It is only after these treatable factors have been corrected and PH is persistent that consideration for pulmonary vasodilators should be made.

None of the approved therapies for PAH have received approval for use in this setting.[36] The use of pulmonary vasodilators without the relief of MS is potentially dangerous as it may lead to pulmonary edema from an inability of the lungs to drain through a stenosed MV. Most of the data regarding the use of pulmonary vasodilators in MS are from the postoperative setting (usually after MVR). Following MVR, inhaled nitric oxide (NO) and inhaled prostacyclin

have been shown to reduce PAP, PVR, and TPG in a dose-dependent manner accompanied by an increase in cardiac output with no significant change in PACP.[54] Inhaled NO has been shown to reduce the length of ICU stay and the need for vasoactive drugs.[55] Sildenfail citrate, a phosphodiesterase-5 inhibitor, has also been shown to reduce PAP and PVR after cardiac surgery enabling weaning of inhaled or intravenous pulmonary vasodilators.[56] Preliminary studies have demonstrated an additive effect of combining sildenafil and inhaled NO in lowering PVR and PAP after cardiac surgery.[57]

Data on the long-term use of pulmonary vasodilators for persistent PH are limited. A case report demonstrated the efficacy of long-term intravenous epoprostenol in reducing PVR and mean PAP in a patient with persistent severe PH after MVR for severe MS.[58]

Similarly, the role for chronic sildenafil therapy following relief of MS (by MVR/PTMC) is not backed by any strong evidence, although its use in such scenarios is becoming increasingly common. Recently, the results of the randomized SIOVAC trial[59] were reported. This study evaluated the effect of sildenafil in patients with successfully corrected valvular heart disease and residual PH (mean PAP >30 mmHg more than 1 year after surgery). Two hundred patients were randomized to sildenafil or placebo, with 91% of patients having undergone mitral surgery (MVR 80%, MV repair 11%). After 6 months, patients in the sildenafil group had a worse clinical composite score (almost double) and greater number of hospitalization for heart failure. The authors concluded that off-lab usage of sildenafil PH due to valvular heart disease should be discouraged.

Given the role of endothelin-1 in the pathogenesis of PH in MS, bosentan was evaluated in a small prospective non-blinded study of ten patients with MS and severe PH (mean PAP >40 mmHg).[60] Bosentan therapy was associated with an increase in six-minute walk distance, a reduction in mean PAP, and a marked reduction in BORG dyspnea index and serum proBNP levels. Paradoxically, the maximum oxygen uptake (a co-primary endpoint) was significantly reduced as compared to baseline. Another limitation of this study was that all the patients had uncorrected MS.

Finally, there has been some debate regarding the role of β-blockers in MS patients with PH. Some authors have suggested caution in their use in patients with severe PH and especially right-heart failure as they may further aggravate RV dysfunction and impaired cardiac output.[61] Wisenbaugh et al.[62] studied the effect of IV atenolol in patients with MS with PH undergoing PTMC. After IV atenolol infusion, transmitral gradient and LAP were reduced significantly. However, the PVR increased and this increase was more marked in the subgroup with severe PH (PVR >7.5 WU, N = 17). This subgroup also experienced a fall in systemic blood pressure accompanied by an inappropriate fall in systemic vascular resistance. The authors recommended that in MS complicated by severe PH, especially those with right-heart failure, β-blockers should be cautiously used with gradual up-titration of dose as in dilated cardiomyopathy. An alternative for patients with severe RV dysfunction could be digoxin or ivabradine for rate control.

VIDEOS

Video 22.1 Successful re-redo PTMC in a 41-year-old male (P/CMV, P/PTMC) with splitting of both commissures. https://youtu.be/d_R4SvpGSQY

Video 22.2 Transthoracic echocardiography one year after re-redo PTMC shows bilateral split commissures. https://youtu.be/ewuckThIE14

Video 22.3 & 22.4 Color Doppler across mitral valve in apical four-chamber and parasternal long axis view shows laminar flow across the mitral valve without subvalvular disease. https://youtu.be/e_7r2zGGedU; https://youtu.be/2Q8akJfD-7Q

Video 22.5 Apical four-chamber view showing dilated right atrium and right ventricle with reduced RV systolic function. https://youtu.be/RNPgqZcla3k

Video 22.6 Color flow across tricuspid valve shows trivial-mild tricuspid regurgitation. The tricuspid regurgitation jet velocity was recorded as 68 mmHg. https://youtu.be/G96z-fxUsr8

REFERENCES

1. Wood P. An appreciation of mitral stenosis: II. Investigations and results. Br Med J 1954; 1:1113–24.
2. Simonneau G, Gatzoulis MA, Adatia I et al. Updated clinical classification of pulmonary hypertension. J Am Coll Cardiol 2013;62:D34–41.
3. Galiè N, Humbert M, Vachiery JL et al. 2015 ESC/ERS Guidelines for the diagnosis and treatment of pulmonary hypertension. Eur Heart J 2016;37:67–119.
4. Hoeper MM, Bogaard HJ, Condliffe R et al. Definitions and diagnosis of pulmonary hypertension. J Am Coll Cardiol 2013;62:D42–D50.
5. Emanuel R, Ross K. Pulmonary hypertension in rheumatic heart disease. Prog Cardiovasc Dis 1967;9:401–13.
6. Gamra H, Zhang HP, Allen JW et al. Factors determining normalization of pulmonary vascular resistance following successful balloon mitral valvotomy. Am J Cardiol 1999; 83:392–5.
7. Levine MJ, Weinstein JS, Diver DJ et al. Progressive improvement in pulmonary vascular resistance after percutaneous mitral valvuloplasty. Circulation 1989;79:1061–7.
8. Emanuel R. Valvotomy in mitral stenosis with extreme pulmonary vascular resistance. Br Heart J 1963;25:119–25.
9. Ribeiro PA, al Zaibag M, Abdullah M. Pulmonary artery pressure and pulmonary vascular resistance before and after mitral balloon valvotomy in 100 patients with severe mitral valve stenosis. Am Heart J 1993;125:1110–14.
10. Pourafkari L, Ghaffari S, Ahmadi M, Tajlil A, Aslanabadi N, Nader ND. Pulmonary hypertension in rheumatic mitral stenosis revisited. Herz 2016:1–6.
11. Yang B, DeBenedictus C, Watt T et al. The impact of concomitant pulmonary hypertension on early and late outcomes following surgery for mitral stenosis. J Thorac Cardiovasc Surg 2016;152:394–400.e1.
12. Fawzy ME, Hassan W, Stefadouros M et al. Prevalence and fate of severe pulmonary hypertension in 559 patients with severe mitral stenosis undergoing mitral balloon valvotomy. J Heart Valve Dis 2004;13:942–8.
13. Ward C, Hancock BW. Extreme pulmonary hypertension caused by mitral valve disease: Natural history and results of surgery. Br Heart J 1975;37:74–8.

14. Bahl VK, Chandra S, Talwar KK et al. Balloon mitral valvotomy in patients with systemic and suprasystemic pulmonary artery pressures. *Cathet Cardiovasc Diagn* 1995;36:211–5.

15. Cruz-Gonzalez I, Semigram MJ, Inglessis-Azuaje I et al. Effect of elevated pulmonary vascular resistance on outcomes after percutaneous mitral valvuloplasty. *Am J Cardiol* 2013;112:580–4.

16. Wood P. Pulmonary hypertension with special reference to the vasoconstrictive factor. *Br Heart J* 1958;20:557–70.

17. Roy SB, Bhatia ML, Lazaro EJ, Ramalingaswami V. Juvenile mitral stenosis in India. *Lancet* 1963;2;1193–5.

18. Olesen KH. The natural history of 271 patients with mitral stenosis under medical treatment. *Br Heart J* 1962;24:349–57.

19. Selzer A, Malmborg RO. Some factors influencing changes in pulmonary vascular resistance in mitral valvular disease. *Am J Med* 1962;32:532–44.

20. Otto CM, Davis KB, Reid CL et al. Relation between pulmonary artery pressure and mitral stenosis severity in patients undergoing balloon mitral commissurotomy. *Am J Cardiol* 1993;71:874–8.

21. Magne J, Pibarot P, Sengupta PP et al. Pulmonary hypertension in valvular disease: A comprehensive review on pathophysiology to therapy from the HAVEC Group. *JACC Cardiovasc Imaging* 2015;8:83–99.

22. Zener JC, Hancock EW, Shumway NE, Harrison DC. Regression of extreme pulmonary hypertension after mitral valve surgery. *Am J Cardiol* 1972;30:820–6.

23. Hart SA, Krasuski RA, Wang A et al. Pulmonary hypertension and elevated transpulmonary gradient in patients with mitral stenosis. *J Heart Valve Dis* 2010;19: 708–15.

24. Whitaker W. Clinical diagnosis of pulmonary hypertension in patients with mitral stenosis. *Q J Med* 1954;23:105–12.

25. Guazzi M, Borlaug BA. Pulmonary hypertension due to left heart disease. *Circulation* 2012;126:975–90.

26. Jordan SC. Development of pulmonary hypertension in mitral stenosis. *Lancet* 1965;286:322–4.

27. Mahoney PD, Loh E, Blitz LR, Herrmann HC. Hemodynamic effects of inhaled nitric oxide in women with mitral stenosis and pulmonary hypertension. *Am J Cardiology* 2001;87:188–92.

28. Yamamoto K, Ikeda U, Shimada K. Endothelin production in mitral stenosis. *N Engl J Med* 1993; 329:1740–1.

29. Snopek G, Pogorzelska H, Rywik TM et al. Usefulness of endothelin-1 concentration in capillary blood in patients with mitral stenosis as a predictor of regression of pulmonary hypertension after mitral valve replacement or valvuloplasty. *Am J Cardiol* 2002;90:188–9.

30. Goodale Jr F, Sanchez G, Friedlich AL et al. Correlation of pulmonary arteriolar resistance with pulmonary vascular changes in patients with mitral stenosis before and after valvulotomy. *N Engl J Med* 1955;252:979–83.

31. Tandon HD, Kasturi J. Pulmonary vascular changes associated with isolated mitral stenosis in India. *Br Heart J* 1975;37:26–36.

32. Jorge E, Baptista R, Calisto J et al. Pulmonary vascular remodeling in mitral valve disease: An optical coherence tomography study. *Int J Cardiol* 2016;203: 576–8.

33. Mubeen M, Singh AK, Agarwal SK et al. Mitral valve replacement in severe pulmonary arterial hypertension. *Asian Cardiovasc Thorac Ann* 2008;16:37–42.

34. Langleben D, Lamoureux E, Marcotte F et al. Mitral stenosis obscuring the diagnosis of plexogenic pulmonary arteriopathy and familial pulmonary hypertension. *Thorax* 2000;55:247–8.

35. Mackinnon J, Wade EG, Vickers CF. Mitral stenosis with very high pulmonary vascular resistance and atypical features. *Br Heart J* 1956;18:449–57.

36. Davila CD, Forfia PR. Management of severe pulmonary hypertension in patients undergoing mitral valve surgery. *Curr Treat Options Cardiovasc Med* 2015;17:382.

37. Bossone E, D'Andrea A, D'Alto M et al. Echocardiography in pulmonary arterial hypertension: From diagnosis to prognosis. *J Am Soc Echocardiogr* 2013;26:1–14.

38. Arkles JS et al. Shape of the right ventricular Doppler envelope predicts hemodynamics and right heart function in pulmonary hypertension. *Am J Respir Crit Care Med* 2011;183:268–76.

39. Camara ML, Aris A, Padro JM, Carolps JM. Long term results of mitral valve surgery in patients with severe pulmonary hypertension. *Ann Thorac Surg* 1988;45:133–6.

40. Vincens JJ, Temizer D, Post JR et al. Long-term outcome of cardiac surgery in patients with mitral stenosis and severe pulmonary hypertension. *Circulation* 1995;92(Suppl II):37–42.

41. Wisenbaugh T, Essop R, Middlemost S et al. Effects of severe pulmonary hypertension on outcome of balloon mitral valvotomy. *Am J Cardiol* 1992;70:823–5.

42. Fawzy ME, Mimish L, Sivanandam V et al. Immediate and long-term effect of mitral balloon valvotomy on severe pulmonary hypertension in patients with mitral stenosis. *Am Heart J* 1996;131:89–93.

43. Alfonso F, Macaya C, Hernandez R et al. Percutaneous mitral valvuloplasty with severe pulmonary artery hypertension. *Am J Cardiol* 1993;72:325–30.

44. Dalen JE, Matloff JM, Evans GL et al. Early reduction of pulmonary vascular resistance after mitral-valve replacement. *N Engl J Med* 1967;277:387–94.

45. Braunwald E, Braunwald NS, Ross JJ, Morrow AG. Effects of mitral valve replacement on the pulmonary vascular dynamics of patients with pulmonary hypertension. *N Engl J Med* 1965; 273:509–14.

46. Ramírez A, Grimes ET, Abelmann WH. Regression of pulmonary vascular changes following mitral valvuloplasty. An anatomic and physiologic case study. *Am J Med* 1968;45:975–82.

47. Dev V, Shrivastava S. Time course of changes in pulmonary vascular resistance and the mechanism of regression of pulmonary arterial hypertension after balloon mitral valvuloplasty. *Am J Cardiol* 1991;67:439–42.

48. Sarmiento RA, Blanco R, Gigena G et al. Initial results and long-term follow-up of percutaneous mitral valvuloplasty in patients with pulmonary hypertension. *Heart Lung Circ* 2017;26:58–63.

49. Vahanian A, Alfieri O, Andreotti F et al. Guidelines on the management of valvular heart disease (version 2012). *Eur Heart J* 2012;33:2451–96.

50. Bonow RO, Carabello BA, Kanu C et al. ACC/AHA 2006 guidelines for the management of patients with valvular heart disease. *Circulation* 2006;114:e84–231.

51. Nishimura RA, Otto CM, Bonow RO et al. American College of Cardiology/American Heart Association Task Force on Practice Guidelines. 2014 AHA/ACC guideline for the management of patients with valvular heart disease. *J Am Coll Cardiol* 2014;63:e57–185.

52. Kulik TJ, Harris JE, McElhinney DB. The impact of pulmonary venous hypertension on the pulmonary circulation in the young. *Congenit Heart Dis* 2011;6:603–7.

53. Nair KK, Pillai HS, Titus T et al. Persistent pulmonary artery hypertension in patients undergoing balloon mitral valvotomy. *Pulm Circ* 2013;3:426–31.

54. Fattouch K et al. Inhaled prostacyclin, nitric oxide, and nitroprusside in pulmonary hypertension after mitral valve replacement. *J Card Surg* 2005;20:171–6.

55. Fernandes JL, Sampaio RO, Brandão CM et al. Comparison of inhaled nitric oxide versus oxygen on hemodynamics in patients with mitral stenosis and severe pulmonary hypertension after mitral valve surgery. *Am J Cardiol* 2011;107:1040–5.

56. Trachte AL, Lobato EB, Urdaneta F et al. Oral sildenafil reduces pulmonary hypertension after cardiac surgery. *Ann Thorac Surg* 2005;79:194–7.

57. Matamis D, Pampori S, Papathanasiou A et al. Inhaled NO and sildenafil combination in cardiac surgery patients with out-of-proportion pulmonary hypertension: Acute effects on postoperative gas exchange and hemodynamics. *Circ Heart Fail* 2012;5:47–53.

58. Elliott CG, Palevsky HI. Treatment with epoprostenol of pulmonary arterial hypertension following mitral valve replacement for mitral stenosis. *Thorax* 2004;59:536–7.

59. Bermejo J, Yotti R, García-Orta R, Sánchez-Fernández PL et al. Sildenafil for improving outcomes in patients with corrected valvular heart disease and persistent pulmonary hypertension: A multicenter, double-blind,

randomized clinical trial. *Eur Heart J.* 2017 Dec 21. doi: 10.1093/eurheartj/ehx700.

60. Vlachogeorgos GS, Daskalopoulos N, Blatsiotis P et al. Bosentan for patients with echocardiographic evidence of pulmonary hypertension due to long-standing rheumatic mitral stenosis. *Hellenic J Cardiol* 2015;56:36–43.

61. Klein HO, Sareli P, Schamroth CL et al. Effects of atenolol on exercise capacity in patients with mitral stenosis with sinus rhythm. *Am J Cardiol* 1985;56:598–601.

62. Wisenbaugh T, Essop R, Middlemost S et al. Pulmonary hypertension is a contraindication to beta-blockade in patients with severe mitral stenosis. *Am Heart J* 1993;125:786–90.

23

Left-ventricular dysfunction in mitral stenosis

RAVI S. MATH

INTRODUCTION

In mitral stenosis (MS), the inherent pathology is obstruction to inflow of blood into the left ventricle (LV) from the left atrium (LA). As such, it has been believed that the LV systolic function should be normal as the pathology is upstream to LV. A number of studies have documented the presence of LV systolic dysfunction (usually defined as an LV ejection fraction of <50%[1,2]). The importance of these findings relates primarily to the outcomes of relief of the mechanical obstruction (either by surgery or percutaneously). If the LV systolic dysfunction is indeed related to an inherent myocardial pathology, then the mere relief of valve obstruction may not lead to complete relief of symptoms. On the other hand, if the LV systolic dysfunction is related primarily to hemodynamic abnormalities, then the relief of MS should reverse the LV dysfunction. Thus, the debate regarding the presence and causality of LV systolic dysfunction is more than a matter of semantics.

The prevalence of LV systolic dysfunction in MS has varied, with some studies performed a few decades ago quoting figures as high as 31%.[1] These studies relied primarily on angiography and two-dimensional (2D) echocardiography. With the advent of strain echocardiography, subclinical LV systolic dysfunction has been reported in most patients (85%) despite normal LV ejection fraction (LVEF).[3] These studies have excluded other causes of LV systolic dysfunction such as coexistent coronary artery disease, significant mitral regurgitation or aortic valve disease, diabetes mellitus, hypertension, other structural heart disease, etc.

ASSESSMENT OF LV SYSTOLIC DYSFUNCTION IN MITRAL STENOSIS

Anatomic studies

It was in 1929 that Kirch[4] first pointed out that the posterior wall of the LV was markedly shortened in nearly all patients with pure MS at autopsy. This finding was subsequently substantiated by Grant in 1953.[5] He noted that the inflow tract of the LV was markedly shorter than the outflow tract in patients with MS at autopsy. The mitral ring was markedly tilted and no longer perpendicular to the inflow tract. He hypothesized that this was due to selective atrophy of the posterior wall of the heart. Thickening of the mitral valve leaflets and fibrosis of chordae converted the valve into a dense scar tissue that immobilized the posterior wall leading to its selective atrophy. Histopathology of this area did not reveal any reduction in myocardial fiber diameter to support this hypothesis. It was presumed that the myocardium was completely resorbed. However, Sunamori et al.[6] did note fibrosis of the myocardium at the base of papillary muscles removed at the time of mitral valve replacement (MVR).

Pathologic studies

Two pathological studies of myocardial biopsies have been reported using electron microscopy.[7,8] They arrived at slightly differing conclusions. In the first study, LV biopsies were performed at the time of surgery in 11 patients with pure MS.[7] Of these, only four patients had a normal LV function (LVEF >55%). Electron microscopy showed normal myocyte cell diameter. There was a moderate interstitial fibrosis and moderate histiocytic reaction. The correlation between LV function and fibrosis was poor. Although five out of six patients with reduced LV function showed considerable fibrosis, in other cases, the LV function was normal despite notable fibrosis, or the LV function was reduced with discrete fibrosis. Thus, the authors concluded that myocardial abnormalities (possibly due to healing from rheumatic myocarditis) could be one of the factors responsible for reduced LV function but were not sufficient to explain these changes.

In the second study,[8] 15 patients with isolated MS (nine with normal LV function, six with reduced LV function) underwent LV endomyocardial biopsy during cardiac catheterization. They noted a varying degree of pathological changes in the myocardium in all patients. These changes were not related to the severity of MS. Rather, patients with reduced LV function had more extensive loss of myofibrils resulting from either disproportion of the mitochondria:myofibril ratio or myofibrillar degeneration. The myofibril diameter was reduced. They concluded that the extent of myocardial involvement by the rheumatic process rather than hemodynamic derangement was the basic pathologic mechanism responsible for LV dysfunction.

Cardiac catheterization

In 1955, Harvey et al.[9] first reported a series of eight patients with "myocardial insufficiency" based on hemodynamic data at rest and during exercise. All patients had moderate to severe symptoms. They noted that half of these patients had low cardiac output at rest and there was an abnormally low response to exercise in all patients. The pulmonary artery pressure was normal in most cases but rose with exercise in the majority of cases. Two of these eight patients underwent closed commissurotomy (both had a narrow mitral valve at surgery) with no improvement in symptoms or hemodynamic parameters. The authors concluded the existence of a group of MS patients whose symptoms were primarily related to "myocardial insufficiency," which would not be relieved by commissurotomy. Except for the two patients who underwent surgery, an assessment of the mitral valve area (MVA) was not performed in the rest of the patients.

It was subsequently pointed out that the low cardiac output and normal pulmonary pressure in such patients may be due to a readjustment of the cardiac output to lower operating levels through potent (yet unidentified) flow-regulating factors rather than "myocardial insufficiency."[10,11]

Through detailed evaluation of hemodynamic tracings, Feigenbaum et al.[12] studied diastolic filling in patients with pure MS (mean MVA 1.2 cm^2, range 0.5–2.3 cm^2). Three-quarters of cases had cardiac output below normal at rest. The LV end-diastolic pressure (LVEDP) was normal at rest in most cases, but it did increase with exercise in 25% of cases. More than half of the patients showed a reduction in $\Delta v/\Delta p$ (the mean increase in LV diastolic volume per mmHg increase in LV pressure during ventricular filling) during exercise indicative of an abnormal LV in MS. They suggested that this abnormality may be related to reduced left-ventricular compliance, which could reflect the abnormalities noted by Grant.[5] Of the 24 patients who underwent surgery, 20 patients showed evidence of carditis in the left atrial appendage (Aschoff nodules).

Subsequently, Heller et al.[13] used cineangiography to assess quantitative and qualitative abnormalities of the LV in patients with pure MS (MVA = 0.4–2.1 cm^2). They noted that the LV end-diastolic volumes (EDV) were normal but the LV end-systolic volumes (ESV) were significantly larger in patients with MS than in controls. As a result, LVEF was significantly lower in MS patients (LVEF = 55%) as compared to normal subjects (LVEF = 76%). Qualitative analysis of the LV angiogram revealed abnormal contraction patterns in 20 out of 25 patients. The posterobasal area was rigid, distorted, and immobile as compared to the rest of the LV. This was confirmed at autopsy in one patient. This, once again, supported the Grant hypothesis that, in MS, the mitral valve ring, leaflets, chordae, and papillary muscles form a rigid complex, restricting the mobility of the adjacent LV, leading to fibrosis of that area. Horwitz et al.[14] demonstrated reduced contraction in the anterior wall. This may be due to limitation in motion due to adherence of the scarred, shortened anterior papillary muscle to the contiguous ventricular wall. Curry et al.[15] noted anterolateral wall motion abnormality of the LV, which they suggested may be the result of abnormal right-ventricular enlargement and pulmonary hypertension in MS. Other authors have demonstrated diffuse hypokinesia of the LV as well.[16,17]

Finally, Gash et al.[1] studied LV systolic performance in patients with isolated MS. They studied indices of preload, afterload, ejection fraction, and LV contractile function independent of loading conditions (end-systolic wall stress/end-systolic volume index [ESS/ESVI]). Thirty-one percent of MS patients had an LVEF of <50%. They noted that LV preload was reduced, LV afterload was increased, and the latter was not compensated for by an increase in preload. The increased LV afterload was due to inadequate end-systolic wall thickness (leading to high LV wall stress at normal LV systolic pressure) and elevated systemic vascular resistance. LV ejection indices in the form of EF, velocity of circumferential fiber shortening (Vcf) and stroke work index (SWI) were reduced. However, the ratio of ESS:ESVI, which is independent of loading conditions, was normal, indicating that LV muscle function per se was normal.

In normal hearts, the LV diastolic pressure always remains positive and never falls below zero. Sabbah et al.[18] using micromanometers, demonstrated that the LV pressure falls below zero in patients with MS during early diastole. This LV diastolic suction leads to less reliance on atrial contraction for LV filling but at the same time contributes to abnormal septal motion. Conditions associated with increased LV diastolic pressure (such as hypertensive heart disease) cause this mechanism to be lost. This could lead to an increase in symptoms.

To summarize, based on cardiac catheterization studies, patients with severe MS have a reduced cardiac output and normal LVEDP. The preload is reduced, afterload is increased, and EDV are normal, whereas the ESV is increased, leading to reduced EF. Regional wall motion abnormalities are seen in a significant proportion of patients, in the form of reduced contraction of the posterobasal area, and in some cases, the anterior wall as well.

Echocardiography

Echocardiography enables noninvasive assessment of the LV geometry and contractility. Initial studies used M-mode echocardiography.[19,20] They found that indices of LV performance such as cardiac output, ejection fraction, and Vcf were reduced in patients with severe MS. Mohan et al. noted[21] that the LV tended to be more spherical than ellipsoid in patients with isolated MS. Measurement of EF and LV volumes is highly subjective and variable. Load-independent indices such as tissue Doppler imaging (TDI) and strain rate imaging have been studied. Using TDI, Ozdemir et al.[22] demonstrated that myocardial velocities of the LV in the long axis were reduced even in patients with normal ejection fraction. Subsequently, Dogan et al.[23] using Doppler-derived strain rate imaging demonstrated that in patients with mild to moderate MS with normal global systolic function, the peak-systolic strain rate and end-systolic strain was significantly reduced as compared to controls. The impaired long-axis function despite normal systolic function indicated subclinical LV dysfunction. Since Doppler-derived strain is angle-dependent, Aydan et al.[24] used 2D strain and strain rate imaging with speckle tracking, which is angle-independent. Among patients with mild to moderate MS with normal LV systolic function, the mean global longitudinal strain (GLS) and global longitudinal strain rate (GLSR) were significantly reduced in patients with isolated MS. Regional analysis demonstrated significantly reduced longitudinal peak strain and strain rate in all the basal segments and in some of the mid-segments (inferior, anteroseptal, interventricular septum) of the LV. The authors felt that a possible extension of the rheumatic process from the mitral valve to the basal segments could explain the reduced strain and strain rate in these areas. Bilen et al.[25] included cases of severe MS (in addition to mild and moderate MS) with normal LV function as well. They noted similar reduction in LV global strain and strain rate in MS patients and this was independent of the hemodynamic severity of the obstruction. They felt that the most probable reason for this was rheumatic myocardial involvement.

MS restricts LV filling in early diastole whereas the unobstructed tricuspid valve allows rapid RV filling. This leads to a brief posterior or leftward motion of the interventricular septum in early diastole just after the mitral valve opens.[26] Pulmonary hypertension or RV enlargement can further lead to abnormal septal movement.[27]

Natriuretic peptides

Natriuretic peptides have been used in the diagnosis and prognosis of heart failure. BNP and NT-proBNP levels are elevated in MS and are positively correlated with the severity and symptoms of MS.[28–31] They have been shown to be useful in risk stratification of MS patients who are asymptomatic[32] or have equivocal sysmptoms.[28] Following successful PTMC, levels of BNP and NT-proBNP have been shown to fall and they may be used to predict the success of PTMC in sinus rhythm[33,34] and a fall in PA pressure after PTMC.[35] Currently, data on their role in the assessment of LV function in MS is not available.

OUTCOMES AFTER RELIEF OF MITRAL STENOSIS

Many studies have been performed to evaluate LV function before and after relief of mitral stenosis. An immediate improvement in LV function indicates that the mechanical obstruction was the proximate cause for LV dysfunction whereas a failure/delayed improvement in LV function would indicate

a myocardial cause. Limitations of these studies have been that they have been performed over differing time frames, used different methods to assess LV function (angiography vs. echo), and have enrolled patients with and without LV dysfunction with limited follow-up. Moreover, studies involving open-heart surgery are confounded by the effects of surgical technique, cardiopulmonary bypass, and anesthesia on LV function.

Outcomes following surgery

A few studies have evaluated the surgical outcomes of MS patients with LV systolic dysfunction.[36–38] These studies (except one) are retrospective in nature. These studies found that the overall in-hospital mortality was no different among patients with or without depressed LV function.[36–38] One study noted a higher incidence of thromboembolism in patients with LV dysfunction in the postoperative period.[38] This contributed to poor survival in the long-term at 15 years.[38] Another study with long-term follow-up (mean 9 years) found a higher incidence of heart failure and heart failure-related deaths in patients with LV systolic dysfunction.[37] However, overall mortality was not different.[37]

These studies concluded that moderate depression of LV function should not be a contraindication to MVR. However, data regarding evolution of LV function after surgery was missing in all these studies.

Outcomes following PTMC[3,39–48]

Studies that have evaluated the effect of percutaneous transvenous mitral commissurotomy (PTMC) on LV function have the advantage that PTMC relieves mitral obstruction without many other confounding factors (no anesthesia or cardiopulmonary bypass). However, these studies are limited by the fact that the most severely deformed valves would not be subjected to PTMC. These patients are the ones in whom a myocardial rather than a mechanical cause for LV dysfunction is likely due to an extension of the scarring process. Other limitations mentioned earlier apply to PTMC studies as well.

Overall, most studies found a reduced LVEDV before PTMC or an improvement in LVEDV after PTMC, indicating reduced LV filling. Some studies noted an increased LVESV in patients with LV dysfunction (Table 23.1). There was an increase

Table 23.1 Studies evaluating outcomes of PTMC on hemodynamics

Author, year, number, modality	Pre-PTMC	Post-FTMC	Follow-up	Conclusion
Wisenbaugh et al., 1992,[39] N = 10 EF >0.55, N = 11 EF <0.55, LV angiogram, pressure data	ESV ↑, CO ↓, SVR ↑, PVR ↑, MVA ↓ in LV dysfunction group, LVEDP, LVEDV, EDWS ↔	LVEDF ↑, LVEDV ↑ in LV dysfunction group, CO ↑, SVR ↓ in both groups, compliance ↔, EF ↔	NA	Excessive vasoconstriction account for higher afterload, lower ejection performance and lower CO
Liu et al., 1992,[40] N = 9 (all normal EF), micromanometer with transient IVC occlusion	Compared to controls CO ↓, LVEDP ↓, LVEDV ↓, afterload ↑, LVEDPVR shifted to left with increased slope	CO ↑, LVEDV ↑, end-systolic elastance ↓	EF ↑, LVEDV ↑, elastance maintained at three months ↓	Reduced LV compliance from functional restriction caused by ventricular attachment to a thickened and immobile valve apparatus; acutely reversed by PTMC
Goto et al., 1992,[41] N = 11 (all normal EF), LV angiogram, pressure data		LVEDV ↑, CO ↑, EF ↑, mean systolic ejection rate ↑		Insufficient preload could affect ejection performance
Yasuda et al., 1993,[42] N = 22 (EF >50%), N = 10 (EF <50%), LV angiogram, pressure data at baseline, echo at FU	LVEDVI ↑, LVEF ↓ in LV dysfunction	LVEDP ↑ immediately normalized in normal EF group at 20 min only LVEDVI ↑, SVI ↑, EF ↑ in normal EF group only	Further increase in LV diastolic dimension in normal LV function, no increase in LVDD or FS in LV dysfunction	Internal characteristics of LV chamber rather than reversal of LV restraint explain LV volumetric data
Lee et al., 1996,[43] N = 27, all EF <0.50 LV angiogram, pressure data		In 20 pts, LVEF improved to >0.5, 7 pts EF did not improve; no reduction in SVR in group 2; LVESV, contractility, and wall motion scores improved in group 1		Both myocardial and mechanical factors play an important role

(Continued)

Table 23.1 (Continued) Studies evaluating outcomes of PTMC on hemodynamics

Author, year, number, modality	Pre-PTMC	Post-PTMC	Follow-up	Conclusion
Mathur et al., 1996,[44] N = 16 (EF <50%), N = 44 (EF >50%), 2D echo		LVEDV, LVESV & EF ↔	LVEDV, LVESV & EF ↔	No specific conclusions
Fawzy et al., 1996,[45] N = 11 (EF >50%), N = 4 (EF <50%), LV angiogram, pressure data	LVEDVI ↓	LVEDP ↑, LVEDVI ↑, SVI and EF ↑, systolic ejection rate ↑, SVR ↓, LVESVI ↔	LVEDP returned to baseline. LV EDVI ↑, SVI ↑, EF ↑, and systolic ejection rate ↑, SVR ↓, LVESVI ↓	LV ejection performance improves due to increase in preload and reduction in afterload
Pamir et al., 1997,[46] N = 21 (EF >50%), N = 2 (EF <50%), LV angiogram, pressure data		LVEDP ↑, LVEDV ↔, EF ↔		LV diastolic performance is impaired and LVEF does not change with PTMC
Sengupta et al., 2014,[3] N = 49 (EF >50%) N = 8 (EF <50%) 2D echo, speckle tracking strain, prospective study	LVEDV ↓, SV ↓, EF ↓ compared to control, GLS and GCS ↓	LVEDV ↑, LVESV ↑, LV ↑, SV ↑, GLS and GCS ↑, 8/9 pts in group 2 had improved		LV diastolic filling responsible for LV systolic dysfunction
Roushdy et al., 2016,[47] N = 32 (normal EF), 2D echo, speckle tracking strain, prospective study	LVEDD ↔, EF ↔, LV and RV GLS ↓	LVEDV ↑, EF ↑, LV and RV GLS ↑		Support mixed etiology theory
Esteves et al., 2017,[48] N = 142 (LVEF <40% excluded), 3D echo, prospective study		LVEDV ↑, SV ↑, LVEF ↑ and LVEDP ↑, SVR ↓, LVESV ↔		Loading conditions responsible for LV function

Abbreviations: N, Number; EF, ejection fraction; LV, left ventricle; LVESV, left ventricle end-systolic volume; CO, cardiac output; SVR, systemic vascular resistance; PVR, pulmonary vascular resistance; MVA, mitral valve area; LVEDP, left ventricle end-diastolic pressure; LVEDV, left ventricle end-diastolic volume; EDWS, end diastolic wall stress; EDPVR, end-diastolic pressure volume relation; LVEDVI, left ventricle end-diastolic volume index; SVI, stroke volume index; LVDD, left ventricle diastolic diameter; FS, fractional shortening; LVESVI, left ventricle end-systolic volume index; GLS, global longitudinal strain; GCS, global circumferential strain; ↓, decreased; ↑, increased; ↔, no change.

in LVEDP and an improvement in stroke volume and ejection fraction after PTMC. The increased LVEDP subsequently returned to baseline in patients with normal LV function. A few studies found increased afterload in the form of increased systemic vascular resistance, whereas others have noted reduced LV compliance. Most studies noted an improvement in LV function and contractility after PTMC, but in a minority of patients' the impairment of LV function persisted. In patients with persistent LV dysfunction after PTMC, the LVEDP continued to remain elevated and did not return to baseline. Further, there was no increase in LVEDV in this group of patients. Sensitive measures of LV function such as strain rate have found widespread subclinical LV systolic dysfunction, even when the LV function was found to be normal.[3, 47]

MILD MITRAL STENOSIS WITH LEFT-VENTRICULAR DYSFUNCTION

This was initially described by Fleming and Wood in 1958.[49] About 3% of their cases had evidence of mild MS with low cardiac output. Patients were predominantly female (M:F was 7:1) of middle age (mean age 43 years). All were in atrial fibrillation (AF). Their symptoms were that of left- and right-ventricular failure (exertional dyspnea, orthopnea, pedal edema). The symptoms were intermittent but incapacitating, lasting a long period of time (mean duration 9 years). Almost half had systemic embolism. Hemodynamic studies revealed a low cardiac output, almost-normal LA pressure and normal to mildly raised pulmonary vascular resistance. Clinical, radiological, operative, and autopsy data revealed little evidence of left-ventricular abnormality. Atrial fibrillation and the accompanying fast ventricular rate most likely accounted for the symptoms, low cardiac output, and high incidence of embolism. Good functional status could be achieved through rate control and anticoagulation. Mitral valvotomy did not improve the cardiac function in such cases.

MEDICAL THERAPY

Data regarding medical therapy in patients with LV dysfunction and MS is limited. Anemia, infections, and hyperthyroidism should be corrected. Loop diuretics and salt restriction are useful in relieving congestive symptoms. Aldosterone antagonists have been shown to improve survival in patients with heart failure and LV dysfunction. These can be added to loop diuretics in MS patients with LV dysfunction. They have the added advantage of counteracting the hypokalemia that develops with loop diuretics. Digoxin is useful in MS with left- and/or right-ventricular dysfunction, especially in the presence of AF. β-blockers are commonly used in patients with symptomatic MS and have been shown to improve symptoms and mortality in patients with LV systolic dysfunction and heart failure. However, heart failure trials have consistently excluded patients with significant valvular heart disease (including MS). Thus, their usage in patients with MS with LV systolic dysfunction is not evidence-based but rather a matter of extrapolation. Likewise, ivabradine (a pure negative chronotropic agent) has been shown to reduce hospitalization for heart failure among heart failure patients with high heart rates (>75 bpm). It improves exercise capacity in patients with mild to moderate MS in sinus rhythm.[50,51] It may be considered where β-blockers are not tolerated. Anticoagulation is indicated for patients with MS in AF even in the absence of embolic event/LA clot irrespective of LV function.[52] It is not clear whether MS patients with LV dysfunction in sinus rhythm should receive anticoagulation. One may consider anticoagulation in such patients in the presence of large LA (>55 mm) or spontaneous echo contrast.[53] In the absence of the latter, use of the CHAD2VASC score may be considered.

Finally, the use of angiotensin-converting enzyme inhibitors (ACEI) has often been contraindicated in patients with significant MS for the fear of precipitating hypotension in the setting of a fixed obstruction. Chockalingam et al.[54] studied the safety and efficacy of ACEI (enalapril) among 109 patients with significant MS (MVA <1.5 cm²) in NYHA class III–IV. While 35 patients had isolated MS, others had multivalvular disease. LV function was preserved in the majority of patients, with only ten patients having an EF of <50%. Enalapril was well tolerated, without development of hypotension or worsening of symptoms. There was an improvement in NYHA class, Borg Dyspnea Index, and six-minute walk distance. Thus, patients who have MS and reduced ejection fraction can benefit from ACEI. This may be due to the reduction in the elevated afterload that is seen in some of these patients. However, a priori identification of this subgroup without hemodynamic assessment is very difficult.

CAUSES OF LV DYSFUNCTION IN MS[27,36,55]

Finally, the factors responsible for LV dysfunction in MS can be summarized as below (Table 23.2):

1. Inadequate LV preload
   a. Reduced LV filling in diastole from severe valvular obstruction; data supporting this comes for a number of studies that have shown improvement in reduced LVEDV after commissurotomy.
   b. Reduced LV compliance
   c. Abnormal septal motion due to RV pressure overload may impinge on the LV, leading to reduced LV filling
2. Myocardial insufficiency; primary LV systolic dysfunction due to an intrinsic abnormality. This may be due to smoldering rheumatic carditis resulting in LV systolic dysfunction or it may be due to scarring of the subvalvular apparatus leading to wall motion abnormalities. Studies supporting this hypothesis have shown that:
   a. LV contractile function does not improve completely even after corrective surgery
   b. Depressed LV function is not necessarily seen in those with severe MS alone

Table 23.2 Causes of left-ventricular dysfunction in mitral stenosis

Reduced reload	Reduced LV filling
	Abnormal IVS motion
Myocardial insufficiency	Smoldering rheumatic carditis
	Scarring of subvalvular apparatus
Increased afterload	Reduced LV wall thickness
	Increased systemic vascular resistance
Other	Tachycardiomyopathy due to atrial fibrillation and fast ventricular rate
	Coronary embolism of LA/LAA clot

c. Larger LV systolic volumes are seen in patients with depressed EF, indicating that LV contractile function is diminished
d. Widespread subclinical LV systolic dysfunction has been demonstrated by strain echocardiography in MS patients with normal LV ejection fraction
e. There is myofibrillar degeneration in pathological studies.
3. Excessive LV afterload, which has been demonstrated in patients with severe MS. This is due to diminished LV wall thickness or increased systemic vascular resistance.

Results from intervention studies have demonstrated that most patients with LV dysfunction in MS have an immediate improvement in EF, indicating that the predominant mechanism is mechanical obstruction of mitral rather than myocardial inflow. However, the fact that a minority of patients do not have an improvement in EF indicates that the myocardial aspect is also operational. The prognosis of the latter patients is reasonably good and such patients should not be denied surgical/percutaneous therapy on the grounds of poor LV function.

REFERENCES

1. Gash AK, Carabello BA, Cepini D et al. Left ventricular ejection performance and systolic muscle function in patients with mitral stenosis. *Circulation* 1983;67(1):148–54.
2. Snyder RW II, Lange RA, Willard JE et al. Frequency, cause and effect on operative outcome of depressed left ventricular ejection fraction in mitral stenosis. *Am J Cardiol* 1994;73(1):65–9.
3. Sengupta SP, Amaki M, Bansal M et al. Effects of percutaneous balloon mitral valvuloplasty on left ventricular deformation in patients with isolated severe mitral stenosis: A speckle-tracking strain echocardiographic study. *J Am Soc Echocardiogr* 2014;27:639–47.
4. Kirch E. Alterations in size and shape of individual regions of heart in valvular disease. *Verh Deutsch Kong Inn Med* 1929;41:324–36.
5. Grant RP. Architectonics of the heart. *Am Heart J* 1953;46:405–31.

6. Sunamori M, Suzuki A, Harrison CE. Relationship between left ventricular morphology and postoperative cardiac function following valve replacement for mitral stenosis. *J Thorac Cardiovasc Surg* 1983;85:727–32.

7. Perennec J, Herreman F, Ameur A, Degeorges M, Hatt PY. Ultrastructural and histological study of left ventricular myocardium in mitral stenosis. Correlations with angiocardiographic indices of left ventricular function (in 11 observations). *Basic Res Cardiol* 1980;75:353–64.

8. Lee YS, Lee CP. Ultrastructural pathological study of left ventricular myocardium in patients with isolated rheumatic mitral stenosis with normal or abnormal left ventricular function. *Jpn Heart J* 1990;31:435–48.

9. Harvey RM, Ferrer MI, Samet P et al. Mechanical and myocardial factors in rheumatic heart disease with mitral stenosis. *Circulation* 1955;11:531–51.

10. Carman GH, Lange RL. Variant hemodynamic patterns in mitral stenosis. *Circulation* 1961;24:712–9.

11. Hugenholtz PG, Ryan TJ, Stein SW et al. The spectrum of pure mitral stenosis. Hemodynamic studies in relation to clinical disability. *Am J Cardiol* 1962;10:773–84.

12. Feigenbaum H, Campbell RW, Wunsch CM et al. Evaluation of the left ventricle in patients with mitral stenosis. *Circulation* 1966;34:462–72.

13. Heller SJ, Carleton RA. Abnormal left ventricular contraction in patients with mitral stenosis. *Circulation* 1970;42:1099–1119.

14. Horwitz LD, Mullins CB, Payne PM et al. Left ventricular function in mitral stenosis. *Chest* 1973;64:609–14.

15. Curry GC, Elliott LP, Ramsey HW. Quantitative left ventricular angiographic finding in mitral stenosis. *Am J Cardiol* 1972;29:621–7.

16. Holzer JA, Karliner JS, O'Rourke RA, Peterson KL. Quantitative angiographic analysis of the left ventricle in patients with isolated rheumatic mitral stenosis. *Br Heart J* 1973;35:497–502.

17. Silverstein DM, Hansen DP, Ojiambo HP, Griswold HE. Left ventricular function in severe pure mitral stenosis as seen at the Kenyatta National Hospital. *Am Heart J* 1980;99:727–33.

18. Sabbah HN, Anbe DT, Stein PD. Negative intraventricular diastolic pressure in patients with mitral stenosis: Evidence of left ventricular diastolic suction. *Am J Cardiol* 1980;45:562–6.

19. Mcdonald IG. Echocardiographic assessment of left ventricular function in mitral valve disease. *Circulation* 1976;53:865–71.

20. Ibrahim MM. Left ventricular function in rheumatic mitral stenosis. Clinical echocardiographic study. *Br Heart J* 1979;42:514–20.

21. Mohan JC, Agrawala R, Calton R, Arora R. Cross-sectional echocardiographic left ventricular geometry in rheumatic mitral stenosis. *Int J Cardiol* 1993;38:81–7.

22. Ozdemir K, Altunkeser BB, Gok H et al. Analysis of the myocardial velocities in patients with mitral stenosis. *J Am Soc Echocardiogr* 2002;15:1472–8.

23. Dogan S, Aydin M, Gursurer M et al. Prediction of subclinical left ventricular dysfunction with strain rate imaging in patients with mild to moderate rheumatic mitral stenosis. *J Am Soc Echocardiogr* 2006;19:243–8.

24. Ozdemir AO, Kaya CT, Ozcan OU et al. Prediction of subclinical left ventricular dysfunction with longitudinal two-dimensional strain and strain rate imaging in patients with mitral stenosis. *Int J Cardiovasc Imaging* 2010;26:397–404.

25. Bilen E, Kurt M, Tanboga IH et al. Severity of mitral stenosis and left ventricular mechanics: A speckle tracking study. *Cardiology* 2011;119:108–15.

26. Weyman AE, Heger JJ, Kronik G et al. Mechanism of paradoxical early diastolic septal motion in patients with mitral stenosis: A cross-sectional echocardiographic study. *Am J Cardiol* 1977;40:691–9.

27. Klein AJ, Carroll JD. Left ventricular dysfunction and mitral stenosis. *Heart Failure Clinics* 2006;2:443–52.

28. Sharma V, Stewart RA, Zeng I et al. Comparison of atrial and brain natriuretic peptide for the assessment of mitral stenosis. *Heart, Lung and Circulation* 2011 Aug 31;20(8):517–24.

29. Eryol NK, Dogan A, Ozdogru I et al. The relationship between the level of plasma B-type natriuretic peptide and mitral stenosis. *Int J Cardiovasc Imaging* 2007;23:569.

30. Iltumur K, Karabulut A, Yokus B et al. N-terminal proBNP plasma levels correlate with severity of mitral stenosis. *J Heart Valve Dis* 2005;14:735–41.

31. Arat-Özkan A, Kaya A, Yiğit Z et al. Serum N-terminal pro-BNP levels correlate with symptoms and echocardiographic findings in patients with mitral stenosis. *Echocardiography* 2005;22:473–8.

32. El Zayat A. Potential use of Brain Natriuretic Peptide in patients with asymptomatic significant mitral stenosis. *The Egyptian Heart Journal* 2014;66:269–75.

33. Chadha DS, Karthikeyan G, Goel K et al. N-terminal pro-BNP plasma levels before and after percutaneous transvenous mitral commissurotomy for mitral stenosis. *Int J Cardiol* 2010;144:238–40.

34. Shang YP, Lai L, Chen J et al. Effects of percutaneous balloon mitral valvuloplasty on plasma B-type natriuretic peptide in rheumatic mitral stenosis with and without atrial fibrillation. *J Heart Valve Dis* 2005;14:453–9.

35. Selcuk MT, Selcuk H, Maden O et al. The effect of percutaneous balloon mitral valvuloplasty on N-terminal-pro B-type natriuretic peptide plasma levels in mitral stenosis. *Int Heart J* 2007;48:579–90.

36. Snyder RW, Lange RA, Willard JE et al. Frequency, cause and effect on operative outcome of depressed left ventricular ejection fraction in mitral stenosis. *Am J Cardiol* 1994;73:65–9.

37. Mangoni AA, Koelling TM, Meyer GS et al. Outcome following mitral valve replacement in patients with mitral stenosis and moderately reduced left ventricular ejection fraction. *Eur J Cardiothorac Surg* 2002;22:90–4.

38. Park KJ, Woo JS, Park JY, Jung JH. Clinical effect of left-ventricular dysfunction in patients with mitral stenosis after mitral valve replacement. *Korean J Thorac Cardiovasc Surg* 2016;49:350.

39. Wisenbaugh T, Essop R, Middlemost S et al. Excessive vasoconstriction in rheumatic mitral stenosis with modestly reduced ejection fraction. *J Am Coll Cardiol* 1992;20:1339–44.

40. Liu CP, Ting CT, Yang TM et al. Reduced left ventricular compliance in human mitral stenosis. Role of reversible internal constraint. *Circulation* 1992;85:1447–56.

41. Goto S, Handa S, Akaishi M et al. Left ventricular ejection performance in mitral stenosis, and effects of successful percutaneous transvenous mitral commissurotomy. *Am J Cardiol* 1992;69:233–7.

42. Yasuda S, Nagata S, Tamai J et al. Left ventricular diastolic pressure-volume response immediately after successful percutaneous transvenous mitral commissurotomy. *Am Heart J* 1993;71:932–7.

43. Lee TM, Su SF, Chen MF et al. Changes of left ventricular function after percutaneous balloon mitral valvuloplasty in mitral stenosis with impaired left ventricular performance. *Int J Cardiol* 1996;56:211–5.

44. Mathur A, Agrawal VV, Thatai D et al. Percutaneous transvenous mitral commissurotomy for rheumatic mitral stenosis with impaired left ventricular function: An echocardiographic follow-up study. *Int J Cardiol* 1996;56:217–21.

45. Fawzy ME, Choi WB, Mimish L et al. Immediate and long-term effect of mitral balloon valvotomy on left ventricular volume and systolic function in severe mitral stenosis. *Am Heart J* 1996;132:356–60.

46. Pamir G, Ertaş F, Oral D et al. Left ventricular filling and ejection fraction after successful percutaneous balloon mitral valvuloplasty. *Int J Cardiol* 1997;59:243–6.

47. Roushdy AM, Raafat SS, Shams KA et al. Immediate and short-term effect of balloon mitral valvuloplasty on global and regional biventricular function: A two-dimensional strain echocardiographic study. *Eur Heart J Cardiovasc Imaging* 2015;17:316–25.

48. Esteves WAM, Lodi-Junqueira L, Soares JR et al. Impact of percutaneous mitral valvuloplasty on left ventricular function in patients with mitral stenosis assessed by 3D echocardiography. *Int J Cardiol* 2017 Jun 23. doi: 10.1016/j.ijcard.2017.06.078.

49. Fleming HA, Wood P. The myocardial factor in mitral valve disease. *Brit Heart J* 1959;21(1):117–22.

50. Parakh N, Chaturvedi V, Kurian S et al. Effect of ivabradine vs atenolol on heart rate and effort tolerance in patients with mild to moderate mitral stenosis and normal sinus rhythm. *J Card Fail* 2012;18:282–8.

51. Saggu DK, Narain VS, Dwivedi SK et al. Effect of ivabradine on heart rate and duration of exercise in patients with mild-to-moderate mitral stenosis: A randomized comparison with metoprolol. *J Cardiovasc Pharmacol* 2015;65:552–4.

52. Nishimura RA, Otto CM, Bonow RO et al. 2014 AHA/ACC guideline for the management of patients with valvular heart disease: A report of the American College of Cardiology/American Heart Association Task Force on Practice Guidelines. *J Am Coll Cardiol* 2014;63:2438–88.

53. Whitlock RP, Sun JC, Fremes SE et al. American College of Chest Physicians. Antithrombotic and thrombolytic therapy for valvular disease: Antithrombotic Therapy and Prevention of Thrombosis, 9th ed. American College of Chest Physicians Evidence-Based Clinical Practice Guidelines. *Chest* 2012;141:e576S–e600S.

54. Chockalingam A, Venkatesan S, Subramaniam T et al. Safety and efficacy of angiotensin-converting enzyme inhibitors in symptomatic severe aortic stenosis: Symptomatic Cardiac Obstruction–Pilot Study of Enalapril in Aortic Stenosis (SCOPE-AS). *Am Heart J* 2004;147:740.

55. Gaasch WH, Folland ED. Left ventricular function in rheumatic mitral stenosis. *Eur Heart J* 1991;12(suppl_B):66–9.

24

Subvalvular deformity in mitral stenosis

VIVEK CHATURVEDI

INTRODUCTION

The affliction of the subvalvular apparatus in rheumatic MS is almost universal in the current era. The inflammation and scarring consequent to the rheumatic process involves the subvalvular structures of chordae tendineae and the papillary muscles (PM) to a variable degree and has a significant impact on outcomes for both percutaneous and surgical treatment procedures. In this section we discuss in brief the clinical anatomy, pathology, diagnosis, and management approaches to subvalvular disease (SVD) in rheumatic MS.

ANATOMY, FUNCTION, AND RHEUMATIC PATHOLOGY

The mitral apparatus consists of the mitral leaflets (anterior and posterior), commissures, chordae tendinae, and two papillary muscles: anterolateral (APM) and posteromedial (PPM). The papillary muscles form a fairly large part of the left-ventricular musculature and play an important part in coordinated contraction. The papillary muscles (with adjacent left-ventricular free wall) and chordae tendinae together constitute the subvalvular component of the mitral apparatus. Both the papillary

muscles are attached to the middle third of the left-ventricular free wall, more apical than basal. The APM is a single muscle trunk, while PPM consists of one to three muscle heads.[1] In terms of orientation, they lie in a similar plane as the mitral commissures. The APM is the larger papillary muscle and is supplied by a branch from the left circumflex (LCX) or the left-anterior descending (LAD) artery. The PPM is mostly supplied by the posterior descending branch of the right coronary artery (RCA). The chordae tendineae are stringlike structures arising from the tips of the papillary muscles. As the papillary muscles lie below the respective commissures, chordae tendineae arise from each papillary muscle and connect to the ventricular surface of the ipsilateral halves of *both* leaflets. There is a large variation in their length, number, course, and place of insertion on the leaflets. But broadly, after a certain distance, each chordae tendineae divides into two to four "functional units" that then insert on the leaflet. The point of insertion is usually the leaflet edge (rough zone) on the AML while it is away from the edge towards the annulus on the PML.[2] A functional classification of the chordae tendineae was proposed by Lam et al., keeping in mind the morphology and location of the chordae.[3]

The opening and closing of the mitral valve is not merely a passive phenomenon determined by pressure gradients. Rather, it is an energy-consuming process requiring contraction of the entire mitral apparatus, especially the subvalvular component.[2] The principal function of the chordae tendineae and the papillary muscles is to prevent the prolapse of the leaflets into the atrium during ventricular systole and proper apposition of the rough zones of the two leaflets to ensure valve competence.

The involvement of the subvalvular apparatus in rheumatic heart disease (RHD) is a consequence of direct inflammation and scarring due to valvulitis as well as fibrosis induced by flow disturbances due to mitral stenosis. While the papillary muscles are hardly involved directly in the rheumatic inflammation, the chordae are commonly involved. The scarring leads to thickening, fusion, retraction, shortening, nodularity, and calcification of the chordae. With extensive scarring, the interchordal space is drastically reduced and the leaflets tend to be pulled downwards due to retraction of chordae. The distorted (but mildly affected) leaflets and the fused thickened chordae then constitute a funnel-shaped outlet below the leaflet level, termed submitral or chordal MS.[4]

DIAGNOSIS OF SUBVALVULAR DISEASE

While theoretically the classical auscultatory findings of MS require a pliable valve and good-sized chordal length practically, clinical examination cannot reliably differentiate purely valvular MS from subvalvular involvement. The cornerstone for diagnosis of SVD is transthoracic (and in certain situations, transesophageal and transgastric) echocardiography. This has been covered in detail in the chapter on echocardiography (see Chapter 8). Several echocardiographic scores have been published that include assessment of SVD as one of the parameters evaluated, primarily for deciding eligibility for percutaneous intervention and subsequent outcomes. None is superior to another, and the default method has usually been the Wilkins Score.[5] While measurement of chordal length can be done to assess the severity of subvalvular involvement,[6] it is cumbersome. We prefer to describe in detail the involvement of individual

papillary muscles and the corresponding chordae in general with semi-quantitative terms such as mild, moderate, and severe. As mentioned in the chapter on echocardiography, it is important to assess the subvalvular apparatus in modified and tilted views in more than one plane. Mostly this involves the tilted parasternal long-axis view, parasternal short-axis view, and the apical two-chamber view. Fluoroscopy can also be used to detect calcification in the chordae.

In the past, invasive left-ventricular angiography has been used to evaluate papillary muscles and SVD. A "mitral subvalvular ratio" was devised in the pre-echo era to assess the need for mitral valve replacement instead of open commissurotomy.[7] On cardiac catheterization, the absence of a c-wave on the left-atrial pressure trace is commonly associated with rigid, thickened, and short chordae tendineae preventing the billowing of the AML into the left-atrial cavity in diastole.[8] Conversely, the presence of a c-wave on the trace implies, at best, only mild subvalvular thickening. During percutaneous transvenous mitral commissurotomy (PTMC), subvalvular involvement manifests as a "balloon impasse" and "balloon compression" sign (see Chapter 12).

PREVALENCE OF SUBVALVULAR DISEASE IN RHEUMATIC MITRAL STENOSIS

The involvement of SVD in rheumatic MS has been noted in 40% of autopsy specimens.[4] It has been observed surgically in up to two-thirds of patients undergoing open mitral commissurotomy (OMC).[9] The prevalence among patients undergoing PTMC has been variable depending on how the subvalvular apparatus was studied. In a study from India which assessed subvalvular disease angiographically among patients undergoing PTMC, the prevalence of severe SVD was 40%.[10] In Iung's series, the presence of extensive SVD among 1024 patients was 55%[11] by Cormier's score.[6] In the Cormier score, pliable non-calcified anterior mitral leaflet with thickened chordae <10 mm in length are scored as extensive SVD. A recent study from India focusing on careful evaluation of individual papillary muscles for SVD found severe SVD of both muscles (and corresponding chordae) in 11% of cases.[12]

OUTCOMES AFTER INTERVENTION IN MITRAL STENOSIS WITH SUBVALVULAR DISEASE

The symptomatology and clinical features of subvalvular disease are similar to predominantly valvular MS with mild SVD. However, it does impact the outcomes and management approach of percutaneous or surgical intervention for MS. According to some investigators, the presence of severe SVD in both papillary muscles is a contraindication for PTMC because the risks of acute severe mitral regurgitation or failure to open the valve are unacceptably high. In the recent study by Bhalgat et al.[12] (where SVD was evaluated individually for each papillary muscle and attached chordae tendineae) of 356 individuals undergoing PTMC, 43 patients had acute adverse outcome in terms of inability of the valve to open (14 patients) or the development of acute severe MR (29 patients). Of these, 41 patients had a SVD score of III (severe) on echo grading. The findings were subsequently corroborated in the 39 patients who underwent mitral valve replacement. In contrast, in a much larger series earlier among 1514 patients,[6] with 59% having extensive SVD by Cormier classification, the complication rate was approximately 2.5 times higher when compared to those with absence of significant SVD. However, 92.6% of the patients with SVD still achieved good outcomes (valve area ≥ 1.5 cm^2 with mitral regurgitation at ≤ 2 on the Sellers grade). These differences in outcomes may be partly explained by the different methods of assessment of SVD. While failure to open the valve may in general be more related to excessive rigidity and thickening in any component of mitral annulus, including subvalvular apparatus, the reason for development of severe MR may be different (see Chapter 8).[13] This is due to unevenness of fibrosis/calcification in the valvular apparatus that will predispose certain points (interfaces of the mitral valve complex) for tearing. As the thicker portions refuse to give way, the brunt of asymmetric and large forces generated during balloon dilatation is borne by these weaker areas, especially with an inappropriately large balloon or a balloon in a high-pressure zone.[39] This asymmetry can exist within the leaflets and commissures, as well as on the interface between two components, for example, excessive thickening in commissures and/or subvalvular tissue in relation to leaflets, with the latter being less thick. It is the AML that mostly tears at a "hinge" point.

Subvalvular disease also influences the long-term outcomes of interventions for severe rheumatic MS. In a study by Iung et al.,[11] among the 912 patients who achieved good immediate results after PTMC, late outcomes were assessed after a mean follow-up of 49 months. The ten-year actuarial rate of good functional results (survival with no cardiovascular death and no need for surgery or repeat dilatation and in NYHA class I or II) was 56% in the entire population. The presence of extensive SVD at baseline increased the likelihood of unfavorable outcome by 1.5 times, as compared to less extensive SVD at baseline. Similar results have been reported by other investigators worldwide. SVD has an influence on surgical commissurotomy procedures as well. In a large series of patients (N = 1280) undergoing OMC in the contemporary population, Choudhary et al.[14] found that baseline subvalvular disease was the single most important predictor for mitral restenosis following the surgical procedure. The presence of severe SVD usually leads to mitral valve replacement rather than a conservative procedure.

Sometimes, the SVD itself can be the site of obstruction causing MS rather than the valve per se. While attempts have been made to address this obstruction by PTMC or open commissurotomy, the results are underwhelming and such patients often require mitral valve replacement (MVR). As the subvalvular apparatus contributes significantly to left-ventricular geometry and performance, several surgeons perform total or partial chordal preservation during MVR (see Chapter 14). This has been shown to improve left-ventricular function after mitral valve replacement.[15] However, others have reported no difference in actual outcomes with preservation of subvalvular apparatus in patients with rheumatic aetiology undergoing mitral valve replacement.[16]

PTMC IN SUBVALVULAR DISEASE

(See Chapter 13.)

REFERENCES

1. Du Plessis LA, Marchand P. The anatomy of the mitral valve and associated structures. *Thorax* 1964;19:221–7.
2. Turgeman Y, Atar S, Rosenfield T. The subvalvular apparatus in rheumatic mitral stenosis. Methods of assessment and therapeutic implications. *Chest* 2003;124:1929–36.
3. Lam JHC, Ranganathan N, Wigle ED et al. Morphology of the human mitral valve: I. Chordae tendineae: A new classification. *Circulation* 1970;41:449–58.
4. Rusted IE, Scheifly CH, Edward JE. Studies of the mitral valve: Certain anatomic features of the mitral valve and associated structures in mitral stenosis. *Circulation* 1956;14:398–406.
5. Wilkins GT, Weyman AE, Abascal VM, Block PC, Palacios IF. Percutaneous balloon dilatation of the mitral valve: An analysis of echocardiographic variables related to outcome and the mechanism of dilatation. *Br Heart J* 1988;60:299–308.
6. Iung B, Cormier B, Ducimetie're P et al. Immediate results of percutaneous mitral commissurotomy: A predictive model on a series of 1514 patients. *Circulation* 1996;94:2124130.
7. Akins CW, Kirklin JK, Block PC et al. Preoperative evaluation of subvalvular fibrosis in mitral stenosis: A predictor factor in conservative vs replacement surgical therapy. *Circulation* 1979;60:71–6.
8. Turgeman Y, Suleiman K, Freedberg NA et al. Balloon mitral valvuloplasty and the echocardiographic score: Do we have a better alternative [abstract]? *Isr J Med Sci* 1995;31(Suppl):269.
9. Vega JL, Fleitas M, Martinez R et al. Open mitral commissurotomy. *Ann Thorac Surg* 1981;31:266–70.
10. Bahl VK1, Chandra S, Talwar KK et al. Influence of subvalvular fibrosis on results and complications of percutaneous mitral commissurotomy with use of the Inoue balloon. *Am Heart J* 1994;127:1554–8.
11. Iung B, Garbarz E, Michaud P et al. Late results of percutaneous mitral commissurotomy in a series of 1024 patients. Analysis of late clinical deterioration: Frequency, anatomic findings, and predictive factors. *Circulation* 1999;99:3272–8.
12. Bhalgat P, Karlekar S, Modani S et al. Subvalvular apparatus and adverse outcome of balloon valvotomy in rheumatic mitral stenosis. *Indian Heart J* 2015;67:428–33.
13. Chaturvedi V, Gupta MD, Girish MP. Subvalvular disease in patients undergoing balloon mitral valvotomy: A strong base is not always good. *Indian Heart J* 2015;67:416–8.
14. Choudhary SK, Dhareshwar J, Govil A, Airan B, Kumar AS. Open mitral commissurotomy in the current era: Indications, technique, and results. *Ann Thorac Surg* 2003;75:41–6.
15. Morimoto N, Aoki M, Murakami H, Nakagiri K, Yoshida M, Mukohara N. Mid-term echocardiographic comparison of chordal preservation method of mitral valve replacement in patients with mitral stenosis. *J Heart Valve Dis* 2013;22:326–32.
16. Coutinho GF, Bihun V, Correia PE, Antunes PE, Antunes MJ. Preservation of the subvalvular apparatus during mitral valve replacement of rheumatic valves does not affect long-term survival. *Eur J Cardiothorac Surg* 2015;48:861–7.

Index

Page numbers followed by f and t indicate figures and tables, respectively.

T - #0173 - 111024 - C384 - 254/178/18 - PB - 9780367571399 - Gloss Lamination